GW00976035

INNOVATIONS

in End-of-Life Care

Practical Strategies & International Perspectives
Volume 3

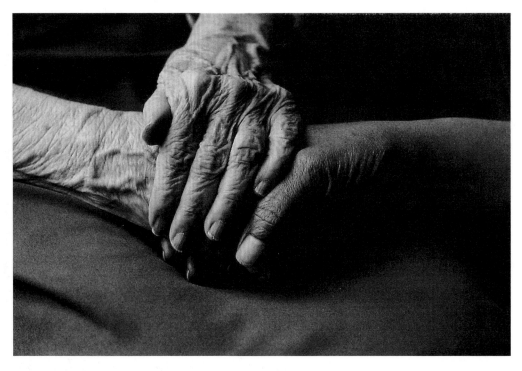

"Old and Young Hands"
©1988 Nita Winter.

INNOVATIONS

in End-of-Life Care

Practical Strategies & International Perspectives
Volume 3

Edited by

Anna L. Romer, EdD
Karen S. Heller, PhD
David E. Weissman, MD
Mildred Z. Solomon, EdD

Foreword by Kathleen M. Foley, MD

Center for Applied Ethics & Professional Practice
Education Development Center, Inc.

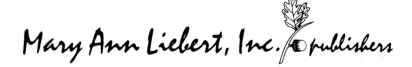

Mary Ann Liebert, Inc. publishers

Copyright ©2002 by Education Development Center, Inc.

ISBN: 0–913113–93–X

All rights reserved.

No part of this book may be reproduced, stored in a retrieval system, or transmitted in any form or by any means, electronic, mechanical, photocopying, microfilming, recording, or otherwise, without written permission from the publisher.

Parts of this book appeared in a slightly different form in the electronic journal *Innovations in End-of-Life Care* at **<www.edc.org/lastacts>** and in the ***Journal of Palliative Medicine***.

Cover image courtesy of NASA Space Photography.

All papers, comments, opinions, findings, conclusions, or recommendations in *Innovations in End-of-Life Care* are those of the author(s) and do not constitute opinions, findings, conclusions, or recommendations of the Publisher, the Editors, and the editorial staff.

Printed in the United States of America.

Photograph Acknowledgments:

Frontispiece: "Old and Young Hands" ©1988 Nita Winter.

Part One: Building Bridges for Better Continuity of Care. "Conversation" ©1995 Susie Fitzhugh. All Rights Reserved.

Part Two: Institutionalizing Palliative Care. "Passing Time." ©1985 Nita Winter.

Part Three: Supporting Family Caregivers. ©1998 Roger Lemoyne and Living Lessons.

Part Four: On Grief and Bereavement. ©1998 Roger Lemoyne and Living Lessons.

Part Five: Promoting Better Pain Management in Long-Term Care Facilities. "Learning New Skills." ©1992 Susie Fitzhugh. All Rights Reserved.

Part Six: Quality of Life. ©1998 Roger Lemoyne and Living Lessons.

Part Seven: Appendices, Contributors, and Interviewees. "Set Adrift." ©1992 Eleanor Rubin. Woodcut medium, 18" × 26". Photo by Louise Webber.

CONTENTS

Innovations in End-of-Life Care: Volume 3

Core Editorial Team

Mildred Z. Solomon, EdD, Editor
Anna L. Romer, EdD, Editor
Karen S. Heller, PhD, Editor
David E. Weissman, MD, Editor
Holly D. Sivec, Staff & Art Editor

•◆•

Contributors to Volume 3

Mary Arata, BSN, RN, OCN
Ellen Bartoldus, MSW, CSW
Mariela Bertolino, MD
Douglas Bishop
Marilyn Bookbinder, PhD, RN
Nereida Borrero, RN, MSN, GNP
Carleen Brenneis, RN, MHSA
David Browning, LICSW, BCD
Christian Juul Busch
Kathy Carroll, BSN, RN
Yvette Colón, MSW, ACSW, BCD
Richard Della Penna, MD
John E. Ellershaw, MA, FRCP
Robin L. Fainsinger, MBchB,
  CCFP
Kathleen M. Foley, MD
Julie Griffie, RN, MSN, CS,
  AOCN, CHPN
Stein Kaasa, MD, PhD
Robin F. Kramer, MS, RN, PNP

John Larkin, MD
Carol Levine
Neil MacDonald, CM, MD
Sandra Matson, BSN, MA, RN, C
Sandra Muchka, RN, MS, CS,
  CHPN
Jeffrey N. Nichols, MD
Mimi Pattison, MD
Russell K. Portenoy, MD
Alison Ryan
Phyllis R. Silverman, PhD
Samantha Libby Sodickson
Judith A. Spross, PhD, RN,
  AOCN, FAAN
James A. Thorson
Georganne Trandum, RN, OCN
Vittorio Ventafridda, MD, PhD,
  MCRP
David E. Weissman, MD
Carol Wogrin, RN, PsyD

Innovations in End-of-Life Care

www.edc.org/lastacts

Mildred Z. Solomon, EdD
Editor-in-Chief

Anna L. Romer, EdD
Associate Editor

Karen S. Heller, PhD
Associate Editor

David E. Weissman, MD
Associate Editor

Holly D. Sivec
Staff Editor

Editorial Board

Susan D. Block, MD
United States

Linda Kristjanson, PhD
Australia

Eduardo Bruera, MD
United States/South America

Neil MacDonald, MD
Canada

Ira Byock, MD
United States

Juan Núñez Olarte, MD, PhD
Spain

Thomas Delbanco, MD
United States

Laurence O'Connell, PhD
United States

Betty Ferrell, RN, PhD, FAAN
United States

Carla Ripamonti, MD
Italy

Alan Fleischman, MD
United States

Robert Ubell
United States

Irene J. Higginson, PhD
United Kingdom

Michael Zenz, MD
Germany

Stein Kaasa, MD, PhD
Norway

Zbigniew Zylicz, MD, PhD
The Netherlands

A Last Acts Initiative
Supported by The Robert Wood Johnson Foundation

Foreword

In 1990, the World Health Organization (WHO) defined palliative care as follows:

> The active total care of patients whose disease is not responsive to curative treatment. Control of pain, of other symptoms, and of psychological, social, and spiritual problems, is paramount. The goal of palliative care is achievement of the best quality of life for patients and their families. Many aspects of palliative care are also applicable earlier in the course of the illness in conjunction with anticancer treatment.[1]

Reading this definition, all will agree that palliative care, like its embedded element, quality of life, is a worthy goal, something each of us would wish for our loved ones and for ourselves. The challenge—socially, medically, economically, and culturally—is to transform the goals of palliative care into practice.

The WHO concept of palliative care is set within a framework of developing a public health approach to the care of patients with serious life-threatening illness. For example, the WHO recommended that every country developing a cancer control program should include palliative care as one of its essential aspects, along with prevention, early diagnosis, and treatment. This same approach is now being integrated into international HIV/AIDS initiatives, as exemplified by the UN-AIDS program, which now integrates palliative care approaches into its community-based treatment models.[2] The WHO, together with an international palliative care group, is developing a monograph on "Solid Facts of Palliative Care" to further emphasize the role of palliative care as a public health issue.

In the United States, the field of palliative care is rapidly expanding. A series of national reports has advocated the integration of palliative care into the US health care delivery system. These reports include the 1997 Institute of Medicine (IOM) report *Approaching Death: Improving Care at the End of Life*,[3] which identified serious inadequacies in end-of-life care for Americans and called on both governmental and nongovernmental organizations to address the barriers. In addition, two reports from the National Cancer Policy Board (NCPB), *Ensuring Quality Care for Cancer*[4] and *Improving Palliative Care for Cancer*,[5] strongly supported palliative care initiatives. The 1997–1998 President's Cancer Panel, in its report *Cancer Care Issues in the United States—Quality of Care, Quality of Life*,[6] supported the need for the National Cancer Institute to fund research and training across the continuum of care from prevention to palliative care. In addition, the Medicare Payment Advisory Commission, in its 1999 report,[7] recommended that the Medicare Program and the Department of Health and Human Services make end-of-life care a national quality improvement priority and support research and demonstration projects to bridge the existing gaps between hospice and palliative care.

More than 17 professional organizations have signed on to the Principles and Practices of Palliative Care. These groups have agreed to help to support palliative care programs, as well as the education and training of health care professionals and improved health care delivery systems. The Department of Veterans Affairs system, in which one in seven Americans dies, has made a commitment to integrate palliative care into its health care delivery system. It has developed both a residency education program and a faculty development program.[8]

CHALLENGES FOR THE FIELD

Two questions will help us to focus on the important challenges facing the field of palliative care: (1) How are we supporting the development of new science? (2) How are we translating that science into clinical practice? The first question was addressed in the 1997 report by the Institute of Medicine (IOM), which challenged the National Institutes of Health (NIH) to look at this domain from a research perspective. Attracting the interest of the NIH was an important step in setting a research agenda for palliative and end-of-life care, and the NIH has now identified the important issues. Over the last five years, through the development of a trans-NIH initiative on end-of-life care, a series of conferences has been sponsored by multiple NIH agencies, often developed by the National Institutes of Nursing Research (NINR), to address research agenda issues. In 1997, the NINR held "Symptoms in Terminal Illness."[9] In 2000, the NIH end-of-life interest group convened a meeting, "The End of Our Lives: Guiding the Research Agenda."[10] In 2001, the National Institute of Aging and the NCI held a meeting, "Exploring the Role of Cancer Centers to Integrate Aging and Cancer Research," to address issues of end-of-life care affecting the elderly. In July 2002, there will be a state-of-the-science meeting on symptom control in patients with advanced disease.

This concise volume, *Innovations in End-of-Life Care: Practical Strategies & International Perspectives*, Volume 3, addresses and expands the second question of translating science into practice. With detailed descriptions of successful institutional change, the reader can see what was involved and how local context shaped the process.

Innovations offers the opportunity for colleagues to share practical information and knowledge gained from clinical experience. These articles serve, in a way, as a written form of "grand rounds." To date, we have not had a forum like this in the field of palliative care. This volume presents the reader with information about an extraordinary group of people who are expanding this field either through research, quality improvement programs, or clinical care. Readers also gain access to the personal reflections of family members and professionals exploring the ways that their personal experiences have helped them to better understand grief, bereavement, and the complex task of being a family caregiver.

This third volume of *Innovations in End-of-Life Care* focuses on a specific institutional approach called quality improvement, which has a standard process and a set of methods that lead to cooperation, collegiality, and change. In Part Two, "Institutionalizing Palliative Care," the quality improvement approach is harnessed to improve end-of-life care. This represents one way to translate scientific knowledge, as exemplified by a set of standards, into clinical care. The Palliative Care for Advanced Disease (PCAD) pathway featured in this part is an example of just this kind of approach. The Franciscan Health System West program featured in Part One, "Building Bridges for Better Continuity of Care," and the Beth Israel program described in Part Two, "Institutionalizing Palliative Care," are both examples of moving to a quality improvement method. Yet the full impact of each of these ongoing projects is difficult to assess. These approaches need to be coordinated and assessed in ways that examine the program outcomes. For example, are they cost effective? These narratives of change expand our knowledge base of the practice of palliative care in the details and processes that they report and the questions that innovators' experience uncovers.

MODELS OF CARE

The work featured in this volume offers unique examples of how individual institutions have approached problems of integrating palliative care into their service offerings. Moreover, these essays and interviews are candid reports of both the barriers to implementing the projects and the limitations of what the innovators have done. Each one of these initiatives required the institution to uncover new sources of funding from various sources, including private philanthropies, through creative reallocation of resources within the institution, and from the government. Some required substantial volunteer efforts. In some cases, an innovative system of care was grafted onto an existing system to minimize the need for new resources or major systemic change. However, each of these efforts required a greater use of staff resources or donated time to provide the new services.

The importance of securing funding sources is an important reality that affects our ability to create new innovative programs to improve care. What are some of the innovative ways of funding such valuable programs? How should financing mechanisms evolve so that everyone has access to quality care? The examples in this volume demonstrate that, when an institution invests money in this effort, clinicians can often demonstrate effective service-delivery programs that enhance care for patients.

This group of articles shows that developing a field of palliative care may require both a hospital-by-hospital and a systems-by-systems approach. Developing the field in this way requires respect for the culture of each individual institution. Each will find a distinctive way to incorporate palliative care into its system.

THE VALUE OF CONCEPTUAL FRAMEWORKS

Clinicians working to improve palliative care should understand how to frame their own efforts in relation to the larger context of the problem. By becoming familiar with the underlying theories of change, culture, and socialization of health care professionals, they may be able to make more informed choices about the ways that they choose to implement their ideas. In Part Five, "Promoting Better Pain Management in Long-Term Care Facilities," Judith Spross explicates the value of a conceptual framework for understanding institutional change as leaders design and implement initiatives to improve care. She reviews the institutional change literature and shares her experience with clinicians working to promote better pain management policies and practice. These case studies provide a framework for evaluating and understanding the success or failure of efforts to institutionalize new practice. David Weissman, Julie Griffie, and their colleagues map their experience working with 87 long-term care facilities to improve pain management practices through a series of educational and quality improvement steps. Their educators' perspective is complemented by an interview with workshop participant Mary Arata, who reflects on the process of carrying out these activities in her own work in the long-term care setting. These multiple perspectives on the same process provide the reader with a greater understanding of what is involved in changing pain management practices in extended care settings.

The importance of having an explicit theory or conceptual framework underlying one's work is addressed in Part Six, "Quality of Life." Each of these contributors defines quality of life somewhat differently in this section, illustrating the inherent challenge of measuring and implementing improvements in this domain. Stein Kaasa approaches quality of life from a research perspective, Robin Fainsinger approaches it from a clinical perspective, Mariela Bertolino discusses quality of life from both a clinical and cultural perspective, and Vittorio Ventafridda connects it with national policy.

Robin Fainsinger discusses how the Edmonton Palliative Care Program, in Edmonton, Alberta, Canada, uses the Edmonton Symptom Assessment Scale (ESAS) as a way to assess quality of life. Fainsinger acknowledges at the outset that one of the most challenging aspects of those addressing quality of life is that the elements that are easiest to measure may not be the most important features of quality of life for the patient. Balfour Mount is critical of the concept of health-related quality of life when a person is dying. He advocates for the use of quality of life measures with a much richer range of topics than the ESAS; these include domains that patients who are dying think are important—spiritual, psychosocial, and existential issues. Yet, in the world of clinical practice, a tool that can promise rapid assessment of factors that staff members feel that they have some control over may be perceived as the most "useful" tool.

The middle sections of the book turn squarely to the experience of patients and their families. Part Three, "Supporting Family Caregivers," draws our attention to an area central to palliative care. Jeffrey Nichols's acute care dementia unit at Cabrini Medical Center in Manhattan exemplifies the creativity found in many of these innovative programs. This program was inspired by the observation that patients suffering from dementia were coming to the hospital with a broken hip and were leaving in worse medical and cognitive states. Nichols and his colleagues listened to the concerns and experience of families and consulted experts in dementia to institute a series of small but significant changes in the environment and care systems for patients suffering from dementia. These changes appear to have made a great difference to the families' and patients' quality of life during and after hospitalization.

Alison Ryan in the United Kingdom also focuses on how changing the family caregivers' (or carers' as they say in the United Kingdom) experience through support and the existence of a local community-based network can improve patients' and caregivers' quality of life and lighten the burden on professional caregivers.

The essays in Part Four, "On Grief and Bereavement," demonstrate the enormous need for research, especially large, epidemiological and longitudinal studies that frame and test hypotheses about grief and bereavement. There is concern by some that grief will be overmedicalized; others worry that particular psychological and psychiatric disorders will not be anticipated and appropriately treated. The papers in this section lay out the range of theories underlying different approaches to the care of bereaved people. The authors demonstrate that how we frame bereavement has policy implications, particularly in the United States, because many bereavement services are underfunded and therefore not widely available. How do we determine the policy agenda? Who should provide services? How should they be trained? What should be the standards of care? Again, answering these questions requires a conceptual framework and knowledge of what we know works and does not work.

Currently, the Project on Death in America (PDIA) is supporting the Center for the Advancement of Health to bring together a group of experts to look at the challenge of research in grief and bereavement,[11] defined initially in a 1984 Institute of Medicine report on grief.[12] This group is examining the underlying science, including the mind–body–behavioral components and then will frame the major research agenda.

CONCLUSION

Anyone interested in better understanding the multidimensional aspects and the interdisciplinary components of palliative care would benefit from reading this volume of *Innovations in End-of-Life Care*. Those who are attempting to frame a research agenda and develop a research priority need only to look at this book to get a sense of the extraordinary opportunities available and the questions that still need to be answered.

Kathleen M. Foley, MD
Director, Project on Death in America, The Open Society Institute
Attending Neurologist, Memorial Sloan–Kettering Cancer Center
January 2002

REFERENCES

1. *Cancer Pain Relief and Palliative Care*. Technical Report Series 804. Geneva: World Health Organization, 1990.
2. World Health Organization. *Fact Sheet 8 palliative and terminal care.* ⟨www-nt.who.int/whosis/statistics/factsheets_hiv_nurses/fact-sheet-8/index.html⟩ (accessed 26 Jul. 2002).
3. Institute of Medicine Committee on Care at the End of Life, Field MJ, Cassel CK (eds.). *Approaching Death: Improving Care at the End of Life*. Washington, DC: National Academy Press, 1997.
4. Hewitt M, Simone JV (eds.) and the National Cancer Policy Board of the Institute of Medicine. *Ensuring Quality Cancer Care*. Washington, DC: National Academy Press, 1999. Visit ⟨www.iom.edu⟩ and click on "Reports released 1999" to acces this document.
5. Foley KF, Gelband H (eds.) and the National Cancer Policy Board of the Institute of Medicine. *Improving Palliative Care for Cancer*. Washington, DC: National Academy Press, 2001. Visit ⟨www.iom.edu⟩ and click on "Reports released in 2001" to access this document.
6. National Cancer Institute. *Cancer Care Issues in the United States—Quality of Care, Quality of Life*. Baltimore, MD: National Cancer Institute, 1998. ⟨deainfo.nci.nih.gov/ADVISORY/pcp/pcp97-98rpt/pcp97-98rpt.htm⟩ (accessed 26 Jul. 2002).
7. Medicare Payment Advisory Commission. *Improving Care at the End-of-Life*. Washington, DC: Medicare Payment Advisory Commission, 1999. ⟨www.medpac.gov/publications/congressional_reports/Jun99%20Ch7.pdf⟩ (accessed 26 Jul. 2002).
8. Program on the Medical Encounter and Palliative Care. *Program of Resident Education to Promote Awareness and Respect at the End of Life* (PREPARE). Durham, NC: Program on the Medical Encounter and Palliative Care. ⟨hsrd.durham.med.va.gov/PMEPC/Projects/prepare.htm⟩ (accessed 26 Jul. 2002).
9. National Institutes of Nursing Research. *Symptoms in Terminal Illness: A Research Workshop*. Rockville, MD: National Institutes of Health, 1997. ⟨www.nih.gov/ninr/wnew/symptoms_in_terminal_illness.html⟩ (accessed 26 Jul. 2002).
10. NIH End-of-Life Interest Group. *The End of Our Lives: Guiding the Research Agenda*. Bethesda, MD: National Institutes of Health, 2000. ⟨www.nih.gov/ninr/news-info/eol_trans.pdf⟩ (accessed 26 Jul. 2002).
11. Center for the Advancement of Health. *Grief Research: Gaps, Needs and Actions*. Washington, DC: ⟨www.cfah.org/programs/grief_research.cfm⟩ (accessed 26 Jul. 2002).
12. Osterweis, Marian et al. (eds.). *Bereavement: Reactions, Consequences and Care*. Washington, DC: National Academy Press, 1984.

Acknowledgments

We would like to thank the many leaders in palliative care and other colleagues and friends whose efforts have contributed to this third volume of *Innovations in End-of-Life Care: Practical Strategies and International Perspectives*.

Innovations in End-of-Life Care, the online journal, has now been active since January 1999 and continues to publish bimonthly thematic issues at ⟨www.edc.org/lastacts/⟩. The journal came into being through the collaborative vision of Victoria Weisfeld, senior communications officer at The Robert Wood Johnson Foundation (RWJF), and Mildred Z. Solomon, EdD, editor-in-chief of the journal, director of the Center for Applied Ethics and Professional Practice, and vice president at Education Development Center, Inc. (EDC), in Newton, Massachusetts. Vicki Weisfeld and Millie Solomon put their heads together to come up with the idea of an online journal to disseminate promising practices in end-of-life care. We continue to be grateful to Vicki for her leadership in helping us forge this unique vehicle for promulgating new ideas and considering complex issues in end-of-life care and for her imagination and support in envisioning ways to sustain the journal over time. Vicki and the foundation, through its Last Acts initiative, now led by Karen Kaplan, have encouraged the efforts of more than 950 partner organizations to work together to improve the care of dying persons and their families. Working as a member of this larger effort to improve care of the dying has extended the reach of *Innovations* and led to a number of fruitful collaborations.

Innovations has now grown into three distinct products. Since January 1999, we have been publishing bimonthly thematic issues on the Web. In 2000, we began a productive partnership with David E. Weissman, MD, and the *Journal of Palliative Medicine* such that *Innovations* has since been a standing section in each issue of *JPM*. We are grateful to Lisa Pelzek-Braun, managing editor of *JPM*, for orchestrating the smooth coordination of *Innovations* and *JPM* manuscripts and material. That same year, Mary Ann Liebert, Inc., published the first of this annual series of print compendia of the online journal. With this current and third volume, the series now includes 16 complete issues of the journal, edited and reorganized for the book format, as well as several additional pieces never published online or in *JPM*.

We wish to thank all the members of our editorial board for their ongoing guidance and support, as they continue to lead us to innovative work, share insights, and serve as reviewers of submitted manuscripts. Neil MacDonald, CM, MD, and Stein Kaasa, MD, PhD, have each authored essays in this volume. We also appreciate the support and interest of Kathleen Foley, MD, who wrote the foreword to this volume. Dr. Foley has generously responded to our queries and suggested promising practices since the inception of the journal.

In this volume, we feature the work of two recipients of the American Hospital Association's Circle of Life Award, one in 2000 and one in 2001, as well as publishing a list of all the winners and recipients of Citations of Honor in 2001. (Volume 2 of this series features the work of the other year 2000 winners.) We appreciate the collaborative spirit and actions of Gail Lovinger, director, Association Governance, and assistant secretary of the American Hospital Association, for introducing us to the work of these outstanding innovators.

We are grateful for the dedicated and talented journal staff at EDC. Holly D. Sivec, current staff and art editor of *Innovations*, has painstakingly edited every page of this book, improving our consistency and collective style as well as attending to the numerous details of production, including managing the selection process for art in this volume with grace and aplomb. Holly's patience, keen eye and ear for language, and excellent time management skills have been invaluable to the production of this volume.

Samantha Libby Sodickson served ably as staff editor and key member of the editorial team during the creation and production of the six issues that make up this book. She conducted four of these interviews and authored a book review in Part Three. We are grateful to Sam for her many contributions to the overall quality of this volume, including her design of the cover of this series.

Stacy Piszcz-Shaw, management associate at the Center for Applied Ethics, manages the website database and responds to the needs of our more than 10,000 registered users, as well as overseeing many other aspects of the project. We are grateful to her attention to all these logistical details.

Pamela Metz, of Interactive Web Design, has served as technical consultant to the journal since its inception. This past year she created a much more detailed system for tracking Web use that has provided us with essential information about reader interest and use. Her flexibility, professionalism, and timeliness continue to enhance the effectiveness of our production team.

We wish to thank all our colleagues at the Center for Applied Ethics and Professional Practice at EDC. In particular, we wish to thank Judith A. Spross, RN, PhD, for her editorial in Part Five and Perryne O'Reilly, who has cheerfully and accurately transcribed many interviews on short notice. Ellen Clarke, RN, EdD, Erica Jablonski, MA, Deborah Sellers, PhD, and Alan Stockdale, PhD, have all offered advice and feedback. Erica has lent her quantitative skills to implementing and analyzing our annual reader survey, which has enabled us to gain a much more fine-grained understanding of our readers' concerns and interests.

We also wish to thank Stephanie Vrattos, MA, who transcribed many of the telephone interviews that we conducted with innovators and other contributors.

We are most grateful to those who have helped to bring *Innovations*, in both online and print editions, to the attention of health care providers worldwide. In particular, we wish to acknowledge the efforts of Karen Long and Jill Stewart of Stewart Communications, Ira Byock, MD, and Julie Emnett at The Robert Wood Johnson Foundation's Promoting Excellence in End-of-Life Care, and Kevin Harris, online editor of the Last Acts website.

The vision and support of our colleagues at EDC continue to inspire our efforts. Tony Artuso, director of publishing at EDC, has provided valuable advice and ongoing support since we started the journal. Diane Barry enhanced our marketing efforts with her guidance and wrote a press release for the Supporting Family Caregivers issue (Part Three in this volume). Erik Peterson has provided technical assistance to the project. We are grateful for the encouragement and support of Janet Whitla, Cheryl Vince-Whitman, and Dan Tobin.

Thank you to Vicki Cohn, Mary Ann Liebert, and the publications staff at Mary Ann Liebert, Inc., which has published this series of *Innovations* compendia and the *Journal of Palliative Medicine*. In particular, we wish to acknowledge the fine work of Larry Bernstein, Susan Jensen, and Paula Masi on the design, layout, and production of the book. We are especially pleased that Susan Jensen was inspired by David Browning's essay in *Innovations*, which is included in Part Four of this volume, to contribute her moving Personal Reflection to the Coping with Loss issue of the journal, which was published on the Web in November 2001.

Thank you to the artists whose beautiful work illustrates these pages: Susie Fitzhugh, Roger Lemoyne, and Nita Winter for their photographs and Eleanor Rubin for her woodcut.

This book would not exist without our contributors, whom we thank for sharing their wisdom and experience as change agents in the evolving field of end-of-life care. Their innovative approaches and thoughtful perspectives provide inspiration for other health care providers around the world who are working to improve the care of the dying and their families. Some contributors have granted permission for their tools or forms to be reprinted in this volume. We are pleased and privileged to present their work here.

Anna L. Romer, EdD
Karen S. Heller, PhD
David E. Weissman, MD*
Mildred Z. Solomon, EdD

Center for Applied Ethics and Professional Practice
Education Development Center, Inc.
Newton, Massachusetts

*Palliative Medicine Program
Department of Medicine
Medical College of Wisconsin
Milwaukee, Wisconsin

Part One

Building Bridges for Better Continuity of Care

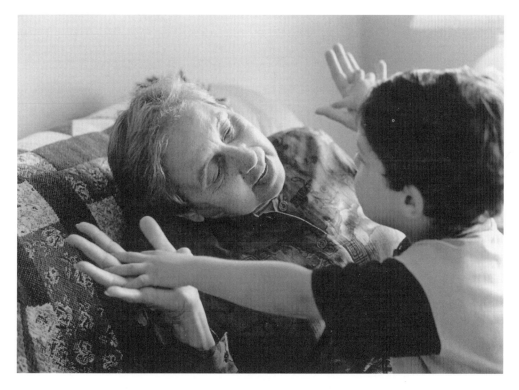

"Conversation"
©1995 Susie Fitzhugh. All Rights Reserved.

Asking the Right Question

RICHARD DELLA PENNA, MD

Kaiser Permanente Aging Network
San Diego, California

The American Hospital Association's (AHA) *Circle of Life Award* reflects the increasing awareness of a need to afford each of us an opportunity to discuss, plan, and define the kind of care that we want as we approach death. The recognition of Franciscan Health System West's *Improving Care through the End of Life* is noteworthy, as this program possesses key elements required to build systems of care that are reliably responsive to our needs and wishes when we become seriously ill and approach the end of life. It is important to understand the program's key features, as well as the context of health care in the new millennium.

Health professionals, insurance companies, and care systems continue to focus on episodic and acute interventions. Much of this care is breathtaking. Most people want state-of-the-art care that will truly benefit them, but also want more than what technology alone can offer. They desire personalized, responsive care that is respectful of their concerns, fears, culture, and values.

Moving from concept to change in clinical practice is often difficult. Mixed incentives, shifting reimbursement methodologies, realignments among traditional allies, and declining revenue make change especially challenging as payers and regulators require physicians and other health professionals to do more in less time.[1] Innovation in the current environment is difficult if it cannot fulfill the mandate to have a clear and immediate return on investment.[2] Any new program that does not have a rapid and obvious payback faces considerable barriers. Promising innovations in areas where there is strong professional or cultural resistance face even greater obstacles. *Improving Care through the End of Life* is an example of how a small group of individuals successfully met these challenges and made a difference.

The actual moment of death is brief, but most of us will spend months to years in predictable steady decline. This period is punctuated by losses, but it can be a time for growth, development, and closure. Few today would disagree that we each should have the opportunity to know our diagnosis and prognosis, decide what treatments we want, complete unfinished business, express where we want to die, and appoint someone who will make health care decisions for us when we no longer want to or cannot participate in making them. The Franciscan program provides its participants with the opportunity to accomplish these tasks.

Many provider groups are developing population management programs. Pop-

> *Few today would disagree that we each should have the opportunity to know our diagnosis and prognosis, decide what treatments we want, complete unfinished business, express where we want to die, and appoint someone who will make health care decisions for us when we no longer want to or cannot participate in making them.*

ulation management is based on the understanding that the traditional delivery system does not do a particularly good job at identifying and managing people at high risk from particular diseases or conditions. Health care insurers, systems, and providers are investing considerable resources in this approach because individuals with diabetes, congestive heart failure, renal failure, and other conditions are typically high cost. Population management relies on evidence-based medicine and introduces additional elements into the traditional approach to care. It usually has elements that ensure better continuity. Significantly less attention and fewer resources have been devoted to developing population management programs that do not have an immediate return on investment and on conditions that do not have an obvious medical responsibility. Programs for frail older adults, people with dementia, or those approaching the end of life fall into this category. Why then has the Franciscan program met with success when other similar attempts often fail? What are its core features?

Sustained organizational change and innovation require champions and people with the technical and leadership skills to effect the change. It also requires senior management-level commitment. The Franciscan program meets these requirements. The change team's members were the vice president of mission and ethics, the regional hospice director, the medical director, and a nurse versed in ethics and caring for gravely ill patients.

Physicians and systems do not reliably address the needs of people approaching death.[3] The Franciscan program identifies people in a primary care setting who are at risk of dying soon. (Population management jargon refers to this process as risk stratification.) Unlike most other population management programs, it does not depend on laboratory values, medications, or strict service utilization algorithms to target individuals. Instead, it relies on physician perceptions. Early on, the program asked primary care physicians to refer gravely ill patients who would benefit from its supportive services. Physician prediction of death in serious illness is actually reasonably accurate when compared to the use of more formal guidelines.[4] However, this general request was too vague and too difficult to incorporate into practice. There was difficulty getting physician referrals. Dr. Mimi Pattison's insightful question, "Would you be surprised if any of these patients died in the next 12 months?" made all the difference. Physicians were much more comfortable and willing to answer this question and so began to target patients who would benefit from a discussion about treatment choices as well as being linked to supportive services available in the community. The referrals came in. Physicians are key in starting discussion and without their cooperation little will change. Gaining physician acceptance and participation removed a barrier.

Furthermore, providing physicians with the language skills to open the dialogue and engage in this difficult conversation with patients made the task less onerous.

An important program element is the activity to heighten physician awareness and sensitivity to the issues and the apprehension people have as they approach the end of life. A physician continuing medical education (CME) program presents an overview that includes dying in America, pain and symptom management, and ways to support gravely ill people. But information alone has little impact. The formal and informal educational efforts of this program clearly convinced physicians that referrals to this program were of value to their patients. Without this physician buy-in, success would have been difficult even with Dr. Pattison's question.

Awareness, education, and demonstrating value, however, are insufficient to change established clinical practice. This has become evident to me as a physician who has spent the last 23 years working in a large, well-established, prepaid integrated delivery system. I have had the opportunity to develop and implement programs that serve vulnerable older adults. These populations include the "frail," people with dementia, the depressed, and those approaching the end of life. This activity has been with Kaiser Permanente locally in San Diego (57,000 aged 65+ members), regionally in Southern California (300,000 aged 65+ members), and nationally (800,000 aged 65+ members). This experience has provided me with a practical appreciation of the complexities and difficulties of bringing about clinician- and system-level change and improved performance. This is an especially challenging task in areas that medical culture does not traditionally value.

Our efforts at Kaiser Permanente to improve the care of members with dementia have many parallels with the Franciscan program. Earlier efforts, which used the traditional CME approach, were inadequate to change practice. There was no gain simply by asking physicians to do a better job in diagnosing dementia. What made a difference were focused activities geared at heightening physician awareness of dementia, as well as the importance of making the diagnosis and the value of the action plan that follows diagnosis. Successful programs typically introduced dementia care specialists, who worked with physicians in gathering assessment data and took responsibility for ensuring that members and caregivers were linked with educational, support, and planning services within Kaiser and in the community. Physician and caregiver satisfaction showed significant improvement, the care process for people with dementia had less variation, and cost offsets have been demonstrated.[5]

Both the Kaiser and Franciscan programs target largely invisible populations, people with dementia and gravely ill people who are likely to die within a year, respectively. Both programs had champions with visions of how care could be improved. They increased primary care physician awareness of a condition, improved their understanding of the value in addressing it, and introduced another team member to provide follow-up and continuing care. Successful programs to improve the care of depressed older adults have met similar obstacles and have similar program elements to overcome them.

Evidence-based practice guidelines abound and fill volumes, bookshelves, and pockets. Most, while terribly important, are too complex for primary care physicians to reliably follow, given the pressures of office practice. Innovators must recognize this and make the desired change uncomplicated for physicians. Change must be easy for those who are linchpins in the process.

The Donabedian model emphasizes structure, process, and outcome as a conceptual framework for looking at quality.[6] Improvement often requires introducing structural changes in the process of care. Effective changes assist physicians in caring for their patients and make it easier for them to do the right thing. Examples include automated decision support and the introduction of other health professionals as team members to collaborate with physicians. Given the demands of clinical practice, primary care physicians have become more receptive to the idea that they cannot and do not have to do it all. Collaboration with nurses, social workers, and others is necessary if their patients are to receive more reliable care. Improving performance in end-of-life care is complex, and a team is better equipped to meet the challenge than a lone clinician.

> *Improving performance in end-of-life care is complex, and a team is better equipped to meet the challenge than a lone clinician.*

In the Franciscan Health System West's program, the inclusion of the clinical nurse specialist is a structural change that increases the likelihood of achieving the program's desired outcomes. It is also the most obvious cost to the program. This additional resource makes it less onerous for physicians to raise the issue of prognosis with appropriate patients. Physicians start the discussion and then seamlessly introduce the patient to the nurse specialist, who has the skills and time to continue it. The office setting seems more natural for discussing preferences for treatment and care at the end of life. This contrasts with the hospital, with its frenzied pace and crisis orientation. The clinical nurse specialist also provides continuity and acts as a point of contact.

The program empowers patients. Gravely ill people become very dependent on their physicians and look to them for guidance about treatments. Truly informed consent easily fades into the shadows. Hurried physicians offer treatments that may offer hope and meaningful life prolongation. They often fall short in realistically explaining the goals, risks, and outcomes of the treatments of serious illnesses. The Franciscan program provides patients with time to discuss these matters and better understand what is happening. This feature has the potential to turn patients into informed consumers who can make better choices. The unknown and the dreaded become more evident and less unmanageable.

There seem to be some positive outcomes of *Improving Care through the End of Life*. Patients like it. Referrals to the hospice program are improving and hospice length of stay has increased. Physicians seem to value the program as indicated by more ready referral. The clinical nurse specialist fits into the pace of everyday practice. Many questions, however, remain. What are the key leverage points in the program? Why did it succeed when other interventions have failed?[3] Will the program continue when grant support ends? What are the direct and indirect program costs? Are there downstream cost offsets? Do physicians honor treatment preferences as patients move through different sites of care? How stable are these preferences? Does the program use validated instruments? What aspects of the program are most meaningful to patients, families, and physicians? Will it work in specialty settings? Will it work in the offices of physicians who are not part of a large provider group or in a large system? Is it replicable? Can social workers be as effective as nurses in the role of care coordinator? What changes in health care financing and public policy are necessary to make replication easier and provide people with the support that they require? Can accrediting bodies ease replication? Answering these questions will require further study and rigorous analysis.

In his International Perspective piece, Neil MacDonald reflects on how the challenges addressed by the Franciscan program play out in the Canadian context. Dr. MacDonald identifies structural aspects of the Canadian health care system that lend themselves to the promotion of such an initiative, as well as how recent governmental budget cuts have put quality at risk in the Canadian system. As an oncologist and expert in palliative medicine, his reflections on the strengths and challenges to adequately implementing such a program in another health care delivery system are illuminating.

Improving Care through the End of Life is an important step in bringing about change. Providers and systems of care can never truly be responsive to the people that they care for unless they are able to reliably identify those at risk, provide them with the chance to discuss their treatment preferences, and develop programs to honor these choices. This is particularly true for those people whose physicians "would not be surprised if they were to die in the next 12 months."

REFERENCES

1. Gold M. The changing US health care system: Challenges for responsible public policy. *Milbank Quarterly*. 1999;77(1):3–37, iii.
2. Cassel CK, Jameton AL. Dementia in the elderly: An analysis of medical responsibility. *Annals of Internal Medicine*. 1981;94(6):802–807.
3. Lynn J, De Vries KO, Arkes HR, Stevens M, Cohn F, Murphy P, Covinsky KE, Hamel MB, Dawson NV, Tsevat J. Ineffectiveness of the SUPPORT intervention: Review of explanations. *Journal of the American Geriatrics Society*. 2000;48(5 Suppl):S206–S213.
4. Fox E, Landrum-McNuff K, Zhong Z, Daewson NV, Wu AW, Lynn J. Evaluation of prognostic criteria for determining hospice eligibility in patients with advanced lung, heart, or liver disease. SUPPORT Investigators. Study to Understand Prognoses and Preferences for Outcomes and Risks of Treatments. *Journal of the American Medical Association*. 1999;282(17):1638–1645.
5. Della Penna R, Rosenthal M. Fulfilling the promise of managed care: A joint project between Kaiser Permanente and the Los Angeles Alzheimer's Association. *Drug Benefit Trends*. April 1998.
6. Donabedian A. Evaluating the quality of medical care. *Milbank Quarterly*. 1966;44:166–203.

Featured Innovation: Part I

Improving Care through the End of Life

An Interview with MIMI PATTISON, MD

Franciscan Health System West
Tacoma, Washington

In the following interview with Anna L. Romer, EdD, Dr. Mimi Pattison, medical director for Palliative Care Services and the Improving Care through the End of Life *program of Franciscan Health System West, describes the key concepts underlying the program; the processes of identifying, contacting, and referring patients to it; and factors that impede or facilitate acceptance of this kind of bridge to supportive services for people with grave prognoses who are not yet eligible for hospice care.*

Anna L. Romer: *What are the key concepts that underlie the* Improving Care through the End of Life *program?*

Mimi Pattison: The first key concept is that one must have a true understanding of the dying process today. Dying is different from what it used to be. Today few people die suddenly; rather, the majority of people die slowly, with multiple chronic illnesses. From a physician's point of view, we get so focused on the individual condition or symptom that is causing the patient problems that we forget to look at the whole picture. During the process of developing the program, *Improving Care through the End of Life*, and in our work with the Center to Improve Care of the Dying, not only did we learn a rapid quality improvement process, but also we gained a much better understanding of what living near the end of life involves today.*

The second important concept is a willingness to talk about death and the process of dying. Once we understand the process of dying, it is easier to identify those patients who are likely to die, and then we must be able to have the difficult conversations with these patients and families. Only then can we refer patients to supportive services and begin to improve care.

---

*Center to Improve Care of the Dying (CICD) <www.medicaring.org> is an interdisciplinary team of committed individuals engaged in research, public advocacy, and education activities to improve the care of the dying and their families. Joanne Lynn, MD, director of CICD, and other CICD staff provided leadership and served as core faculty for the Institute for Healthcare Improvement's collaborative, Improving Care at the End of Life, which convened in 1998. Franciscan Health System West was a member of this collaborative.

In our program, *Improving Care through the End of Life*, I think the biggest challenge was to identify those patients who are entering that dying phase. When I say "dying phase," I don't mean active dying or being within hours or days of death. I am talking about weeks or months. The program, then, is about changing the experience of this last phase of life for seriously ill patients and their families. It begins with conversation and planning with the patient, family, and physician. A key aspect of this conversation is what the physician expects will happen with the patient during the next weeks to months. Our goal is to find out what is important to each patient and family, to understand what their values are, and to look at spiritual issues. We want to look more closely at symptom management and the ongoing monitoring of symptoms and to assure continuity of care. Continuity—the follow-up and ability to resolve problems once they have been identified—is central to the program. The nurse care coordinator is the keystone of the program; she has direct access to the primary care doctor and is right in the same clinic.

ALR: *Can you walk us through the process of contacting and referring patients to the program? How does the primary physician become involved in this process?*

MP: The first problem was how to get physicians to identify patients who were dying, not tomorrow, but those who were gravely ill and could benefit from supportive services right now. We tried a number of different interventions that did not work. Then we came up with a screening question that has made all the difference. Initially, we were looking at just certain diagnoses—heart disease, Alzheimer's disease, cancer, and advanced lung disease. So we distributed lists of patient names to individual physicians, patients that they have seen over the last month or two, with these particular diagnoses. At the top of the list, we asked the question, "Would you be surprised if any of these patients died in the next 12 months?" If the answer to that question was "No, I would not be surprised," then we encouraged the physician to refer the patient to our program.

> At the top of the list, we asked the question, "Would you be surprised if any of these patients died in the next 12 months?" If the answer to that question was "No, I would not be surprised," then we encouraged the physician to refer the patient to our program.

ALR: *What proportion of patients for whom the answer is "No, I wouldn't be surprised if this patient died in the next year" does the physician actually refer to the program? Is it every single person for whom the answer is "No"? Or are there other factors that the physician is considering before referring patients to the program?*

MP: That is a key question. Other criteria, for example, the hospice criteria for pulmonary disease, often are really difficult to meet or even to remember. So, I think the question really taps into physicians' clinical sense of what is happening for that patient. The only other factors that a physician might consider would be family caregiving factors; for example, if the primary caregiver's health also has taken a downward turn, or if he or she has been diagnosed with something new, or is failing. Otherwise, it is a one-question referral process.

Now, occasionally, some patients will enter the program in crisis, or at the time of diagnosis of a serious or terminal illness. But the majority of our patients are coming to the program through the physicians asking themselves, or being asked, "Would you be surprised if this patient dies in the next twelve months?" This question seems to allow physicians to think in a new way about their patients and these patients' needs. It is as if a switch has been flipped. We've worked with our physicians so that now they will say to the gravely ill patients whom they have identified something like "My expectation is that this condition is going to continue to worsen over the next few weeks to months, and we need to plan for that. I have a program that I'd like to refer you to, or I have special support in our clinic that I'd like to refer you to." With that, the program is introduced, and the nurse comes in, takes over right there, and talks to the patient and family. After that initial meeting, which we try very hard to have occur in the clinic, the nurse does a formal interview and evaluation process over the phone. It probably takes about an hour.

ALR: *Who is at the meeting that occurs in the clinic?*

MP: When the patient comes in for a routine visit, or problems are identified, or the decision is made to refer, the nurse care coordinator often will come and meet the patient and family that day. It may be a brief meeting, depending on time schedules. It may last fifteen or thirty minutes or so. It varies. This meeting either occurs with the physician or just after the physician has seen the patient.

ALR: *How is this meeting framed for the patient?*

MP: We tell the patient that this is about identifying his or her needs and offering the support that he or she needs. The nurse's goal in this initial face-to-face meeting is just to provide a name, title, and phone number, with the implication that one can gain immediate access to her. In addition, she wants to communicate that she will be calling the patient, or the family member who is going to be the spokesperson, to ask for more information.

ALR: *How have families been reacting to that initial opening: "We've targeted you for special services"?*

MP: In general, extremely well. Initially, however, we had some physicians in the program who were really reluctant to begin to have that "bad news" talk and asked us to just go ahead and call the patients. We didn't call and say, "We're from *Improving Care through the End of Life*," but referred to the program as "Improving Care" or a "special program in your clinic." We tell them, "Your doctor has asked me to call you." We identified the program by name only a couple of times because it was such a disaster. The patients and families want to hear bad news from the physician. They don't want to hear it from anybody else.

ALR: *So, you've learned that you have to have the physician in person, speaking directly to their patients about the prognosis and need for supportive services.*

MP: Absolutely! Physicians *have* to be involved, *have* to give that information, bad news, if you will, and then refer the patient. It's nice to have that referral the very same day, or very soon. That works the best. We've taught them some language skills. We use the word "expectations." We don't say, "This is what's going to happen. You're likely to die in three months." Rather, something like "Based on what has happened to your condition over the last few weeks or months, this is what I see. These are my expectations of what may happen in the future." If the physician wants to define this future, that's fine.

ALR: *You mentioned that you started out with target diseases in generating the list of patients to inquire about with the doctor. Do you include diseases for which the prognosis is really more clear, such as pancreatic cancer or some forms of lung cancer?*

MP: We do. In general, these patients are referred very quickly on to hospice. We do include these patients for whom the trajectory is much clearer so as to capture them all in our clinic. We start them in the *Improving Care* program because we can provide something right away. For example, if the patient comes in with abdominal pain and is found to have a mass that looks very suspicious, during that work-up period, the patient will be offered some support from the program. In fact, I have a patient like this right now, who for the last two weeks has been going through diagnostic testing, and some cells have been shown to be cancer. Obviously, a very small tumor has been hard to find on CAT scans or MRIs. So I enrolled this patient in the program a couple of weeks ago. In the next week or ten days, the situation will be clarified as to exactly what's going to happen, how quickly things are going to go. But I didn't feel comfortable referring to hospice yet. Fortunately, I have this other program for awhile. So this patient likely won't be in our program long, but will move on to hospice. With this particular patient the cells were from the bile duct; this tumor is very hard to resect surgically, does not respond to chemotherapy, and is in an anatomical place where it does not have to be very large to do a lot of damage.

ALR: *So, you do not frame this program as purely a confirmation of a downward trajectory?*

MP: No. In fact, with pancreatic cancer, it's pretty clear-cut. We're very honest. But it's less clear with someone who comes in, for example, with worsening heart failure or worsening lung disease and maybe has been in the hospital two or three times. What's really quite interesting is that, once support is offered and things are improved at home, often patients' conditions stabilize, and they get better for awhile. This has not been an uncommon experience in the program.

ALR: *Do those patients whose conditions improve leave the program?*

MP: We never really discharge anybody from the program. We may put them on inactive status, in which they're only checked on every three months.

ALR: *What work did you do with physicians to get them to the point of referring these patients?*

MP: I think the important thing is that we started our program in a clinic where I actively practice. It's a matter of being there, being present, "talking the talk" at every opportunity, whether it is just a brief visit in the hall, a formal presentation, or an item on regular meeting agendas. We call it "being in their face all the time." They can't forget about us. We set up our office, initially, wherever we could find space in the clinic, which happened to be with the OB/GYN nurse practitioner, but the office was on the way to the lunch room, where there was a lot of traffic. As physicians walked by, they would often run into Georganne Trandum, RN, OCN, the program director. This physical presence in the clinic is very important.

ALR: *It sounds as though you do a lot of informal networking.*

MP: Probably more informal than formal. We found that formal training is less effective. However, we also conducted targeted continuing medical education (CME) offerings for the primary care doctors who were going to refer patients to the program. We required these doctors to have a minimum of five to six hours of CME credits. Basically, we offered an overview of dying in America today, including some statistics that stick in people's minds, and highlighted the differences between dying today and in earlier eras. Then we explained the process of the program. We did sessions on pain management, symptom management when patients are actively dying, giving bad news, and advance care planning. We modeled the process of breaking bad news and doing advance care planning for them.

ALR: *What kinds of changes had to occur in the primary care clinic for this program to take hold? In particular, as you think about how physicians and nurses work together, were there any issues you had to address?*

MP: I go back to helping physicians to identify appropriate patients and then encouraging the doctor to take a broader look at the patient and family and how they are doing. Changing how physicians think about these patients allows them to consider whether these patients would benefit from greater support. We aren't asking the physicians themselves to offer greater support, just to think about the patients in a slightly new way and speak to them about their prognoses. Then we can link these patients with existing community services, as well as to the nurse care coordinator as a personal contact for support.

Implementing this change requires working with the physicians and their nurses, informally, in addition to identifying the appropriate patients. We've worked with the physicians' own nurses because they are the ones getting the calls and are often triaging the problems that patients are encountering. We encourage the nurses for these patients to ask the physicians with whom they are working whether this patient would be appropriate for the *Improving Care through the End of Life* program.

ALR: *Did you do anything to enhance the relationship between the nurses who are coordinating the supportive care and the physicians?*

MP: No. I think the personality of the nurse care coordinator is really critical. It has to be somebody who is passionate, experienced, and whom the physician can immediately recognize as a resource. For example, Georganne Trandum, the program director, is well skilled in pain management and brought substantial oncology and bone marrow transplant experience to this role. She was able to offer them help right away, which made her credible.

ALR: *Were there structural changes in the clinic, such as new meetings, or other events that had to occur to implement this program?*

MP: Not really. We made end-of-life care an agenda item on our regularly scheduled meetings and made it a part of existing routines. You cannot go in and set up new meetings or new requirements for attendance if you want the program to succeed. In our experience, that does not work.

ALR: *Have you tried to track the impact of the program on physicians?*

MP: We've tried to assess physician satisfaction. When I hear some of the stories that our physicians have been willing either to write or tell about the program, there's no question but that they feel supported, as well as being able to offer greater support to their patients. The program allows them to give a different level of care, and individual physician job satisfaction and sense of comfort have improved remarkably.

ALR: *Do you have any ideas about what allows physicians to make this shift that you have clearly made?*

MP: I think physicians need to feel a comfort level, which comes from having positive experiences with patients near the end of life. When a physician has one positive outcome, he or she begins to get some feedback and then begins to have some understanding about how much patients and families appreciate being asked these questions. A couple of times we've had rather dramatic responses from families, once we've called them and they have really begun to understand what the program offers. For example, patients have said things like "You're calling me from Dr. Smith's office? I can't believe he cares about me that much to have referred me to this special program. That is wonderful!" And we make it very clear when we call that we are calling from the physician's office. We're not calling from a program that's separate, but on behalf of the patient's physician. This link is key.

ALR: *Are there incentives or disincentives for physicians to be involved in this program?*

MP: If anything, there may be a disincentive because of the extra time that is involved, particularly in the advance care planning sessions. Dealing with this extra time issue is another key challenge. There is still not good reimbursement for the physicians for that type of counseling activity. There also may be a disincentive to participate in terms of time spent and income lost because the participating physician does more care coordination, which, today, has no reimbursement unless the patient is in home health or hospice. Many of these patients are not being served by either of those programs.

ALR: *Does the physician end up doing more coordinating for patients even though a nurse care coordinator is involved?*

MP: For patients enrolled in the *Improving Care* program, more care coordination is being done, and the physician has oversight of this activity. In the end, this coordination makes care easier. But the physician doesn't get reimbursed for this time.

Right now this program is costing our clinic money. Once the program is totally funded by the clinic, at certain times *less* money will be coming to physicians because this money will have to pay for program staff salaries, including the nurse care coordinator. However, the reality is that if we keep patients out of the emergency room and keep them out of the hospital, where they *don't* want to be, then there's going to be more money left in the pot, if you will. So during this time of transition and in a mixed payer system, it is hard to really sort out the financial piece. Lack of appropriate reimbursement is a barrier.

ALR: *Is there any kind of financial relationship between patient enrollment in the program and what the physician earns?*

MP: I would say probably not. Right now we have a mix of capitated care and fee for service. We don't separate these patients in any way.

ALR: *As medical director of the program, what have you learned from this experience?*

MP: My greatest learning has been that the physicians are often the biggest barrier to good end-of-life care. I say this in front of groups of physicians or in front of anyone. They *are*. There is no question about it. I do not say this in a critical fashion but in a practical sense, given the way modern medicine has evolved. The

> *The reluctance to begin to have that difficult conversation is a key barrier to good care.*

reluctance to begin to have that difficult conversation is a key barrier to good care. I think this is true the majority of the time. There are exceptions—physicians who are more skilled and so perhaps able to be more sensitive. But in my experience in implementing this program over the last three years, working with a variety of physicians in different settings in the hospital and the clinics, I have found that the physician often is the biggest barrier. Physicians frequently want to hold out more hope and to look at more medical treatment interventions, as opposed to being able to ask the patient questions such as, "What is it that you want at this point? What's the most important thing to you?"

ALR: *What are you still curious about as you continue to do this work?*

MP: I think that there are cultural barriers among patients and families that are the same as the ones the physicians are encountering, such as fear of death, lack of understanding about death, lack of familiarity with death, with the exception of a lot of high-tech death. Most people today in this country have not experienced a loved one dying at home. So I'm curious about the best ways to overcome these barriers and to get the culture, if you will, or the community to be more willing to talk about death and dying. I think the Bill Moyers series that aired in September 2000 created a tremendous opportunity.[†] At Franciscan Health System West, we convened community members in public forums for open dialogue about these issues, which offered an opportunity to speak about dying in America.

I think we need to work with the community, and our health care systems need to reach out in ways that we have not done before. People today are fascinated by technology in medicine, by new technical innovations. And yet people are desperate for a sense of compassion and caring. The challenge is how to integrate this compassion into our care. How do we overcome the intrigue and allure of technological fixes?

ALR: *Do you think the allure of technology is related to financing issues?*

MP: Absolutely! Technical procedures are reimbursed. The second greatest barrier to our program is reimbursement. There is no good reimbursement for advance care planning or other conversations about treatment goals with patients. A few months ago I led a session for staff in cardiac services in our system. We invited all the cardiologists, the cardiovascular surgeons, the nurses, all the people associated with their programs.

Attendance by cardiologists was disappointingly poor. Our program has the

---

[†]*On Our Own Terms—Moyers on Dying* <www.pbs.org/wnet/onourownterms/>. This four-part PBS series led by Bill Moyers and Judith Davidson Moyers reported on the end-of-life issues facing Americans and was first aired on September 10–13, 2000.

strong support of one cardiovascular surgeon, who commented that it was a lot more attractive to be in the cath lab that morning than here talking about caring for the dying. It is important to remember in this context the number one cause of death in America—cardiovascular disease. I have learned this from colleagues in other parts of the country who are promoting change in end-of-life care. This experience is not unique to our particular medical community.

ALR: *If other physicians are interested in replicating your efforts, what do they need to consider?*

MP: I still see that the biggest issues are getting comfortable with having *that conversation* and learning how to conduct it. A related issue is for clinicians to be willing to admit what they don't know, that is, that they have gaps in their knowledge in this domain. There are tremendous resources available to physicians today—hospice educational efforts and the Education for Physicians in End-of-Life Care (EPEC) program,[‡] as well as the End-of-Life Physician Education Resource Center (EPERC).[§] We can all upgrade our skills to improve our everyday practice of medicine.

[‡]See Education for Physicians in End-of-Life Care at <www.epec.net/> for more information about this training effort.

[§]See End-of-Life Physician Education Resource Center (EPERC) at <www.eperc.mcw.edu/>.

Implementation of Coordinated Care: Improving Care through the End of Life

An Interview with GEORGANNE TRANDUM, RN, OCN

Franciscan Health System West
Tacoma, Washington

Georganne Trandum, RN, OCN, directs Franciscan Health System West's Improving Care through the End of Life, *a primary care clinic-based program in Washington state. In this interview with Samantha Libby Sodickson, Ms. Trandum speaks about the genesis and development of this program, as well as continuing barriers to providing exemplary end-of-life care for patients seen in a clinic setting.*

GENESIS OF THE PROGRAM

Samantha Libby Sodickson: *Please tell us about the history of the* Improving Care *program.*

Georganne Trandum: The program developed as an outreach from the Franciscan Health System Ethics Committee. Most of the ethical dilemmas that came to our committee were regarding end-of-life care in the intensive care unit (ICU). Problematic situations occur when patient wishes are unknown and aggressive treatments have been started in emergency departments, after which the patient is then transferred to the ICU. Families across this country are faced with making difficult decisions regarding continued intubation, possible surgeries, feeding tubes, or other aggressive care options for their loved ones. We felt that we had to do something to learn about patients and families' advance directive wishes *prior* to an acute hospital episode.

At the same time, the opportunity to become part of the Institute for Health Care Improvement's (IHI) Collaborative, Improving Care at the End of Life,* came across the desk of our medical director, Dr. Mimi Pattison. The vice-president of

---

*Since July 1997, Improving Care at the End of Life, an initiative of the Institute for Health Care Improvement (IHI), has involved 48 health care institutions in collaborative efforts to improve the quality of care for the dying in the United States, while also reducing unwanted, nonbeneficial care. For more information, visit the IHI website at <www.ihi.org/collaboratives/breakthroughseries/bts-endoflife.asp>.

mission and ethics, the regional director of hospice, Dr. Pattison, and myself formed the team from Franciscan Health System West that participated in the IHI Collaborative. Of the 48 participating organizations in the IHI Collaborative, ours was one of only two teams that worked on an end-of-life program out in the community. The four of us attended all the IHI learning sessions and, through the course of the year, met among ourselves weekly or every other week to discuss what we were doing, what was working, and where to go next.

I had been an oncology bone marrow transplant nurse. We needed to have someone who could be the Collaborative team leader and actually do the day-to-day work, so I took a leave of absence to assume that role. I *wanted* to do it and was excited to do it. We spent a year in the IHI Collaborative. First, we learned the model for rapid quality improvement, which we implemented. Early on, we decided we would do something at a clinic, rather than in the hospital or hospice. So, over the course of that year, we created a clinic-based program in one pilot clinic, and I've been with it ever since.

EARLY IDENTIFICATION OF PEOPLE IN NEED OF SUPPORTIVE CARE SERVICES NEAR THE END OF LIFE

SLS: *What did you decide to do in the pilot program?*

GT: In the pilot clinic in Gig Harbor, Washington, there were nine physicians with whom we wanted to work and to whom we wanted to provide continuing medical education and training. We wanted to give them some really good information about how to take care of patients at the end of life, how to have conversations to break bad news, and how to do better pain management. So we concentrated on those nine doctors, offering all of that, *plus* I made myself available to them to offer any kind of triage help with patients who might be dying. I sat at a desk that they had to pass by in order to get coffee. Seeing me helped to spark their memory of an appropriate patient referral or a question about palliative care. We also offered lunchtime videos from the EPEC curriculum[†] and time just to talk about end-of-life care in a relaxed atmosphere.

SLS: *In designing the program, how did you identify the patients who needed your services?*

GT: We realized that identifying which patients were dying was the very first problem we had to solve. We spent, probably, three months coming up with different ideas that might help the clinic physicians to identify patients who were dying. We tried all kinds of fancy things: graphics, trifold brochures, flyers, more

---

[†]Education for Physicians on End-of-Life Care (EPEC) was developed by the American Medical Association's Institute for Ethics and is funded by a grant from The Robert Wood Johnson Foundation. For more information about EPEC, see their website at <www.epec.net>.

education. None of them worked, until we finally came up with the idea of asking them the question, "Would you be surprised if this patient (whom you saw in the last two months) died in the next year?" If they were "not surprised" about a given patient, this was the patient who would be appropriate to have some special attention, special triaging, and connection to community resources. So, that was, like, "bingo!" It just turned out to be an excellent question because physicians were not threatened by it; they didn't feel as though they were putting their medical judgment on the line. As an example, I could say to a physician, "This person has heart failure. It has been going on for years, exacerbations are more frequent, and the medications are not as effective. Would you be surprised if this person died in the next year?"

This question could also be relevant to patients with chronic obstructive pulmonary disease (COPD), and certainly all of us have followed the trajectory of cancer. A lot of doctors are very good at predicting life expectancy for patients with cancer, but *not* so good with those who have chronic illnesses. Of the five most common causes of death in this country, the two leading causes on which doctors tend to focus are heart disease and cancer. But there are also stroke, dementia, and pulmonary diseases; physicians rarely address end-of-life issues early enough with these patients. We really felt that, before starting this initiative, health care in general was not helping the people with end-stage chronic illnesses.

SLS: *Was the vision of the original program primarily promoting continuity and coordination of care at the end of life? Or was it to target the end-of-life population a little bit earlier?*

GT: Actually, it was all of that. The purpose of the program was, first of all, to identify who is dying and slipping through the cracks. We wanted to find those patients who were not getting the quality end-of-life care that they deserve. We needed to connect dying patients and their families to the community resources that are underutilized, but out there. We also needed to promote honest conversations with physicians so that these patients could have the benefit of quality time with their families. In addition, we needed to inform patients about their hospice benefit so that they could be referred earlier and have a longer time with hospice. Hospice is the gold standard in end-of-life care, but typically patients are not referred early enough, resulting in short lengths of stay and crisis management, instead of meaningful and comfortable time for life closure. While a patient is entitled to 180 days, nationally the mean length of stay in hospice is 49 days, and median length of stay is 29 days.[1] So our initiative aims to promote continuity and coordination of care in a timely manner for patients who are seriously ill.

SLS: *What tools did you need to get this program going?*

GT: As the first doctors referred patients to the program, we created forms to triage these patients. Basically, this was the birth of the program. Over the course of the year, we had enough data, new forms, and material for me to write a training manual on how to duplicate the program. It's 13 chapters, about 220 pages long.[2] When our participation in the IHI Collaborative ended, we were able to say to our organization, "This is what we've created. We would like to put it in another clinic." So, at the request of the physicians, we expanded to two more clinics.[‡] We wanted to know, "Would this kind of program work in a rural setting?" and it has been very successful.

I think that prior to implementing the program in a clinic, it is important to have the physicians *requesting* our type of service. We document the number of Medicare patients, number of physicians, and types of resources in a particular geographical area prior to expanding the program to that location. Over time, physicians and clinic managers have requested that we bring the service to their clinic. We started programs to support six clinics in Washington state in autumn 2000. As of October 2000, clinics in Columbus, Ohio, Little Rock, Arkansas, and Nashville, Tennessee, have shown interest in the program.

SLS: *In the initial pilot program, was it easy to train the nine physicians with whom you first started? Or did it take a while to get people to embrace the project?*

GT: Both. Three physicians jumped on it immediately and were very excited about it. They were internists, physicians whose patient population is predominantly comprised of the elderly, more frail, and chronically ill. Family practitioners did not quite see the value in it for a much longer time, almost up to a year later. In addition, over the course of that year, we had a major system affiliation change, which caused some flux in physician positions. So, in some cases, we had to start over with new doctors and bring them on board. Currently, there are again nine providers and all participate in the program.

CONTACTING PATIENTS AND FAMILIES ABOUT THE PROGRAM

SLS: *Once the doctor made the referral to you and your program, how did you approach the patients and families?*

GT: The doctor was required to tell the patient that he or she wouldn't be surprised if the chronic illness that the patient had would cause death and that it could be within a year or so. The physician could word that message any way that he or she wanted, but we found that it is essential for the physician to tell the news. The patient wants to hear this kind of information from the doctor. Then, a nurse calls or visits the patient, depending on whether the patient is in the clinic at the time that the doctor identifies him or her as eligible for the program. If the patient is in the clinic, the doctor comes and gets the end-of-life nurse. She walks down the hall and spends probably half an hour with the patient and family to talk about the program. If the patient has gone home before the refer-

---

‡See Appendix B, pp. 347–350 for the Opening a Clinic Checklist, one of the tools from this manual.

ral reaches the end-of-life nurse's desk, she calls the patient and says, "Doctor Smith told you that I'd be calling you. I'm the nurse that directs this program. He wants to know how you are doing today." Patients and families feel very validated when their doctor wants them to be contacted to see how they are doing. The dialogue and support begin here. The physician is also supported and feels that his or her patient is not being abandoned. It allows the doctor to move on to the next patient.

SLS: *What do you call the program when you make the initial contact with patients?*

GT: When we talk to patients, we call it *Improving Care*. I'd like us to be able to use the whole program name, but we have scared away a few patients by saying *Improving Care through the End of Life*, because then they think that they are dying imminently. At the point of our first contact with the patient, we just begin the dialogue by asking, "How are you doing?" By reaching out to fix only one small thing, we can build a lot of trust. For example, if the patient's greatest identified need is either a pain issue or some symptom management, we can help triage this and get this issue taken care of. So we call a prescription in to the pharmacy, go get it, and deliver it to the home. This immediate action makes a huge difference to the patient and family.

COORDINATION OF CARE THROUGH COMMUNITY SERVICES

SLS: *What kinds of supportive services are you able to connect your patients with?*

GT: I think, predominantly, the ones that we use are the senior centers, Meals-On-Wheels, Lifeline, shuttle services, prescription delivery, and safety inspections. Then we attend to safety issues in their homes, for example, getting bathroom bars installed, or removing scatter rugs, or getting rid of a lot of clutter that's in the way. Of course, when the time is appropriate we assist in the referral to home health or hospice programs in our area. There are many other supportive services on our list, but I'd say these are the ones that we use most frequently.

We can also address other issues in the home. Maybe the patient lives alone and is afraid. In that case, we may suggest a service called Lifeline, a personal, lightweight, waterproof help button that activates a small in-home monitor connected to an operator who can arrange for help. This service costs $40.00 to install and then $1 per day.[§] Or maybe it's a security issue and the patient needs a deadbolt on the door. Sometimes a patient may need someone to create a connection with a neighbor, someone to say to that neighbor, "If this person's blinds don't go up in the morning, could you please call or visit, go knock on the door and see if

---

[§]For more information on Lifeline Systems see <www.lifelinesys.com>.

she's okay?" We may just do something very simple, but what it does is build some rapport and some trust so that then we can begin talking together, truly, about the end of life, life reviews, spiritual renewal, family connections, and living while dying.

SLS: *Can you tell me about the spiritual component of your program?*

GT: Early on we recognized that patients are grieving about their losses. Loss of health, of course, but they've had many other losses that no one has really addressed. They just figure that it is part of getting old, but they're depressed and sad, they may cry a lot, and they feel hopeless or that they're a burden. Our volunteers call patients at least once a month, and we have trained them to listen for unresolved grief issues so that we can arrange for the appropriate support. We realized very early on that we needed a chaplain to be part of this program. So now there is one chaplain connected to every end-of-life care clinic. Those patients who are identified as having a grief and loss issue, or a spirituality issue, by either the end-of-life nurse, the doctor, the volunteer, or anyone who's interacting with them, are referred to the chaplain. The chaplain makes home visits and follow-up phone contacts, attends advance care planning sessions, and may also facilitate a reconnection to a patient's own faith, church, or synagogue, if desired. Then the chaplain stays connected to these patients throughout the time that the patients are in our program. Later, when patients transfer to hospice, we transfer all our spiritual care to the hospice chaplains.

THE ROLE OF VOLUNTEERS

SLS: *What roles do volunteers in your program tend to play? How do they get involved?*

GT: Most volunteers have come to us because they have read about the program, either in the newspaper or through some community-based circle of knowledge. We try to have volunteers who live in the community surrounding a particular clinic support that clinic. We try to keep everything as community-based as possible. Now we are finding that this is very expensive, so, in time, we may have to centralize some of that. But at this point, and for the last few years, we have had volunteers centered around each clinic, with a volunteer coordinator in each clinic. The volunteers are trained to make phone calls to patients and to be a companion by telephone. Once they've had hospice volunteer training, they *can* reach out and go to the home or go out to coffee with a patient enrolled in the program. The people in our program, of course, are not on their deathbeds. They're still going out for dinner and lunches, and sometimes they are doing quite well. But some of them are more homebound, and they're lonely. If hospice trained, the volunteer can spend time with the patient at home and, if the volunteer wishes, continue with the patient after the patient is admitted to hospice. This relationship with the volunteer allows for great continuity of care.

SLS: *How do you train the volunteers?*

GT: First of all, the people who come to us are always caring, compassionate people or they would not even want to do this work. So, we really build on that foundation. We interview them and do the obvious usual checks on people's references, and so forth. Then they have a three-hour training just to learn about the program and how to do the phone calls. Within six months, we like them to have hospice volunteer training. However, this is not required if they only want to remain a phone volunteer. Every month we have a meeting, one hour of which is continuing education about end-of-life care, dying, spirituality, and the like. Then the last hour of the meeting is to provide support for those volunteers. We ask them to reflect on their experience; for example, "Tell us about a case that either bothered you, or worried you, and let's just discuss that."

SLS: *Do you provide bereavement support for your volunteers?*

GT: Yes. If they are hospice trained, they can stay with the patient when the patient moves on from our program into hospice. In doing so, number one, they stay with the patient until death. But, also, because they're hospice trained, they get bereavement counseling and assistance from the hospices. Our program's bereavement counseling is one-on-one. Each volunteer coordinator handles anywhere from 15 to 20 volunteers. So, when a patient dies, the volunteer coordinator calls that volunteer. They may talk over the phone or meet for coffee, or the volunteer may come in for a hug or just to talk about what went on for the patient. We have a library of books, articles, and videos on bereavement to assist the volunteer through this time.

SLS: *What kind of bereavement support do you offer the families of patients in your program?*

GT: Most of our patients ultimately are admitted to hospice care. That's our goal. To date, approximately three-quarters of our patients receive hospice care (more than three times the national average),[1] so the families of these patients automatically receive a year-and-a-half of hospice bereavement care. For others who did not make it to hospice or for some reason didn't choose hospice, our chaplain calls the family two or three times. The volunteer also calls the family two or three times, and we mail bereavement pamphlets to them. But that's about as far as we can take it because the staff must necessarily remain focused on meeting the needs of other patients who are entering the program.

MAKING THE BRIDGE TO HOSPICE CARE

SLS: *Can you describe the relationship the* Improving Care *program has with hospice?*

GT: We have improved referrals to hospice and the hospice lengths of stay. In this community, we have four hospice companies, and we refer to all of them. The physicians in the Franciscan clinics are aligned with the Franciscan system, so, obviously, there are going to be more referrals to the Franciscan hospice program. But that doesn't preclude us from referring to other hospices, depending on what the patients, families, or doctors prefer. By law, we literally have to tell them about all the hospices in our community, and then we have to ask them, "Which hospice would you like?" The families have to choose, or the physician directly writes an order, but we, at the program, do not make this decision.

Once we help the physician, patient, and family determine that "Yes, hospice is timely," we call the referral and send all the paperwork. In this way, the hospice starts out with a wealth of psychosocial and medical information on this patient, which otherwise they often don't have at their fingertips when they first start out with a patient. They appreciate having this information. Also, the end-of-life nurse in our program continues to provide a triage function in relationship to the clinic. For example, when a hospice nurse needs an order change for medicine or some sort of treatment, she calls the end-of-life nurse, who walks down the hall, gets the order changed, and comes back and tells the hospice nurse the change of order or calls it in herself to the pharmacy. This is a service that we provide for all hospice nurses, with the hope of eliminating calls going through the regular switchboard, waiting on hold, or for a call back. In that sense, it makes for smoother communication and continuity of care with the patient's primary care physician.

In Washington state, the primary care physician (PCP) usually remains the point of contact for the hospice patient's orders. In some other states, the hospice medical director or physician becomes the point of contact. We feel that the best continuity of care is to establish the doctor–patient relationship early on and continue that contact. It does not have to be the PCP, but it does have to be someone who learns all that he or she can about this particular patient and then continues to follow the patient until death. Families and patients feel abandoned if their doctor is not available to take calls or prescribe changes in medications. This is especially true during any crisis. The end-of-life nurse facilitates those calls.

SLS: *What happens if a patient is no longer eligible for hospice or improves after being referred to hospice? Can he or she come back to your program?*

GT: It is very important for us to be good stewards of the Medicare Hospice Benefit money, and we want to be sure that patients preserve their benefits. So we tell patients from the very beginning, "If you stabilize and you are no longer actually failing or actively dying, you may be discharged off hospice." We tell patients, "This is not a bad thing." They all kind of laugh about that and call it graduation. So, if a patient stabilizes and is discharged off hospice, the patient is then transferred back to the *Improving Care* program, where we reconnect him or her with the same nurse, chaplain, and volunteer if possible. Once readmitted to the program, the patient is contacted by his or her volunteer on a regular basis and assessed just as before for any physical, emotional, or spiritual needs. A readmit to hospice is completed when the patient again falls within the hospice guide-lines.

SLS: *So, your program really fills in the gaps.*

GT: Yes. This is called a bridge program. We are a bridge to all those community re-sources, including hospice.

> *This is called a bridge program. We are a bridge to all those community resources, including hospice.*

FINANCING THE PROGRAM

SLS: *How do the clinics support the cost of this program?*

GT: At this point, it's all very creatively financed. Some of the clinics pay for the nurse, some pay for the volunteer coordinator, some pay for the chaplain, and some pay for two or three of these positions. The goal is for the clinics to assume total cost of this program by the end of the third year that the program has been in place. The clinics that have been opened the longest are working toward that.

SLS: *Who is assuming the remaining cost right now?*

GT: The remaining cost is assumed by grants. Mostly, the program has been grant funded and foundation funded. We are doing some studies with some insurance companies and are seeking funds to work on a long-term study that could lead to future reimbursement for this type of care. We are also a member of the National Advanced Illness Coordinated Care Council, an initiative that brings together ac-complished, innovative leaders in end-of-life care, administrators in health systems, and insurance executives to integrate advanced illness coordinated care programs into mainstream medical practice.[||]

Physicians should get paid for taking care of dying patients; for example, they should be paid a fee for advance care planning sessions with patients and fami-lies, which is probably the most important part of the program. An advance care planning session takes an hour and a half of time for the physician, the family, the end-of-life nurse, and the chaplain to discuss the patient's diagnosis, what the ex-pectations are down the road, what treatments are available, and what this pa-tient and family's values and wishes are. We really feel that this conversation is key in allowing the patient to verbalize her or his needs and feel validated and supported.

Insurance companies are interested in our program because they feel that, if these conversations take place, it will make a difference in how patients are cared for and be more cost-effective. The key questions are these: How can we pay these

---

[||]The principal investigator of the initiative is Dan Tobin, MD, of the Life Institute, 113 Holland Av-enue, Albany, NY 12208-0980.

physicians for these activities? Can we get to a point where we receive a per diem per patient? Or should we carve out the costs and care for this particular population in the way Joanne Lynn proposes with MediCaring?[3] Somehow, we need to compensate physicians for taking care of this particular population.

SLS: *Do you have any other thoughts on the relationship between financing care and providing quality end-of-life care?*

GT: I think with 80 million baby boomers coming through we will have to find the money for palliative and supportive care for people near the end of life. With current medical technology, people are living longer with chronic illness. Patients and families have unmet needs prior to hospice. We need to figure out how to pay for that support *when* they need it.

   We know physicians are being asked to increase productivity and this decreases time spent with patients during appointments. We need to support doctors in giving this population the time that they need to process what is happening to them. You cannot do that in ten-minute blocks of appointment time. We just have to figure out how to pay physicians something extra as an incentive to take the time for these patients. Time invested at this stage can avoid those expensive ICU hospitalizations in the last six months of life. Besides, it is the right thing to do! It is just a matter of revamping the current codes, how we bill for services, and how we're reimbursed for them.

OFFERING *IMPROVING CARE THROUGH THE END OF LIFE* IN DIFFERENT COMMUNITY SETTINGS

SLS: *How is* Improving Care *being replicated, and what is the process involved in adapting it to the needs of different communities?*

GT: It is easily replicable because the concept is quite simple: two to three people in a clinic are reaching out to that clinic's dying patient population. Over the first year, we created forms and some training that we can now share with others so that they can get a similar program up and running within a couple of weeks.

   The pilot clinic is in a virtually all white, economically diverse community. Then we have the rural clinic on the plateau that is economically diversified. We've also got a clinic going in the inner city, which has even more diversity in terms of race, ethnicity, culture, and economics. The volunteer component both at the rural setting and at the pilot program was never a problem; we almost have more volunteers than we need. But in the inner city it has been harder to build an adequate volunteer base. Otherwise, the program is virtually the same in all three settings.

   We helped staff at the Providence Health System in Portland, Oregon, start an *Improving Care* program in two clinics. They used our training manuals and adapted the program to fit their needs and patient population, but they are trying a different approach. They are using a social worker instead of a nurse as the point person. In addition, they have a nurse practitioner who floats between the two clinics and who answers medical questions. Truly, I think this is a good test, because a lot of what this nurse care coordinator actually does is social work. But the physicians in the Franciscan clinics seem to prefer having a licensed nurse be the care coordinator so that they can give an order to her, and she can make it happen. Whereas, if it's a social worker, physicians have to write the order, and they don't want to take the time. Actually, the job is probably 50/50 registered nursing and social work. So, it makes sense to try it with social workers serving as care coordinators, as long as they have access to a medical person.

Another model we are trying is a "floating care team" out in the community. This is brand new. Many clinics only have one or two physicians, and it would be prohibitively expensive to have a complete team in a small clinic. So, we have a nurse, a volunteer coordinator, and a chaplain situated in one clinic who actually support two other clinics, as well. We're trying to see whether this floating team can do the same thing more cost effectively than having a team situated in each particular clinic.

ADVANCE CARE PLANNING

SLS: *With a floating team, how would the advance care planning session be handled?*

GT: It wouldn't be any different because the advance care planning session is scheduled far ahead of time. It's not like a hospital conference, in which it's imperative that the family comes together with the physician and you decide "Should we do a feeding tube, or take Mom off the vent?" We're saying, "In three weeks, or a month, we would like to gather your family and the physician together on a Friday, or some other day, and pull in the out-of-town adult kids so that the conversations around the table include *all* the important players." Then you don't get those last-minute changes from brother Joe, who flies in from Minnesota and says, "You have to do everything for Mom. That's what I know she wants," when the rest of the family already knows that isn't what Mom wants.

SLS: *What kind of response have you had to the family advance care planning sessions?*

GT: They have been *extremely* successful. They do take an hour to an hour and a half, but the patients just love them. The physicians really like the information gathered at these sessions as it helps them to formulate a plan of care down the road. The worksheet that we fill out during this whole conference is copied and sent home with the family, so they have the discussion right there, including some quotes, and it also becomes part of the medical record in the clinic. We have done these sessions as consultations for other physicians, who either do not want to have this conversation or cannot. We feel that the patient is still entitled to this frank discussion, even if his or her particular physician is not skilled in talking about end-of-life issues or doesn't want to hold the conversation. So, we offer it to all physicians who are part of this program and tell them, "We'd like you to do it, we would like to support you, or even have you come and watch another physician who *is* talented at it model the process for you. Come be a part of this so that, down the road, you will be comfortable doing it."

Now, some have taken us up on that and some have said, "You know, I'm never going to like that part of my practice, so you people just take care of it." Either way, the outcome is favorable for all players.

SLS: *Do the physicians who feel that they are not skilled at these conversations* let *you conduct them?*

GT: Realize that, with this team right in the clinic, we're very present. So we *know* who's skilled and isn't skilled, just from the history. Then we can help to bring them along, but not in any confrontational way. Every clinic *has* to have a champion end-of-life physician who is really on the side of the patient and is trained and preferably certified in palliative medicine. But, barring that, each clinic has at least one physician who is good at having these conversations and has an interest in doing so. Colleagues then tend to defer to him or her and say, "You're good at this. If you don't mind doing this, please do this for me." We think that's great if the champion physician is willing to do so, and we feel that the physician should be rewarded, financially, for taking on that extra duty.

IMPACT ON THE WORK ENVIRONMENT

SLS: *Can you comment on the impact of the program on the clinic work environment?*

GT: Physicians are being placed in a very good light with their patients, so they like that. They also appreciate having someone watching over this fairly fragile patient population—a group of patients who usually require a lot of time on the part of their regular triaging nurses. Their triaging nurses, more and more, are becoming medical assistants. They are the ones that are just taking phone calls and writing down the information, whereas the doctor is the one who actually has to work with every single patient. So, with their time being at a premium and productivity requests being high, physicians don't have as much time to have these conversations with patients, and they're glad that somebody else on the health team is doing that.

FEEDBACK FROM THE PATIENTS AND FAMILIES

SLS: *What kind of evaluation or measurement of outcomes have you developed for this program?*

GT: We have developed an Access database that we use for collecting patient information. Every month, through the volunteer's call, we learn about patients' satisfaction with respect to five given areas: understanding of medical diagnosis and medications, safety in the home, coping with grief and loss, nutrition, and symptom management. The conversation with the volunteer goes wherever the patient wants it to go, but at some point during the conversation it is the volunteer's job to address at least these five areas of satisfaction. We are also collecting data on advance directives, beginning with something as simple as "Do you know what they are? Do you have one? Where is it? Have you made one to go in your wallet? Who else have you discussed these preferences with? Is it just your spouse, or just your physician?" Then, every month, we follow up with another aspect of advance directives.

The third thing we measure is overall satisfaction. Every month, at the very end of the call, each volunteer asks, "Overall, how is your satisfaction with the care you are receiving from your physician and this program and in any way from your community? Is life looking okay? Are you feeling pretty satisfied with what's going on?" The possible answers to those question are "A lot better," "somewhat better," or "unchanged."

Finally, we collect data on the number of supportive services offered, chaplain contacts, deaths with and without hospice, and hospice length of stay. We know month to month where each clinic stands on these measurements. This information helps to create benchmarks for evaluation on how we are doing.

SLS: *Have you made any changes to your program based on the feedback that you collected?*

GT: Definitely. It has been very beneficial. In fact, this is how the "rapid improvement model" works. We make a change for a small sample of patients and then evaluate if it works. If it works, we build on it, and if it doesn't, we try something else. This is how we created the entire program over the course of the first year. And it is how we continue to evolve as we are expanding. Early on, we found that we had to have a chaplain because the "recent loss" satisfaction area was just terrible. Really, sadly, terrible. Patients and families just did not have any support in this realm. We now talk a lot about grief and loss. We ask about spirituality, "What feeds your spirit?" We ask our patients, "How did you handle difficult situations *before?*" so we can learn what patients' strengths *used to be*, and then we can build on those. If it used to be, for example, a lot of prayer or support groups, we'll get that person into prayer or support groups. If it is "I used to walk on the beach and that's where I took my problems," maybe our job is to get that patient to the beach. This feedback helps to direct the plan of care.

> We ask our patients, "How did you handle difficult situations before?" so we can learn what patients' strengths used to be, and then we can build on those.

Another key area we've learned about has been patient knowledge about diagnosis and prognosis. We ask, "How satisfied are you that you understand your diagnosis? What's going on with this illness, and the medications you've been given?" I'm always sad when I hear that a patient doesn't know a thing about his or her diagnosis or the medicine being prescribed. But, we realize, some patients don't want to know, and that's okay, as long as we know that is what they want. So we try to find out by asking, "Do you want to know more about your diagnosis and what usually happens with the course of this illness?" Some will say, "Absolutely," and some will say, "No." We just want to know so that we can guide the doctor and say to him or her, "This patient wants to know more. You need to *really talk* in the next visit about the trajectory of this illness and where you see this is going with this patient." From these discussions we can create the plan of care.

Other areas we talk about with people are safety and nutrition, which are rarely talked about during exam time in the clinic, unless there's a particular weight loss noticed or gastrointestinal upset problem. So we spend quite a bit of time around "*Are* you eating? *Where* are you eating? With *whom* are you eating? And what *kinds* of foods are you eating? Is it satisfactory? Is it adequate? Are you maintaining weight?" This is how assessing patient satisfaction and other feedback have changed the program.

BARRIERS TO GOOD END-OF-LIFE CARE: CHANGING PHYSICIAN BEHAVIOR

SLS: *What are the main barriers that you've been able to overcome?*

GT: The most challenging areas are tied to physician behavior—identifying patients, getting physicians to change the way that they talk to patients, and not offer aggressive treatment to a patient who either doesn't want it, doesn't feel it is necessary, or for whom aggressive treatment may not be appropriate. It is not that physicians do not want to do a better job. In fact, I think 75 percent of those with whom we have worked have been eager to learn these skills.

SLS: *How does the training that you do affect the behavior of those physicians?*

GT: Seeing results over time changes behavior. We have been available, talking, taking care of patients in the clinic for a few years now. Two or three years later, we actually see changed physician behavior. This process is not rapid. The first year you can get referrals to the program and that's fine. But I didn't see actual *changed* physician behavior until the end of the second year, when they were *really* comfortable starting to have these dialogues, offering advance care planning, and doing good pain and symptom management. It just really depends on how much effort is spent in discussion with these doctors and if there is a good rapport between the end-of-life nurse and the physicians. There needs to be a back and forth exchange, which is different from the kind of communication that takes place in the typical doctor–nurse relationship. The hospice teams are also excellent in care management and make good suggestions to the physician for changes in the plan of care and orders, which is another way of learning.

SLS: *So, if someone were to replicate this program, might they expect that it will take longer than a year to see any changes in physician behavior take hold?*

GT: Well, I hate to say a full year because some physicians are so excited about this program right from the get-go and are just eager to learn. I don't in *any* way want to sound disrespectful of the physicians—I think they've never been trained in this domain. I think they *want* to do better, they are just limited in time and expertise in this, and they'd love to know more.

My feeling is, let's put nurses in there that *do* know how to do it and have had that bedside experience. They and the physician champion in the clinic can help to model it for these doctors and bring them along. I also think it takes a dynamic personality to make this kind of a program work in each clinic. The nurse care coordinators have to be able to speak up, reach out, be sharp, a little savvy, all that sort of thing. If you are a little more quiet and shy, maybe it doesn't work as well. My background in oncology and bone marrow transplant, being older, and having a lot of experience, have made a big difference. I don't have any problem approaching a physician and saying, "You know, we really need to do advance care planning here. We need to talk with this family. You can do that. We'd be happy to be in the room and help to support you, but they need to hear it from you. You are the doctor, the leader of the team, and you've got to take that role." Now, some nurses are not comfortable saying that. So, I just feel that we have to select people to do this kind of work who *do* have that comfort and can help to bring physicians along.

The floating care team is where I think we're going to have the bigger barrier in this regard. I don't think there will be any problem setting up referrals, getting patients connected to volunteers, or with the chaplain visits. I think the problem will be, "Will we really change physician behavior if we are not in the clinic, face to face with that doctor?" My suspicion is it will either not happen or it will be slow. But we have to try it to see.

SLS: *What other thoughts would you like to share with our readers?*

GT: I think we always have to take it back to the patient level. Whenever I get bogged down and feel as though everything is bureaucratic, I have to go touch a patient's hand, sit at a bedside or by a chair, or visit with someone in a clinic, and remember it is *this* patient, *this* little 87-year-old woman who is desperately trying to take care of her 91-year-old husband and keep him at home. They're both failing, their children live hither and yon, how can we help them stay home and be viable? That's very important to me—to remember to take it down to just the individual patient and to keep it all as *simple* as possible.

> *We don't have to do rocket science to be good at taking care of a patient who soon may die. In Europe and many other parts of the world, health care professionals do a much better job at this. Other cultures and health care systems seem to embrace end-of-life care as part of the circle of life, whereas we in the United States don't do a very good job of that.*

We don't have to do rocket science to be good at taking care of a patient who soon may die. In Europe and many other parts of the world, health care professionals do a much better job at this. Other cultures and health care systems seem to embrace end-of-life care as part of the circle of life, whereas we in the United States don't do a very good job of that. I think we need to change our culture and expectations. It is going to happen. With those 80 million baby boomers coming through, we're going to have a lot of chronic illness and a lot of people dying in this country, and this may be what really changes our attitude. I think we have to get back to the very simplistic "What can we do for this patient, this family, *right now?*"

REFERENCES

1. *Facts and Figures on Hospice Care in America*. National Hospice and Palliative Care Organization. August 2000.
2. Trandum, G. *Improving Care through the End of Life Training Manual*. Tacoma, WA: Franciscan Health System, 2000. Contact Ms. Trandum at georgannetrandum@chiwest. com.
3. Lynn J, Wilkinson AM. Quality end-of-life care: The case for a MediCaring demonstration. *Hospice Journal*. 1998;13(1–2):151–163.

The Franciscan Program:
A Canadian Perspective

NEIL MACDONALD, CM, MD

Clinical Research Institute of Montreal
Montreal, Quebec, Canada

"Pain *can* kill" was the title of an editorial by the late John Liebeskind in the journal *Pain*.[1] In this article, he mustered evidence on the nocuous effects of pain and stress on the course of cancer. Depression also kills;[2] while, among the many symptoms that bedevil the last days of patients, the cachexia–anorexia syndrome stands out as not only the common cause of dependency and loss of quality of life, but as a syndrome that directly shortens the lives of patients.[3] The practice of medicine is based on an understanding that the early identification of a problem will lead to either ready alleviation or possibly even prevention of the disastrous outcomes that may occur if the problem is not promptly addressed. Is it not logical that we should apply the same thinking to end-of-life care and apply the principles of palliative care as early in the course of a chronic illness as possible? Nevertheless, this simple concept has been ignored within our health care systems; health professionals, patients, and families usually think of palliative/hospice care only when disease is far advanced and death is imminent.

The Franciscan Health System program *Improving Care through the End of Life*, which is described in this part, can serve as a model to help us to overcome current ignorance about the importance of introducing palliative care concepts at the onset of a chronic, predictably fatal illness. My congratulations to Dr. Pattison, Ms. Trandum, their colleagues, and the administration of the Franciscan Health System for implementing a most innovative program.

It is important for programs of this nature to establish and maintain a compre-

> *The practice of medicine is based on an understanding that the early identification of a problem will lead to either ready alleviation or possibly even prevention of the disastrous outcomes that may occur if the problem is not promptly addressed. Is it not logical that we should apply the same thinking to end-of-life care and apply the principles of palliative care as early in the course of a chronic illness as possible?*

hensive database, which can demonstrate that enrolled patients have a measured improvement in their quality of life, excellent family–professional interaction, and a high degree of satisfaction with professional caregivers. The data generated may convince skeptics that the rhetoric of palliative care can translate into improved care for patients at a reasonable cost. It is also key because we may learn that, as one would expect from a review of symptom biology, impeccable patient care may improve not only the quality of existence, but also the length of life.

Concern has been raised that the application of palliative care in acute care settings may dilute palliative/hospice care, as professionals would be caught up in the urgent activities of the acute care setting, functioning simply as "symptomatologists," that is, technicians who cobble together a pharmacological answer to a symptom, but fail to recognize or address the psychosocial components of illness. Thus, they may fail to provide a "warm envelope of care" for patients and families, an approach characteristic of good hospice care. I presume that our colleagues at the Franciscan Health System are answering this concern through ensuring that excellent support services are married with equally excellent treatment of the biological abnormalities created by the disease and its associated symptoms.

I am asked to comment from a Canadian perspective on the Franciscan Health System program. I wish I could say that we "got there first," but I am not aware of a similar Canadian program that identifies patients dying from a variety of chronic illnesses and provides them with a truly "best supportive care" comprehensive program. In the absence of carrying out a survey, I cannot state this as a certain fact; perhaps Canadian readers will be challenged to correct my impression. In our own setting, we are mounting a pilot program whereby patients with inoperable cancer of the pancreas (a disorder with a median survival in the range of four to six months) have the opportunity to enroll in an integrated cancer program combining traditional oncological approaches with specific approaches to pain management, nutrition, exercise programs, identification of psychosocial issues, and, if necessary, professional psychological counseling.[4] Our program is in its infancy, and, while we hope to expand it to include other advanced forms of cancer, it may struggle and fail if we are dependent on existing resources available to us through our health care system; private foundation support will be required.

Our colleagues at Franciscan Health System West are seemingly able to spend the necessary time with patients to ensure that their needs are clearly communicated and addressed. This luxury is not, at present, commonly available in our health care systems. Recently, we have been carrying out a qualitative research project on ethical issues at the end of life, as perceived by patients, families, and palliative care volunteers and health professionals. Although our analysis is not complete, it is already evident that communication issues surface as among the most important ethical concerns raised collectively by all participants. Many of these issues harken back to earlier periods of the disease trajectory, leading one to consider whether a formal communication protocol, mounted at the earliest possible moment, when one knew that a patient would probably die in a predictable period of time, may have alleviated later distress.

I think the Canadian health care system is, please excuse my chauvinism, the best in the world, but our governments, both federal and provincial, have collectively taken a very dangerous step in the last 10 years. Although the costs of our system have always consumed a considerably lower proportion of our gross national product than equivalent American costs, our governments decided in the 1990s that they must cut back sharply on health care expenditures in order to help to balance their budgets. There is no doubt that Canada and its constituent provinces were profligate spenders on a variety of programs (but not on health initiatives, with the exception of the occasional unjustified capital project) in earlier decades, and serious deficits were incurred. Draconian measures were taken, not only in the realm of health, but also in education and social welfare, to correct this situation. Rapid success was achieved and our federal government and almost all provinces now have balanced budgets. However, we do ask ourselves some questions. Why did our governments, which still engage in the "politics of grandeur" (elaborate new government offices, disproportionate bureaucratic systems, unwise investments in the private sector), not protect health and education? Why did they not cut back sharply on nonessential government expenditures? In part, they were strongly influenced by reports of health economists in the early 1990s, who advised government that reduction of numbers of health professionals and hospitals could be successfully carried out without critical damage to the system. They were wrong. The number of Canadian nurses has dropped dramatically in the past few years, leaving us with a critical shortage. Similarly, the decision of our governments to cut back on the intake of students into medical schools in 1993 (roughly a 10 percent cut across the board) has resulted in a problem that, belatedly, the governments are now attempting to redress with urgent requests that the medical schools increase their student intakes. The epidemiologic evidence that the toll of chronic disease was increasing was clearly apparent to all when the decision to cut back on health professionals was made, but this evidence was seemingly not considered. One predictable outcome: while we now teach communication skills to our health professionals, in practice, they are pressed to apply these skills because of the reduced number of people to do the communicating.

Canadian palliative care has a tradition of establishing its large urban programs on a research and educational base. The first programs, at McGill University and St. Boniface Hospital, started in large teaching hospitals. Perhaps they were just being polite, but many American colleagues have indicated their respect for Canadian palliative care, in some part because many of our programs have created innovative academic–community links. There is no doubt that we have many excellent programs, but we stand the risk of falling behind the United States. We take off our hats to recent palliative care initiatives in that country. Consideration of end-of-life issues has received an enormous amount of interest and support of late in the United States. The manifest interest of their professional societies, the impetus created by the SUPPORT studies, the report on end-of-life care by the National Institutes of Medicine, and the fruits of the investment by the Soros Foundation and other foundations, such as The Robert Wood Johnson Foundation, are starting to provide large dividends for Americans. Canada has yet to develop a dedicated research initiative in end-of-life care (such as that by the National Institutes of Health, albeit with a modest investment of funds), or a dedicated program for training internists (in contrast to the program "Improving Residency Training in End-of-Life Care," initiated by Dr. David Weissman in concert with the American Board of Internal Medicine and with The Robert Wood Johnson Foundation sponsorship). Systems for continuing physician education in palliative care, however, are well developed in a number of Canadian provinces, together with excellent educational websites (one example I frequently use and highly recommend is that of the Edmonton Palliative Care Program, <www.palliative.org>).

I believe that when the Canadian health care system is once again adequately supported, the basic tenets of that system (Figure 1) free us to make enormous progress. Contrary to popular American opinion, the Canadian health care system

---

The five principal features of Canadian Medicare, as originally included in the *Hospital Insurance Act* and reaffirmed in the *Canada Health Act*, derive from the health care system's fundamental principle of equality.[5]

1. **Comprehensiveness:** Coverage extends to all hospital and all physician and surgeon services; some provinces add other health care benefits, such as dental services for children, drugs for the elderly, chiropractic, optometry and physiotherapy treatments.
2. **Universality:** These services are available to all Canadians, regardless of income or other considerations; nor do poor people have to undergo a means test to establish their eligibility for coverage.
3. **Accessibility:** Canadians must have reasonable access to medically necessary services.
4. **Portability:** A resident of one province or territory is covered while traveling in other parts of Canada and, at least partially, in other countries.
5. **Public administration:** Services administered either by an independent commission or by the health department.

Figure 1.   Principle Features of Canadian Medicine. Copyright © 1994 Prentice Hall Canada. Reprinted with permission by Pearson Education Canada, Inc.

is characterized by less red tape than one encounters in dealing with the myriad different insurance systems and health maintenance organizations in the United States. Moreover, government bureaucracies can be exasperating, but at least we are shareholders in the system, and "profits" accrue directly to all citizens.

A few current examples of how the structural aspects of the Canadian health care system lend themselves to the promotion of a community-based initiative such as the Franciscan program include the following:

• The health care services in a number of Canadian provinces have designated palliative care as a special program. Consequences include the provision of salary support for palliative care physicians and special program support for community palliative care services. In a fee-for-service system it is extremely difficult, if one is indeed spending the necessary time with patients, to make a reasonable income.

- As health care is developed on a regional basis in most Canadian cities, it is possible to develop fully comprehensive programs that cover whole regions. Consequently, there is less competition between programs and better opportunities for cooperative endeavors. Many such programs exist in Canada. I am most familiar with the Edmonton Palliative Care Program, which covers an entire city region of more than 800,000 people. Developed on an academic foundation, the community service program is funded through a base budget by the Edmonton Regional Health Authority, with additional support for educational and research projects provided by both provincial and local hospital and university sources. The program provides sophisticated palliative care services, involving a range of health professionals, for the entire city. Special home nursing care and palliative care inpatient units are available, but a great proportion of the work involves consultation and cooperative activity with the excellent family physicians practicing in the Edmonton region.
- In the larger city in which I now live, Montreal (with more than three million people), a regional program has yet to emerge. Our McGill program, also developed on a research and educational base, is carrying out a pilot project in which we interact with five community health centers in Montreal. In the core of our city, private family practice is less developed than in Edmonton, and many patients depend on nursing or physician care offered through the community health centers.
- Many Canadian centers have mobile palliative care teams that visit people at home. An early example, from which we have all learned, is the Victoria Hospice Program. The aforementioned Edmonton program is famous for its interdisciplinary "bus rounds."
- Publicly supported residency programs in palliative care are now available in Canada. Six of our sixteen universities (Alberta, McMaster, Ottawa, Laval, McGill, and Manitoba) now offer yearlong training programs. As a result, we hope to provide a cadre of palliative care specialists who will serve as consultants to physicians with primary responsibility for the care of patients with chronic illness and increasingly involve them in coordinated programs for the early application of palliative care.

In some ways, on both sides of the border, our government health leaders are like World War I generals—overly concerned with the "macro" issues of rear echelon bureaucratic planning and ensuring administrative order, with consequent failure to address the simple needs of patients and families at the end of life.

In some ways, on both sides of the border, our government health leaders are like World War I generals—overly concerned with the "macro" issues of rear echelon bureaucratic planning and ensuring administrative order, with consequent failure to address the simple needs of patients and families at the end of life. All this will change when innovative models of care, such as that exemplified by the Franciscan program, are publicized and our communities and organizations press legislators and medical leaders to reset their priorities.

The diverse and creative palliative care initiatives currently underway in the United States certainly enhance our efforts in Canada. I hope that, in turn, some of our initiatives may continue to interest and influence our American colleagues. While some American legislators have recently expressed concerns about the permeability of the U.S.–Canada border, mutually, we count our blessings that there is no "duty" on advances in palliative care, which freely cross the 49th parallel.

REFERENCES

1. Liebeskind JC. Pain *can* kill. *Pain*. 1991;44:3-4.
2. Wulsin LR. Does depression kill? [editorial; comment]. *Archives of Internal Medicine*. 2000;160(12):1731–1732.
3. MacDonald N, Baracos VE, Plata-Salaman CR, Tisdale MJ. Cachexia–Anorexia review. *Nutrition*. 2000;16(10):1009–1018.
4. MacDonald N, Ayoub JP, Barkun A, Dalzell MA, Gagnon B, Rosenberg L. Carcinoma of the pancreas: An integrated programme. *Cancer Strategy*. 2000;2(1):17-24.
5. Roy DJ, Williams JR, Dickens BM. *Bioethics in Canada*. Scarborough, Ontario: Prentice Hall Canada Inc., 1994, 95-96.

Part One

Selected references by contributors to this part:

Della Penna R, Rosenthal M. Fulfilling the promise of managed care: A joint project between Kaiser Permanente and the Los Angeles Alzheimer's Association. *Drug Benefit Trends*, April 1998.

Doyle D, Hanks GWC, MacDonald N (eds.). *Oxford Textbook of Palliative Medicine*. Oxford, England: Oxford University Press, 1998.

MacDonald N. A march of folly. *Canadian Medical Association Journal*. 1998;158(13):1699–1701.

MacDonald N. Palliative care: An essential component of cancer control. *Canadian Medical Association Journal*. 1998;158(13):1709–1716.

MacDonald N, Ayoub JP, Barkun A, Dalzell MA, Gagnon B, Rosenberg L. Carcinoma of the pancreas: An integrated programme. *Cancer Strategy*. 2000; 2(1): 17–24.

MacDonald N, Baracos VE, Plata-Salaman CR, Tisdale MJ. Cachexia–Anorexia review. *Nutrition*. 2000;16(10):1009–1018.

Trandum, Georganne. *Improving Care through the End of Life Training Manual*. Tacoma, WA: Franciscan Health System, 2000. Contact Ms. Trandum at georgannetrandum@chiwest.com.

References about *Improving Care through the End of Life*:

Enck, RE. Hospice: The next step. *American Journal of Hospice & Palliative Care*. 1999;16(2):436.

Moyers: People want gentle, loving end of life. 8 May 2000. *American Hospital Association News*. 4 January 2002 <www.ahanews.com>.

The Oncology Roundtable. *Culture of Compassion: Best Practices in Supportive Care*. Washington, DC: Advisory Board Company; Best Practices Compendium, 2000, 106–110. Contact www.orders@advisory.com.

Warren R. Improving care at the end of life. *Supportive Voice*. Winter 2000;6(1): 11–12.

Other selected references:

Claessens MT, Lynn J, Zhong Z, Desbiens NA, Phillips RS, Wu AW, Harrell FE Jr, Connors AF Jr. Dying with lung cancer or chronic obstructive pulmonary disease: Insights from SUPPORT. Study to Understand Prognoses and Preferences for Outcomes and Risks of Treatments. *Journal of the American Geriatrics Society*. 2000;48(5 Suppl):S146–S153.

Larson DG, Tobin DR. End-of-life conversations: Evolving practice and theory. *Journal of the American Medical Association*. 2000;284:1573–1578.

Lynn J. Reforming the care system to support those coming to the end of life. *Cancer Control*. 1999;6(2):131–135.

Lynn J, Wilkinson A, Etheredge L. Medicine and money: Financing of care for fatal chronic disease: Opportunities for Medicare reform. *Western Journal of Medicine*. 2001;175:299–302.

Lynn J, De Vries KO, Arkes HR, Stevens M, Cohn F, Murphy P, Covinsky KE, Hamel MB, Dawson NV, Tsevat J. Ineffectiveness of the SUPPORT intervention: Review of explanations. *Journal of the American Geriatrics Society*. 2000;48(5 Suppl): S206–S213.

Lynn J, Ely EW, Zhong Z, McNiff KL, Dawson NV, Connors A, Desbiens NA, Claessens M, McCarthy EP. Living and dying with chronic obstructive pulmonary disease. *Journal of the American Geriatrics Society*. 2000;48(5 Suppl):S91–S100.

Lynn J, O'Connor MA, Dulac JD, Roach MJ, Ross CS, Wasson JH. MediCaring: Development and test marketing of a supportive care benefit for older people. *Journal of the American Geriatrics Society*. 1999;47(9):1058–1064.

Lynn J, Wilkinson A, Cohn F, Jones SB. Capitated risk-bearing managed care systems could improve end-of-life care. *Journal of the American Geriatrics Society*. 1998;46(3):322–330.

O'Connor MA, Lynn J. MediCaring: Comprehensive support services as a Medicare option. *Caring*. 1995(May):72–76.

Rogers AE, Addington-Hall JM, Abery AJ, McCoy ASM, Bulpitt C, Coats AJS, Gibbs JSR. Knowledge and communication of difficulties for patients with chronic heart failure: Qualitative study. *British Medical Journal*. 2000;321:605–607.

Roy DJ, Williams JR, Dickens BM. *Bioethics in Canada*. Scarborough, Ontario: Prentice Hall Canada, Inc., 1994, 95–96.

Part Two

Institutionalizing Palliative Care

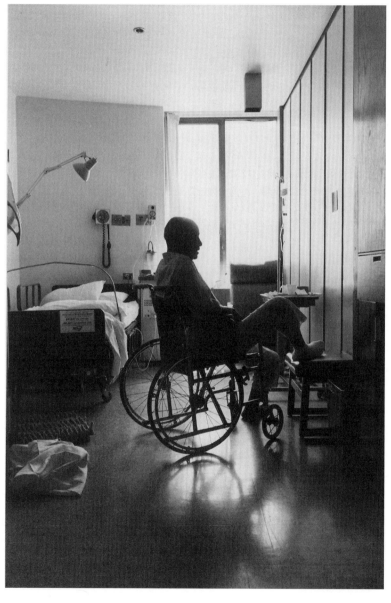

"Passing Time"
©1985 Nita Winter.

Clinical Pathways for Care of the Dying: An Innovation to Disseminate Clinical Excellence

JOHN ELLERSHAW, MA, FRCP

Marie Curie Centre & Royal Liverpool University Hospital
Liverpool, England

Palliative care developed in response to increasing concern about the standard of care for dying patients and their families.[1] There were several widely publicized cases where patients died without dignity and with poorly controlled symptoms. These cases also revealed inadequate support for families and a disregard for the spiritual element of care. Health care professionals trained in a culture of "cure" seemed unable to respond to the needs of dying patients and their families. Dissatisfaction with this situation provided the impetus for the pioneers in palliative care, to demand a fundamental change in attitude toward the care of dying patients and their family/carers. It is imperative that as a palliative care movement we capture this model of excellence in care of the dying and hold it as a beacon to be clearly seen and understood. It can then be translated to other care settings and delivered by other health care professionals.

> *It is imperative that as a palliative care movement we capture this model of excellence in care of the dying and hold it as a beacon to be clearly seen and understood. It can then be translated to other care settings and delivered by other health care professionals.*

Palliative care services include inpatient and outpatient care, day therapy, bereavement care, and a specialist advisory role in both community and hospital settings. This clinical activity is supported by education and research activity. Palliative care services may offer all these elements, but more commonly focus on specific areas. There is an increasing emphasis on rehabilitation and a current trend toward including non-cancer patients. These new developments may give the appearance of a reduced emphasis on the care of the dying. Specialists in palliative care may assume that this aspect of care is well recognized and so are keen to emphasize other aspects of care. This attitude may be complacent. The model of excellence for care of the dying developed throughout the palliative care world has been under-researched and poorly disseminated outside the palliative care unit/hospice setting.

This part of *Innovations* features the development of two palliative care services, those offered by the Beth Israel Medical Center in New York City* and the Trondheim University Hospital in Norway. Drs. Portenoy and Kaasa share their respective experiences, which include the challenges of evolving new services. The interview with Dr. Bookbinder on the Palliative Care for Advanced Disease (PCAD) pathway provides an important example of how best practice for care of the dying can be delivered in all health care settings by empowering health care professionals to deliver high-quality care to dying patients.

INTEGRATED CARE PATHWAYS

Integrated Care Pathways (ICPs), or Clinical Care Pathways, have their origins in the United States.[2] Over the past decade they have gained popularity in the United Kingdom and in Europe.[3-5] An ICP is developed by the multiprofessional team involved in the caring process and should incorporate evidence-based practice and appropriate guidelines.[6,7] The ICP then acts as a template describing the process of care that is generally delivered in a given clinical situation. The ICP outlines both the role of each health care professional involved in the care of patients and their family/carers and details of the expected outcome of such care delivery. These outcomes are then recorded on the ICP. If the expected outcome is not achieved, the reason is documented. This deviation from expected care delivery is called a "variance."

Variances from the pathway are acceptable, but need to be documented along with an explanation for the variance. It is important that health care professionals recognize that the need to record variances and the education to encourage this documentation represent key challenges during the initial implementation of a care pathway. A review of the variances will often identify areas of educational need or resource issues that, when addressed, will improve care delivery. As well as deficits, variances show more effective ways of delivering care, which in turn lead to further modification of the ICP. The ICP is a dynamic document that will evolve over time and may in some circumstances replace all other documentation, becoming a central coordinating document of care.

ICPs AND PALLIATIVE CARE

The philosophy of palliative care emphasizes a holistic approach to an individual and the family/carers. ICPs initially seem at odds with this philosophy, appearing too rigid to facilitate the delivery of care in a palliative care setting. However, several care pathways, including the PCAD pathway, have been developed in a palliative care setting.*[8,9] ICPs do not prevent the delivery of individualized care; in-

---

*The Department of Pain Medicine and Palliative Care at Beth Israel Medical Center is one of three winners of the American Hospital Association's 2001 Circle of Life Award.
†See <www.StopPain.org >, the Beth Israel Medical Center Department of Pain Medicine and Palliative Care.

stead, they allow the clinical freedom to provide care within an evidence-based framework. They are particularly appropriate in palliative care, acting as a multi-professional document that staff can use to coordinate and record the care of the patient.

ICPs AND CARE OF THE DYING

Transferring the palliative care model of excellence for care of the dying into the hospital and community setting is, I believe, one of the greatest challenges for the palliative care movement. ICPs are potentially a powerful tool in the achievement of this goal. A number of important steps in the care of the dying are often considered routine in a palliative care unit or hospice, but are often only partially or poorly performed in other health care settings.

Diagnosing Dying

The hospital setting has a strong emphasis on cure, and the concept of diagnosing dying is almost counterculture. Consequently, doctors are often reluctant to diagnose dying. Instead, they feel that there must always be additional investigations or treatments to make the patient "better." This attitude can be very destructive. The patient and family/carers are led to believe that improvement is possible or likely. When the patient then deteriorates and dies, the family may be left with a feeling of betrayal and lose trust in the health care professionals. The patient's death can appear unexpected and the relatives may be unprepared, often expressing the wish that they had been warned—"If only someone had told us."

As in other aspects of medicine, the diagnosis of dying is a combination of science and art. If we believe that the patient is in the dying phase, then we should care for the patient and family/carers appropriately. One barrier to diagnosing dying is that health care professionals may not know what to do next for dying patients and therefore continue active treatment. An ICP for the dying patient at this point is an important tool.

The very existence of an ICP for the dying patient in a clinical setting makes health care professionals aware that there is a model of excellence for care of the dying and that in order to deliver this, a diagnosis of dying must be made. In some situations a dying patient may occasionally improve, in which case the

> *The very existence of an ICP for the dying patient in a clinical setting makes health care professionals aware that there is a model of excellence for care of the dying and that in order to deliver this, a diagnosis of dying must be made.*

ICP for the dying patient is discontinued. However, to my knowledge, having an ICP in place has never been to the detriment of either the patient or the family/carers.

Initial Assessment and Care of the Dying Patient

When patients enter the dying phase they are generally semicomatose, are unable to take oral medication, and have become bed bound. Given these criteria in cancer patients, the median time to death is two days.[10] This is a common scenario for cancer patients, but cannot be extrapolated to all patient populations. It is of vital importance that the multiprofessional team agree that the patient is dying so that a diagnosis of dying can be made. Disagreement in the team can mean that the patient and family/carers receive conflicting messages.

When the patient enters the dying phase in a palliative care unit/hospice, an active process of care for both the patient and family/carers is initiated. In contrast, particularly in hospital settings, staff may withdraw at this point in time. The active process of care includes reviewing the patient's medication. Nonessential drugs are discontinued, and appropriate medication is prescribed with consideration of the route of administration. Relatives are made aware that the patient is dying and the religious and spiritual needs of the patient are addressed. These and other important aspects of care are identified in the PCAD pathway.

Ongoing Care of the Dying Patient

It is important that an inpatient be reviewed on a regular basis, with at least four observations of symptom control and appropriate action taken if required. Particular attention is paid to pain, agitation, respiratory tract secretions, mouth care, and micturition difficulties. It is also important that appropriate psychological and religious support be given to the patient and family/carers.

IMPLEMENTATION AND EDUCATION PROGRAM LINKED WITH AN ICP

To develop and implement an ICP for the dying patient and subsequently deliver a high standard of care would appear to be straightforward. However, the practicalities of actually achieving this are seismic. If best practice is to be achieved in the care of the dying, it is not just the acquisition of knowledge and skills that is required, but also a change in attitude, especially in the hospital setting.

The educational role of palliative care teams is well recognized, but often poorly achieved. The clinical workload frequently excludes the possibility of an educational program, and even if this can be delivered, exposure to theory often does very little to change clinical practice, as Dr. Portenoy highlights in his interview.

To achieve a change in practice by implementing an ICP involves a major time commitment. First, it needs to be introduced into an organization that has signed up at the executive level to implement it. The next step is to undertake a base review. This is a retrospective review of current practice and establishes a base line from which post-implementation data can be compared. It also encourages the development of reflective practice in the health care professionals who are using the ICP.

It is important not to underestimate the amount of educational commitment required to implement an ICP for the dying patient. It can take from 6 to 18 months before the ICP can be introduced into a new clinical area. Importantly, however, the ICP can be a powerful educational tool for palliative care professionals. So often we educate at a level that merely informs the participants that we know more than they do. As a result, when health care professionals care for a patient with palliative care needs, they automatically refer to the palliative care services. This leads to overall de-skilling of health care professionals. Palliative care advisory teams can never hope, nor should they aim, to be involved in all deaths occurring in the hospital and community. It is essential that generic palliative care, including care of the dying, be delivered by *all* health care professionals. It is of critical importance that an ICP for care of the dying facilitate education at a level appropriate to the health care professionals, to avoid de-skilling and to promote empowerment of staff.

On a broader educational theme, the integration of palliative care ICPs into health care professionals' educational programs (not just at the postgraduate level, but at the undergraduate level as well) is a good opportunity to influence attitudes at an early stage in their training. If nurses and doctors are familiar with such tools when they commence practice, they will provide a powerful model for care delivery. Indeed, in his interview in this issue, Dr. Kaasa describes a vision of an international curriculum of palliative care. Undoubtedly, the components of an ICP for care of the dying patient should be an integral part of any such curriculum.

IMPACT OF AN ICP ON AN ADVISORY PALLIATIVE CARE TEAM

Interestingly, the role of an advisory palliative care team is influenced by the implementation of a care of the dying pathway. At first it may appear as a threat to the team, conveying the message that palliative care is predominantly about care of the dying. In fact, experience proves otherwise. The intense educational process and program that are undertaken around the role of the palliative care services impacts on the understanding of all health care professionals. The knowledge, skills, and attitudes gained during the implementation of the care pathway will have an influence on the care of patients earlier in their disease, including improvements in symptom control and communication skills. Frequently, the experience of palliative care teams is that, following the introduction of a care pathway, health care professionals use the team more appropriately.

The ICP for the Dying Patient in the Palliative Care Unit/Hospice Setting

Introducing an ICP for the dying patient in a hospital or community setting can clearly lead to benefits for patients and their family/carers. However, the benefits of introducing it into a palliative care unit/hospice are perhaps less clear. Why introduce a document into a care setting where we already have a model of excellence for care of the dying?

Outcome-based culture within palliative care is poorly developed. The introduction of ICPs provides the potential to overcome this problem. By documenting the process of care, demonstrable outcomes can be identified, which can then be audited to set standards[10,11] and facilitate reflective practice (e.g., case audit). It has been said, "If you try to measure something that is important, what you measure then becomes important." Therefore, it is important that outcome measures from an ICP capture the physical, psychological, social, and spiritual aspects of palliative care.

CONCLUSION

Clinical pathways are an innovation that can lead to the dissemination of clinical excellence in palliative care. The PCAD pathway is an example of an ICP that leads to the empowerment of health care professionals. It enables them to deliver a model of excellence in care of the dying, which if widely implemented has the potential to improve quality of care for all dying patients. ICPs can be used to promote the educational role in palliative care and to develop the role of specialist palliative care advisory teams. If health care professionals need further convincing of the importance of providing a high standard of care for dying patients, they should consider this comment made by a husband, following the death of his 40-year-old wife: "All the excellent treatment and care that went before meant nothing because she died a painful, undignified death."

ICPs also have the potential to set standards and to be used for quality assurance within palliative care unit/hospice settings. Most of all, they can perhaps achieve what the pioneers in palliative care most desired and society increasingly demands—that the culture for care of the dying be fundamentally changed.

REFERENCES

1. Clark D. Originating a movement: Cicely Saunders and the development of St. Christopher's Hospice 1957–1967. *Morality*. 1998;3:43–63.
2. Zander K. Critical Pathways. In *Total Quality Management: The Health Care Pioneers*, M Melum, M Sinior (eds.). Chicago: American Hospital Publishing, Inc., 1992, 305–314.
3. Overill SA. A practical guide to care pathways. *Journal of Integrated Care*. 1998;2:93–98.
4. de Luc K. *Developing Care Pathways: A Handbook*. National Pathways Association. Oxford, England: Radcliffe Medical Press, 2001.
5. Campbell H, Hotchkiss R, Bradshaw N, Porteous M. Integrated care pathways. *British Medical Journal*. 1998;316:133.
6. Working Party on Clinical Guidelines in Palliative Care. *Changing Gear: Guidelines for Managing the Last Days of Life in Adults*. National Council for Hospice and Specialist Palliative Care Services. Northamptonshire, England: Land & Unwin (Data Sciences) Ltd., 1997.
7. Adam J. The last 48 hours. *British Medical Journal*. 1997;315:1600–1603.
8. Ellershaw J, Foster A, Murphy D, Shea T, Overill S. Developing an integrated care pathway for the dying patient. *European Journal of Palliative Care*. 1997;4:203–207.

9. Gordon DB. Critical pathways: A road to institutionalising pain management. *Journal of Pain and Symptom Management*. 1996;11:252–259.

10. Ellershaw J, Smith C, Overill S, Walker S, Aldridge J. Care of the dying: Setting standards for symptom control in the last 48 hours of life. *Journal of Pain & Symptom Management*. 2001;21:12–17.

11. Kitchener D, Davidson C, Bundred P. Integrated care pathways: Effective tools for continuous evaluation of clinical practice. *Journal of Evaluated Clinical Practice*. 1995;2:65–69.

Developing an Integrated Department of Pain and Palliative Medicine

An Interview with RUSSELL K. PORTENOY, MD

Beth Israel Medical Center
New York, New York

In 1996, the United Hospital Fund awarded planning grants to 12 hospitals to analyze their needs, resources, capacities, and program development strategies. Beth Israel Medical Center in New York City was one of five programs to receive a further implementation grant from UHF in 1998 to continue their efforts.* The Department of Pain Medicine and Palliative Care (DPMPC) was established in 1997–1998 under the leadership of Russell K. Portenoy, MD, a neurologist with expertise in pain management and palliative care. By drawing together the specialized care and resources involved in pain medicine, inpatient and outpatient palliative care, and hospice care, this department is the first of its kind to exist as an integrated department within a hospital system. As such, it provides one of the most comprehensive models for palliative medicine found in the United States. With its focus on multidisciplinary teamwork, symptom management, and pain control and the integration of hospice into the practice of palliative medicine, Beth Israel Medical Center's DPMPC brings together the benefits of expert medical practice and psychosocial care to patients and families in one comprehensive center.

  The Department of Pain Medicine and Palliative Care is one of three recipients of the American Hospital Association's 2001 Circle of Life Award. In the following interview with Karen S. Heller, PhD, Dr. Portenoy speaks about the unique opportunity he has had to create an integrated department within the hospital institution. He discusses the strengths and successes of such a comprehensive and coordinated program, as well as the limitations and challenges that still lie ahead in the field of palliative care.

---

*For the full UHF Report, see Hopper SS. *Building Hospital Palliative Care Programs: Lessons from the Field*. New York: United Hospital Fund of New York, 2001.

HISTORY OF THE DEPARTMENT OF PAIN MEDICINE
AND PALLIATIVE CARE

Karen S. Heller: *When did you first start thinking about developing a pain and palliative care program and how did it happen?*

Russell K. Portenoy: The senior leadership at Beth Israel had a very long history of interest in humanistic care and end-of-life care that dated back many years. In 1997, the administration responded to an RFA (Request for Applications) from the United Hospital Fund (UHF), which was focused on plans to build palliative care infrastructure at various hospitals around New York City. The Beth Israel Medical Center (BIMC) grant was originally designed to provide some education in palliative care to housestaff.

I was contacted by the administration after they received the award and asked if I would consult for the educational program. I went down to BIMC for a preliminary meeting about the program and began to talk a little bit about what palliative care is and where palliative care is going in the United States. The senior medical staff to whom I was speaking literally pushed the grant application aside and said, "What would you want to do here if you could create a model program?" I began to speak to them about things that I had been considering for more than five years in what was then my current position as co-chief of the Pain and Palliative Care Service at Memorial Sloan–Kettering Cancer Center. We had begun to work at Sloan–Kettering to try to bring a more comprehensive palliative care approach to what had been a pain program.

I described a program with inpatient and home care elements, which would be focused on quality-of-life-oriented care throughout the course of an illness, as well as excellence in end-of-life care. They were immediately interested and asked me to put my ideas down in writing, which I did the next day. Four days later, I received a call saying that the administration had decided to go for the package, that they wanted to recruit me and, essentially, give me whatever I wanted in order to try to build this palliative care program.

The recruitment was an incredible adventure for me. It included a personal visit from the chairman of the board of trustees to my office at Sloan–Kettering. During that visit he told me that they were totally committed to this area, they really wanted this activity, that it was entirely in line with the mission and vision of their institution, and that they would support it in any way I wanted.

Well, for an academic physician to be told that there's a true blank check—I was astonished, incredulous—my heart stopped for about an hour! Then I collected myself and began a series of very serious negotiations with the BIMC administration, speaking with both the medical side and the business side of the administration. Early in those discussions, as I learned more about the facilities and resources that Beth Israel Medical Center had, I realized that its pain program was very limited. I had been doing pain management—nonmalignant disorders like low back pain and headache—for many years, and I brought up the possibility of perhaps linking a multidisciplinary state-of-the-art pain management program to the development of this new model of palliative care that we had been discussing. The BIMC administration said, essentially, "Go for it. Show us what you would need in terms of facilities and personnel, and we'll see if we can accommodate it."

PLANNING A CONJOINED PAIN AND PALLIATIVE CARE PROGRAM

Over a period of months, I negotiated with the institution to establish the organizational structure and requirements for this very large program. It would include a multidisciplinary pain management program as it has been traditionally configured for 20 years in the United States and also a model of palliative care that would not be limited to end-of-life care, but would cover a full range of services for inpatients and outpatients.

During those negotiations, the institution pointed out to me that they were already supporting a hospital-based hospice program, one of only two in New York City, the Jacob Perlow Hospice Program. They suggested that the hospice program be administratively moved and linked to the model that I was talking about. I had already planned to use the hospice program as a resource for end-of-life care within a broader model of palliative care, but the opportunity to administratively join the hospice program with this new program that I was developing was a tremendous advantage to the model itself. It provided a way of creating policies and procedures and budgetary devices that allowed real linkages to form.

After the required personnel and other infrastructural issues were agreed on, I was left with the reality that I was being offered an opportunity to build something that included many people in multiple disciplines, an inpatient unit, and space for ambulatory practice in both pain and palliative care, as well as this relationship with the hospice organization. I began to talk with the hospital's senior leadership about what this entity could possibly be within the bureaucracy of the institution. At one point, I said to them, "Something this substantial, if it weren't in this area of medicine, would probably be called a department," and they said, "Well, we have no problem with that, let's call it a department."

There was this long silence while I was trying to restart my heart again, and I said, "Well, you understand that there are no other departments devoted to either pain medicine or palliative care anywhere in the United States. To create one would represent a very significant statement about the status of these fields in the institutional hierarchy, and it would also carry with it a number of very significant obligations over time."

I got a call from the president and CEO of the institution about a day later and he said, "I just want to clarify for you that we have absolutely no concerns about naming this a department. In fact, in my view I would guess that in about five years there will be departments all over the country." With this decision, I was clearly being offered an unprecedented opportunity. I was being provided with personnel, space, and resources to build both a state-of-the-art pain program and a new model of palliative care, which would integrate a well-established and highly respected hospice program. And it included an opportunity to house the entire thing within a departmental structure, which would have me essentially on equal footing with medicine, surgery, pediatrics, obstetrics/gynecology, and every other department in an academic medical center.

KSH: *What, if anything, predisposed this institution to be so welcoming to a department of pain and palliative care?*

RKP: While I was being recruited, I really tried to find out the answer to that question because it was difficult to believe. I came to understand that there was a very long tradition at Beth Israel of humanistic health care and a very strong commitment on the part of a senior leadership that had all worked together for many years.

Beth Israel began as an infirmary on the lower East Side set up to care for first-generation Jewish immigrants, who were not allowed to enter any of the uptown hospitals. There has been a very long tradition of care for the poor and populations that are underserved or excluded. It was the first hospital to do away with isolation approaches for patients suffering from AIDS and one of the few to establish a hospice program. In the early 1990s, a few years before I was recruited, the hospital allowed a reporter for the *New York Times* to review the charts of more than 10 patients who had died in the hospital, interview the family members, and discuss in-hospital deaths in New York City. This ended up being a front-page series, and it occurred at a time when the whole concept of discussing end-of-life care in the media was not happening as it is today. It took tremendous courage for the hospital to be so open about this subject. The concept that people don't go to hospitals to die, but rather to get fixed, was so embedded in the American conscience that it was a really courageous act to actually admit that people die in our institutions and that care of the dying is part of what we do. Parenthetically, I remember reading that series in the *Times*, turning to my wife, and saying, "Boy, this is so unusual for an institution. . . . I wonder if they're interested in palliative care, and would want to hire me to do it?"

> *The concept that people don't go to hospitals to die, but rather to get fixed, was so embedded in the American conscience that it was a really courageous act to actually admit that people die in our institutions and that care of the dying is part of what we do.*

THE CHANGING FINANCIAL ENVIRONMENT OF HEALTH CARE INSTITUTIONS

In discussing the genesis of my program, I think it's very important to note that the difference between 1997 and 2001 in terms of the financial viability of institutions in New York City is like night and day. In 1997, Beth Israel was coming off of a very long period of surpluses in the operations budget. It had an annual investment budget that was between $50 and $60 million for capital improvements and program development. It was pursuing the concept of centers of excellence in a variety of different areas—complementary medicine, cardiac disease, cancer—and the new focus on pain medicine and palliative care was consistent with the vision of growth and investment.

Between 1998 or 1999 and the present, there has been an incredible financial turnaround in the hospitals in New York City. All the major hospitals are losing money on their operations now. The hospitals are refinancing debt, and investment income is way down. I have no question at all that the hospital couldn't even consider starting a program like mine now, and, in fact, it's to their great credit that they're so totally committed to sustaining my program at a time of so many financial challenges. But, unfortunately, the idea that this could happen now on the scale that was originally offered to me seems unrealistic given the current financial environment. Rather, institutions like mine will be seeking ways to start smaller, phasing-in programs as interest grows and the financial implications become clear. If there is commitment, I am sure that this can still happen. The extraordinary "right place, right time, right people" opportunity that I had might be harder to come by, but things can happen if there is willingness to explore the concept of a specialized palliative care model, to think through the financial stakes, and to work together on a viable business model.

Financing a Complex, Comprehensive Program of Care

KSH: *How is your program financed overall?*

RKP: Because of very complex accounting methodology, the lack of cost accounting, the fact that revenue streams originate in so many different places, and the fact that personnel can be placed on many different cost centers that are themselves sustained by different revenue streams, it is incredibly difficult to answer that simply. Speaking in general, all programs are essentially funded through some combination of clinical revenue, philanthropy, and grants, and clinical revenues are generated only by certain personnel within a department—physicians, nurse practitioners, and psychologists. My department has eight physicians, two psychologists, and several nurse practitioners who have limited practices. Staff that do not generate revenue include a social worker, many nurses, a chaplain, and support personnel. I would guess that the clinical revenue from the collections generated by those individuals who can bill for services support only a very small piece of what we provide in terms of services. Other revenue to the institution generated by these clinicians—by admission to the hospital, facility fees for procedures, new patient referrals, and the like—cover some of our work as well.

Some of the staff are being supported by hospital revenues generated directly through our inpatient unit. We have a 14-bed closed inpatient unit that we try to keep occupied with patients who need our services. The patients in that unit are either hospice patients or non-hospice palliative care patients, or patients with pain who are being admitted for some appropriate reason, for example, the trial of intraspinal therapy or treatment of a pain crisis. The hospice patients are paid by the hospital per diem rate, and the others are paid under the DRG (Diagnosis-Related Group) rule. The hospital realizes income from these admissions and the money is used to support the staff of the inpatient unit.

We also have a large amount of philanthropy that we generate from industry, corporate America, and foundations. Much of the philanthropy goes to support educational programs, such as a program to create a clinical guideline for the care of the imminently dying inpatient, a caregiver program, a program on cancer-related fatigue, and a program on Internet educational activities. We have a very large website[†] that has generated millions of dollars in philanthropic revenue in the last few years. It does this because there is a very profound need out there, both among the corporations that sell medications that may be used for symptom control and among philanthropies, to use the Internet in a positive way.

Finally, we also try to obtain government and corporate grants to support our work. The clinical guideline for the care of the imminently dying, which we call the Palliative Care for Advanced Disease (PCAD) pathway, actually began as a grant from New York State. We also do many clinical trials, most of which are industry sponsored.

All our grants, in addition to providing direct revenue to support personnel in my department, provide an indirect payment to the institution. When the institution is making a decision about whether to continue the salary of our social worker, our nurses, our support staff, our administrators, they also look at these contributions to the general operating fund provided through indirect payments from grants and philanthropic contributions. So, our fundraising success has had both direct and indirect benefits for our program.

One last statistic gives a sense of the complexity of funding for the department. About 20 people in the department, those in our Institute for Education and Research in Pain and Palliative Care, are entirely supported by soft money—grants and philanthropy. About 60 to 70 people are entirely supported by our hospice budget, which will only provide support for those who are actually working for hospice patients. The staff of our inpatient unit is partially supported by hospice dollars and partially by hospital operations. And the rest of the department, some clinical people and some support staff, are funded almost half through operations, almost half through grants and philanthropy, and the remainder through the hospice budget. The doctors are all full-time and, in one way or another, are ultimately expected to support themselves. As I said though, the clinical income that we generate still is insufficient to support the clinical work that we do, and it's completely irrelevant to all the programmatic work that we do. We are dependent on grants and philanthropy to support a lot of people.

[†]<www.StopPain.org> is the website. See pp. 353–356 in Appendix B for a description and links to specific tools.

PATIENT REFERRALS AND INTEGRATION WITH OTHER HOSPITAL DEPARTMENTS

KSH: *How do you get your referrals?*

RKP: Our ability to interact with the various departments in the hospital is very much service dependent. So, for example, we have a very strong reciprocal interaction with oncology. This includes not only a large number of inpatient consultations, but also two sessions per week that are devoted to pain and palliative care for ambulatory patients and occur right in the cancer center. Each week the director of cancer supportive services attends the interdisciplinary meeting of our departmental palliative care division. So we have a very strong interaction with oncology. We also have a strong relationship with the AIDS program, and we have set up a weekly ambulatory session right in the AIDS center, which is manned by a physician, who is a palliative medicine specialist, and a fellow. In addition, we have a strong program in sickle cell disease, which includes a specialized monthly treatment session that involves both music therapy and pharmacotherapy for pain, as well as other palliative care interventions needed by this population.

Beyond that, our specific relationships with other departments are very much *ad hoc*, really based more on whether an individual attending physician thinks his or her patient may be appropriate for our service. We have very little integration with the ICUs at Beth Israel, in part because the ICU attending staff has a very strong interest in end-of-life care and actually is widely regarded as having a high level of expertise in this area, which predated my coming here. End-of-life planning, the withdrawal and withholding of life support, the ethical basis for intensive care medicine—all of that's happening on our ICUs at a very high level. In fact, the person who runs the program has contributed a chapter to a new and highly regarded book on end-of-life care in ICUs.[1] BIMC does have an ethics department, which is separate from ours, and ethics consults are sometimes requested in the ICU.

We are involved with the emergency department in terms of pain, but not palliative care. We're not too involved with geriatrics, a historical situation that we've been working to change. We've incorporated our PCAD project into the geriatrics unit as an outreach effort and have begun to train geriatrics fellows.

KSH: *Is this one of the challenges facing you—the need to generate more referrals, to expand into these areas?*

RKP: I think that, as a general rule, health care providers and administrative staff in institutions don't understand what palliative care is. There is still a tendency, which in some places is strong and in some places is very subtle, to link palliative care simply with end-of-life care. As those in hospice organizations have learned, if you link programs specifically to the imminence of death, you have a problem. Because we're not good at predicting when death is going to occur and because of all the psychological, social, and medical reasons that focus on providing aggressive life-sustaining therapies in institutions, this simple linkage tends to work against trying to provide concurrent, comprehensive, coordinated palliative care.

So, I think that we're constantly in a situation of trying to educate about who we are, what we offer, and how we are going to integrate ourselves with the primary team. We do not try to take over the care of every patient, but, rather, want to work with the primary team to assist or to comprehensively manage the quality-of-life-oriented care. We're available to provide a comprehensive team approach to patients who have very far advanced disease, whether or not they decide to opt into hospice. It's a constant, ongoing effort to educate every new generation of house staff and to educate physicians who are disinclined to believe in this new field. The process of education and integration is one that has to be addressed at multiple levels.

LESSONS LEARNED

KSH: *What are some of the lessons that you have learned that you perhaps did not anticipate?*

Outreach

RKP: The first lesson was *outreach*. One thing that I really strongly believe in now is the necessity of outreach. I didn't believe in this so much or didn't understand how important it was when I first started at Beth Israel. By outreach, I mean setting up PCAD-type programs in the cancer center, in the AIDS center, in long-term care facilities, in geriatric units, to actually provide unit-based tools for end-of-life care. The goals are to create models within our model so that palliative care can be "owned" by the clinic, the service, or the unit. Neither the understanding of what we do nor the referral of patients as a consequence of this understanding is going to happen automatically. With growing concern about the economics of health care, the tendency to be "territorial" about patients may be increasing, and this works against the kind of easy sharing of patients between services. There has to be a more compelling reason to make the referral. Having specialists with a high level of expertise at the sites where potential referrals originate facilitates further referrals and education. That's very much what we're trying to do now.

System Change through Quality Improvement Mechanisms

The second lesson is *the power and the necessity of system change through quality improvement mechanisms*. As a physician, I wasn't really imbued with quality improvement (QI), except insofar as I understood that everybody had to collaborate with the people doing the QI projects.

One of the first things that I did when I got to Beth Israel was to hire Marilyn Bookbinder, PhD, RN, who is an honest-to-goodness, bona fide quality improvement expert.[‡] I began to participate in quality improvement activities both in our own department and through an outreach mechanism in other departments. Through this involvement, I began to feel at a very personal level what the literature shows, which is, basically, you don't ever create changes in practice just by telling people things. Lectures don't work, and reading materials don't work. What works is creating changes in a system such that people's behavior is shaped in a way that leads to a higher standard of care. It's raising a standard of care by creating system change. The best way of doing that is by providing people with the tools to take ownership over the change mechanisms that allow them to achieve a higher standard of practice.

This was really a profound lesson for me. I'll give you two examples. When I came to Beth Israel, the Jacob Perlow Hospice program maintained an eight-bed hospice unit that had been in existence for about eight or nine years. Only patients who were hospice patients and only patients who had signed DNR documents were allowed to be admitted there. The standard of care on that unit was very much devoted to providing a dignified and comfortable death. The staff used basic symptom control techniques and provided wonderful psychological support for the patients who were gravely ill and also for families. This was the goal of the unit and that was how it operated.

When I came in, the institution renovated and converted the unit into a 14-bed unit for the department, which would care for hospice patients, non-hospice palliative care patients, and pain patients. On this one unit, we could have a 30-year-old man with low back pain, who is entirely healthy except for chronic pain being treated with a neuraxial therapy, and a person dying of some serious medical illness, who may or may not be a hospice patient.

CHALLENGE OF CONVERTING FROM A HOSPICE TO A PALLIATIVE CARE UNIT

The challenge in converting this unit was enormous. We had significant staff turnover despite repeated in-service training and meetings. We needed to get a new nurse manager. Slowly, however, using QI as the foundation, we made this transition to a wonderful and unique unit. It would have never happened without the emphasis on creating policies and procedures in collaboration with the nurses, so that there was a sense of collegiality, support, and ownership over change. For some people it was too much, and they left. Others have really bought into our model, and they're going to be with us for the duration. That was the first dramatic example of how system change is the stuff by which one raises the standard of care.

Creating a Clinical Pathway for Palliative Care

The second example is PCAD. We had begun to do something like this clinical pathway at Sloan–Kettering. Marilyn Bookbinder and I recognized that there was

---

[‡]See Raising the Standard of Care for Imminently Dying Patients Using Quality Improvement: An Interview with Marilyn Bookbinder, PhD, RN, pp. 69–83.

a need to improve end-of-life care in the institution and that the best mechanism for doing this was one that encouraged system change through quality improvement. We created this clinical guideline, implemented this quality improvement model, and we now have data that really show that after just nine months of piloting we have had significant improvement in a whole variety of outcomes related to end-of-life care.[§]

> *It's very dramatic and also very profound to think of how little is accomplished with all the lecturing and all the writing, unless it is linked to system change.*

It's very dramatic and also very profound to think of how little is accomplished with all the lecturing and all the writing, unless it is linked to system change. All the didactics are needed and may have subtle, culture-changing impact. But if you want to go into a place where people are sick and get them better care, you have to create systemic change.

KSH: *Does the same staff care for the patients who will go home and those who won't? If so, how stressful is that for them?*

RKP: Yes, it's exactly the same staff, and I think that there are no easy answers to this question because the stresses involved in caring for the imminently dying can be very significant. There is clearly a great deal of stress in caring for sick people who are highly symptomatic. I think there's less job stress if the patients that one is dealing with are not so symptomatic. If a patient has pain, depression, and family disruption, there's going to be stress associated with interacting with that patient, whether or not the context is serious medical illness. If there's serious medical illness and death is imminent, sometimes the stress is more difficult, but sometimes there's an acceptance, a sense of support from the family that makes these experiences less stressful for the staff. In our environment of both pain and palliative care, the sources of staff stress can be very complex.

In all honesty, when I started at this institution, I did not really understand the complexity of creating a unit environment that could support the state-of-the-art management of such diverse patients, all of whom have high level of symptoms, distress, and sickness of one type or another. I was naïve in my understanding about how to really approach the creation of a support system for staff. I think what I learned is that, for any program that establishes an inpatient unit as part of that program, attention must be paid. There has to be time, expertise, and reassessment of the status of that unit to make sure that the standard of care continues to be at a high level and that the staff members are supported, because it's a very tough place to work.

[§]See Bookbinder, pp. 69–83.

HOSPICE AS A RESOURCE IN THE INTEGRATED MODEL OF CARE

KSH: *What is the relationship between your program and the Jacob Perlow Hospice? What distinguishes the care provided by the hospice from the care provided by the palliative care division of non-hospice patients, who might receive hospice-like care?*

RKP: With my arrival at BIMC, the Jacob Perlow Hospice (JPH) was administratively placed into the palliative care division of my department. Initially, this didn't mean too much. The hospice has its own executive director, Paul Brenner, MDiv, a very well known figure nationally in hospice. JPH had its own policies and procedures and its own tradition of providing care for both outpatients and inpatients. There was limited physician involvement.

The process of creating an integrated model, in which hospice is considered to be a resource for end-of-life care within a broader model of palliative care, is still ongoing. It has been quite challenging, given the regulatory and procedural realities of the hospice and given that hospice is mostly home care, which means that most of the practitioners have very little interaction with the rest of the palliative care team. But this process has actually begun to create some very interesting outcomes that I do think make it a model worth continuing. When we started, we hoped that the integration would result in both an increase in hospice census and an increase in length of stay. We have succeeded in increasing the census, which averaged about 80 when I arrived at BIMC and is now about 105. Our length of stay bumped for a while, but then settled back where it had been.

One of the most important points was for everybody to get on the same page about what our vision was in terms of this integration. In a variety of settings, the leadership of the hospice and others from the department used both clinical team meetings and administrative meetings to discuss the critical issues, such as continuity of care, involvement of departmental physicians, and staff training. This has continued to take place at our weekly interdisciplinary team meeting, at which hospice and non-hospice professionals sit together to discuss cases. This meeting facilitates referrals into hospice and has worked well.

The first thing that we needed to do to make this happen was to look at the resources provided by the hospice program and the rest of the program in the palliative care division and ask the question, "Is it possible to create uniform services, which, to the extent possible, are provided by the same professionals?" The inherent challenge is that the hospice budget must fund individuals who are doing hospice work, and this necessitates complex accounting mechanisms if we want the same persons to provide both hospice and non-hospice palliative care. Most of the home care nurses, social workers, and so forth, are spending their entire day in the field, and we could not have these people also perform hospital-based work. The logistics, along with the funding mechanisms, are very complicated. Ultimately, we decided that the hospice nurses and social workers would continue to care solely for hospice patients.

When we looked at the non-hospice palliative care part of our work, we realized that we were in need of a chaplain and volunteer services. We convinced one of our hospice chaplains to accept half his salary from the non-hospice budget. The same chaplain is now actively involved in the care of non-hospice palliative care patients and the hospice patients. This provides a beautiful mechanism for continuity of spiritual care.

We also tried to create a joint method for providing volunteers to patients. The Jacob Perlow Hospice program has more than 165 volunteers and a very good volunteer support program. In the hope of providing similar services in the home care environment, we funded, through philanthropy, a half-time volunteer coordinator to try to bring volunteer services to non-hospice palliative care patients. This is something that actually has *not* worked out as we had expected and we ultimately eliminated this position. For a variety of reasons, the number of non-hospice palliative care patients who could be hooked up with a volunteer in the outpatient setting was small and did not appear to be growing as we became busier. In the end, it was more efficient for us to focus outpatient volunteer services on the hospice population and to continue to work on integration of volunteer services for inpatients.

In contrast to our failure to get a vibrant outpatient volunteer program going for the non-hospice patients, we have been successful in using volunteers on the inpatient unit. The volunteers on the unit do a whole range of activities, such as feed patients, provide support, read to patients, that sort of thing. They now work routinely with both hospice and non-hospice patients.

We not only asked how the palliative care program could become more "hospice-like," but we also asked, "What are the things that need to be improved in the hospice?" There were two general areas. The first was the care in the inpatient unit, which needed to be broadened to include the intensive medical piece, particularly for patients who weren't imminently dying. The second was that the home care nurses needed to have access to physicians with palliative care expertise. Like most hospices in the country, the medical piece for the Jacob Perlow Hospice was very limited before my arrival and did not include access to a medical director who was a palliative medicine specialist.

We have been able to offer our hospice home-care patients access to a palliative care physician through telephone contacts with physicians in the department and through a small program that we call "The Drop In Program." Any hospice patient who is visited by a home care nurse and is perceived to have a need for medical evaluation can be brought to our unit by ambulance and be evaluated by a palliative medicine specialist. This includes patients whose care has been transferred to the hospice medical director and those whose care continues to be managed by an outside physician. As long as the primary attending agrees to the consultation, the patient can have at least some access to a specialist in palliative care.

There are other things that we must do. We have plans to begin piloting a physician home visit program for the first time this year. I have no idea yet whether it will be successful or sustainable, but it makes sense conceptually. Hospice programs in various parts of the country have found that physician home visits can be a very powerful way to provide physician input within the interdisciplinary team approach. Linkages between hospice and palliative care can be further engendered and improved by having physician home visits that can go either to palliative care patients or to hospice patients, without regard to how the bills are being paid.

INSIGHTS TO GUIDE OTHERS EMBARKING ON SIMILAR EFFORTS

KSH: *What have been the most difficult and challenging aspects of this whole process, which would give some insight to someone else who is embarking on this road?*

Create a Strategic Business Plan

RKP: The first insight is that individuals who want to do program development in this area have to learn to speak with the business people at the hospital. As a physician, I was never taught to do that, and at Sloan–Kettering I was generally protected from it. I never had to learn how to create a business plan, elaborate a needs assessment in a way that made sense to the business people, or do a resource assessment so that one could determine whether there were existing resources that could be linked to new resources for program development.

Administrators in hospitals think in these terms. As the climate in health care gets more fiscally tight and as money for program development gets harder to come by, people who want to do program development in palliative care must learn how to speak the language of those who are running the institutions. They have to learn how to be fiscally responsible, to monitor profit and loss in a way that helps to demonstrate sustainability of a program. They have to learn some basic tenets of business, or they have to know how to ask for help from appropriate people and bring them into the team.

I've made a very strong effort in my role as department chairman to talk to the administration in the language of the business plan and the strategic plan. I try to communicate in a way that doesn't appear to have me asking for more and more and more, but rather places me in partnership with the institution, aware of my fiscal obligations. The goal lies in trying to create good business opportunities, while providing things that are good for our patients.

I also ask a lot of questions of others who know more about this than I do. I have an administrator who is much more savvy about some of the inside business aspects of the institution. For others who are building programs, it is good advice to strive for both a detailed understanding of the business side and access to those who inevitably have more knowledge and skills in this area.

Try to Mainstream Palliative Care

Palliative care and hospice are not yet mainstream. In the process of creating palliative care programs, particularly those that link in a meaningful way to hospice, we must work to mainstream what we do. What this means is constantly reaching out to other departments, services, units, and individual health care providers. We need to teach them about what we do and to change the systems within which they work, so that they can begin to participate in expert palliative care and know when to make a referral to a specialized service. I think that the process of mainstreaming is going to take at least another decade, but will probably be the difference between sustainable programs and the whole movement being just a flash in the pan.

Define Palliative Care as a Specialist Service

The third thing I've learned is that we who are doing program development have to continue to portray ourselves as offering specialist-level care. We have to work to define what that means in a very clear way and understand that the most likely way that we will be integrated into mainstream medical care is as a specialty service comparable to any other specialty service in medicine, such as cardiology, gastroenterology, or neurology.

What this realization means, in part, is that those of us who are doing program development are obliged not just to develop our own programs, but also to try to do things that raise the overall level of care for those patients who are not being referred for specialist-level care. This obligation will work to our advantage, because a higher standard of generalist-level care will facilitate appropriate referrals and create better ways of integrating with primary teams. We have an obligation to reach out to these teams and encourage them to realize that they actually provide services that fall under the umbrella of palliative care every day. They need to value the quality-of-life interventions that they offer and recognize when specialist-level care is needed to provide help at any point through the course of the disease. As specialist-level teams, we are particularly well suited to offer help at the end of life, because that's when most of the help seems to be needed.

ONGOING CHALLENGES

KSH: *What would you like to improve in your own program?*

RKP: There are several things that we really have to do. The first is to reach out to the long-term care community. We have a grant written, which has not yet been funded, to establish our model in one nursing home in the New York area. We have contracts to provide hospice services in some nursing homes, but have not yet created a broader model of palliative care in any facility. Our hope is to use access to hospice as a first wedge to open the door to program development based on a link between palliative care and hospice. The need for this type of palliative care in long-term care is staggering.

The second thing we must improve is the system for continuity of care for patients on whom we consult in the hospital and who then go home. Too many of these patients could benefit from our case management approach to palliative care in the home environment, but are lost to follow-up until the next time that they are admitted to the hospital.

KSH: *What are some of the barriers to further improvement in this continuity of care?*

RKP: There are many reasons for problems with continuity of care, some of which we cannot solve. The barriers include primary teams that do not encourage the patient to follow up with us and our program and patients who are already so burdened in getting medical care from multiple different venues that the idea of seeing one more service is very difficult for them. Other barriers are financial and systemic. Many of our patients at Beth Israel are indigent; they may lack insurance or have chemical dependency problems. Continuity in general is problematic in these cases. Some patients have insurance, but the coverage makes it difficult for the patient to follow up with us. They may not have money for transportation, or they may have a deductible on their insurance that they haven't met yet, so they can't pay for extra services.

We have enormous system problems to address. As an example, the doctors in my department may participate in something like 23 separate managed care programs, as well as Medicare and Medicaid. The programs have different formularies, different in-network and out-of-network stipulations for what care can be offered, different preauthorization requirements. Every one is different. So, when you think about taking a patient who's already seeing a radiation oncologist and a medical oncologist, and then providing access to a palliative care medicine specialist, a nurse, a social worker and a chaplain, all the while ensuring the ability to obtain drugs for symptom control and maybe equipment—you can imagine the complexities of dealing with multiple reimbursement systems to make this happen routinely.

KSH: *To sum up, with all these efforts that are underway, what do you feel your program does best?*

RKP: I think we have the unique capability of providing both an interdisciplinary model of palliative care to patients who are not hospice candidates and a system for transitioning patients from non-hospice palliative care to hospice care at a specialist level. When this works well, this type of model has the capability to provide people with serious illness a very sophisticated level of care for months or years. This is what we mean when we talk about providing patients with comprehensive, quality-of-life-oriented care, including intensive palliative care at end of life. When we're able to do it well, when the stars align so that we have the support of the primary team and a patient and family in our system with adequate resources, we are able to offer a level of integrated care that provides continuity across venues of care, across reimbursement systems, and across disease trajectory from early to late. This is really state of the art, in my opinion, and when it works, that's what we do best.

REFERENCE

1. Curtiss JR, Rubenfeld GD (eds.). *Managing Death in the ICU: The Transition from Cure to Comfort.* New York: Oxford University Press, 2001.

Featured Innovation: Part II

Raising the Standard of Care for Imminently Dying Patients Using Quality Improvement

An Interview with MARILYN BOOKBINDER, PhD, RN

Beth Israel Medical Center
New York, New York

The Department of Pain Medicine and Palliative Care (DPMPC) at Beth Israel Medical Center developed the Palliative Care for Advanced Disease (PCAD) pathway to guide the interdisciplinary management of imminently dying patients in that hospital setting. Marilyn Bookbinder, PhD, RN, an expert in quality improvement and evidence-based practice, had previously designed similar pathways to improve pain management and to improve the screening for fatigue assessment when she joined this project.[1,2] In this interview conducted by Anna L. Romer, EdD, Dr. Bookbinder identifies the PCAD as a way to raise the standard of care for these patients using quality improvement (QI). The actual pathway is available on the department's website, along with instructions for its use and ancillary tools.*

Dr. Bookbinder describes PCAD, its design and evolution, as well as the initial results from the pilot implementation of the pathway in two treatment and three control units.[†] PCAD is the first such effort of its kind in the United States. The DPMPC is one of three winners of the American Hospital Association's 2001 Circle of Life Award.

THE PALLIATIVE CARE FOR ADVANCED DISEASE (PCAD) PATHWAY

Anna L. Romer: *Can you describe PCAD?*

Marilyn Bookbinder: When you pull all the pieces together, PCAD is both a process and set of tools to raise the standard of care for patients who are likely

---

*The Department of Pain Medicine and Palliative Care website at Beth Israel Medical Center is <www.StopPain.org>. See Appendix B, pp. 353–356 for links to specific pages and tools.

†The department received one year's funding from a New York State Department of Health Quality Measurement Grant to develop and pilot test PCAD.

to die during the current admission to the hospital. Our goal in the hospital is to cure people and send them home. But, as we know, people do die in hospitals. Once clinicians, patients, and families agree that a patient is likely to die, the care should be primarily directed toward comfort and support. We must meet the patient's needs by adjusting the goals of care, optimizing palliative care, and avoiding unnecessary treatments.

PCAD has been one aspect of my broader role in the department. Among other things, I run our QI initiative. Most hospitals have a systematic quality improvement process in place and, in this case, we have mobilized it on behalf of the needs of dying patients. My role is to bring in research methods when I can: better tools, better outcomes assessment, a better approach using theories about the implementation and change process. In this instance, we developed the tools, the pathway, and the education and can now track process and outcome data related to end-of-life care in a hospital setting. To raise the standard of care, it is important to establish a clear benchmark of excellence and then measure behavior against that standard in order to know what level of care we are offering. At this point, clinicians can work to improve care.

This effort is part of the larger effort described by Dr. Portenoy to establish a premier department of pain medicine and palliative care.[‡] I joined Dr. Portenoy a few months after the DPMPC began. One of our goals from the beginning was to bring the continuous quality improvement (CQI) process to this task of establishing and implementing guidelines for care of patients who are dying. First, you decide on a process that needs improvement, then you organize a team that knows that process well, work with the team to clarify current knowledge and understanding of that process, and then in our case, create new guidelines or a pathway that establishes a standard of care. CQI involves a circular process of planning, data gathering, checking results, and acting on the results. It is iterative and one can start at any point. The key is to keep feeding information back, reassessing and adapting behavior based on the information that you collect. It is crucial to link this process to a clear standard of care so that you are, in fact, changing something that is worth changing, in the direction of excellence.

PCAD consists of three components (all available in PDF format at www. StopPain.org). First, the actual PCAD Care Path is a two-page set of guidelines in the form of a chart that lists suggested treatments, consults, and actions to create an interdisciplinary plan of care for imminently dying patients. It also tracks preadmission criteria and discharge outcomes. Second, the MD Order Sheet is a documentation tool used to activate the care path as well as to suggest symptom control approaches. The reverse side of this form includes medications for consideration in treating pain and 13 other frequently experienced symptoms of patients who are dying. Third, the Daily Patient Care Flowsheet is a tool that nurses use to document daily assessments and interventions. For example, there are places on the form to note the presence of advance directives, results of a comfort as-

---

[‡]See Developing an Integrated Department of Pain and Palliative Medicine: An Interview with Russell K. Portenoy, MD, pp. 53–67.

sessment, vital signs as specifically ordered, and results of pain assessment, as well as a space to document any patient and family education.

In addition to these tools, which are essential to the implementation of the PCAD pathway, we also designed several tools to evaluate its use. Specifically, we have a chart audit tool (an outcome measure), a process audit (a process measure), and a palliative care survey or quiz (a knowledge measure). We also used focus groups, feedback from the QI team, and qualitative comments of the study team mentoring the clinicians who were implementing the pathway.

IMPLEMENTATION PROCESS

To set the PCAD into motion, we created a flowchart with five steps:

1. **Patient identification.** Our referral question is based on Dr. Mimi Pattison's work[§] that has been well publicized by Joanne Lynn, MD. We modified Dr. Pattison's referral question, "Would you be surprised if any of these patients died in the next twelve months?" for our purposes. Any staff member (e.g., nurses, house staff physicians and assistants, social workers, chaplains) may suggest candidates for PCAD, based on an affirmative answer to the question "Is this a patient who could die during this admission?" The goal here is to identify the imminently dying, a challenge that physicians have not been all that successful in meeting, according to research on prognostication of death.[3] Yet, in our setting, this question seems to do a pretty good job at identifying an appropriate pool of patients whose goals of care need clarification and would possibly benefit from PCAD. Parenthetically, I should say that our experience in this initial pilot of the PCAD suggests that it may be worthwhile to supplement the referral question we used with another: "Is this patient a candidate for comfort care?"

2. **Interdisciplinary assessment.** An interdisciplinary team, consisting of a nurse, social worker, chaplain, and physician housestaff, discusses the patient as a candidate with the attending physician. Once there is agreement, an order for PCAD is pending by the attending physician or housestaff officer.

3. **Provider clarification: Family meeting.** The attending physician (and usually a social worker or nurse) have a "family meeting" to clarify the goals of care with the patient and family as a first step. The attending physician orders PCAD if end-of-life supportive care is the primary goal of care.

4. **Implementation.** The housestaff physician or nurse practitioner, in the case of the geriatrics unit, initiates the pathway using the MD Order Sheet, rewriting orders for the patients. Nurses complete the demographic information on the PCAD pathway and initiate the tracking of patient symptoms and care with the PCAD Daily Patient Care Flowsheet.

5. **Discharge.** The patient may be discharged, usually to hospice or to an alternative care setting, but sometimes to home. Some patients die on the unit and,

---

[§]See Improving Care through the End of Life: An Interview with Mimi Pattison, MD, pp. 9–17.

after the patient's death, bereavement activities are initiated and staff members conduct a debriefing session.

> *The goals of PCAD were to shape the responses of staff to ensure patient comfort by minimizing symptom distress and unnecessary interventions, reinforcing respect for values and decisions, optimizing the use of consultants and resources that are appropriate for the goals of care, and providing support for the family.*

ALR: *What are the goals of this pathway?*

MB: The goals of PCAD were to shape the responses of staff to ensure patient comfort by minimizing symptom distress and unnecessary interventions, reinforcing respect for values and decisions, optimizing the use of consultants and resources that are appropriate for the goals of care, and providing support for the family.

DESIGNING THE PATHWAY USING QUALITY IMPROVEMENT METHODS

ALR: *Could you take a step back to discuss how you and your team constructed the pathway and the quality improvement process that you are using?*

MB: Prior to implementing the actual pathway and documenting practice in the pilot and control units, we developed a 22 member QI team. As I mentioned, the first step in starting a QI project is to identify the process or the standard that you are trying to improve and then to recruit the people most closely involved in this care to be part of the change process.

We included all the disciplines that are involved in end-of-life care (chaplains, social workers, nurses, physicians, pharmacy, ethics) and key people from the two pilot units. I refer to these key people as the champions, those who are going to lead the effort at the unit level. On the oncology unit, the champions were the clinical nurse specialist, nurse manager, and case manager. On the geriatrics unit we targeted the nurse practitioners, nurse managers, and the case manager.

Then we set out to educate the CQI team. The team met monthly over the year. We broke up into four working groups that met weekly for about four months to develop the evidence-based care path, flow sheet, and order sheet. A second work group developed implementation strategies and a timeline. Brainstorming, another QI technique, was done with unit staff and the QI team to uncover the barriers that we might face. For example, finding extra time for meetings was difficult. We learned that 7:30 A.M. on Wednesdays was the best time for our work groups to meet. The QI team pilot units saw Dr. Portenoy as providing expertise and leadership throughout the project, as evidenced by the good attendance at our meetings. They appreciated his willingness to hear the "nitty gritty" process of getting PCAD going on their units. A third work group developed educational strategies for nurses, assistants, and housestaff, and the last group, composed primarily of our study team, developed the evaluation methods.

The timeline shows you the phases of implementation: planning, introduction, rollout, evaluation, and reporting. Phase Zero is called *planning*. We received approvals from (1) the Institutional Review Board to conduct the study, (2) the medical records committee, because PCAD involved using new forms for documentation, and (3) the hospital's patient care committee, because positive results of the pilot to improve end-of-life care would potentially mean bringing PCAD to other units at our hospital and our two other sites.

The next phase, *introduction*, begins the work of "getting buy in" from clinicians and colleagues in the pilot units. Dr. Portenoy was asked to present at physicians' medical grand rounds about end-of-life care and the pilot study. Dr. Portenoy and I were invited by QI leaders in the oncology and geriatrics units to present the concept of the pathway. We told them that we had the approval of the IRB and described our hopes and expectations for the pilot implementation, including their involvement. They agreed that they wanted to be a part of this effort.

The implementation phase is the *rollout* of PCAD and the evaluation measures. We conducted in-services for all staff on the use of PCAD and determined a weekly schedule on each pilot unit for the study team to meet with leaders and review patients, both those who might be candidates for PCAD and those who died. It took us one month on each unit to assess the nurses' knowledge, conduct the in-service about how to use the tools, and implement the pathway.

ALR: *What kinds of baseline assessment measures did you make on the pilot and control units before you started training and implementation?*

MB: Another QI principle relates to the need for "continual learning" in organizations. In order to measure changes in practice there needs to be an assessment of baseline competency. We used a simple 20-item knowledge quiz.[4] It is validated, reliable, and a great tool. We gave the palliative care quiz to staff on the experimental units. We used it with housestaff and nurses, but I only reported data on the nurses.

We used the palliative care quiz as a teaching tool as well. For example, we often gave it to house staff and fellows before a case study was presented by one of our staff physicians. In this case, we used it as a way to begin dialogue with them about important issues at end of life, such as futility, the DNR discussion, and hydration. The physician leading the case study discussion would then use their responses to the quiz as a starting point to grapple with these thorny issues.

We also used a chart audit tool to look at deaths in all the units—the control (including hospice) and the experimental units—one year prior to implementing the pathway and again after implementing the pathway. We documented length of stay, diagnoses, and patient demographics, such as age, gender, and ethnicity; admission/referral data; end-of-life decision-making; symptom assessment/management; and death and utilization data. The tool tracks more than 100 items.

THE PILOT STUDY

ALR: *Which units did you choose to pilot the PCAD and why?*

MB: We had two experimental units—oncology and geriatrics. Using QI principles to help to direct us to improve the standard of care, we picked units in which
end-of-life care was the most problem-prone, high-risk, or had the most deaths.[5]
The units that had the most frequent deaths were geriatrics and oncology. We
also had two control units, which were medical units that had patients with
chronic illness and were similar in terms of acuity of care to the pilot units. The
inpatient unit of the Department of Pain Medicine and Palliative Care (which includes hospice, non-hospice palliative care, and pain patients) served as the "gold
standard" unit. For purposes of the pilot study, we only targeted the hospice patients for the pathway. We included our inpatient unit along with the two pilot
units (geriatrics and oncology) because they requested it and because we thought
that comparison with a unit that was farther along would yield important com-
parative data. The culture and practice of palliative care was already firmly established on this unit, whereas on the oncology and geriatric units we assumed
that introducing these guidelines for supportive care would be a change in practice.

The hospice staff used PCAD as a standard of care and as a tool to help them
to document their practice. As the nurses and doctors told us, "It helps the team
get on the same page," so to speak. About one-third of the hospice unit patients
were dying, and we targeted these patients for the pathway.

STAFF EDUCATION

ALR: *What kinds of in-services did you conduct?*

MB: The diffusion literature tells us that to implement new ideas or innovative
practices successfully we need to have champions to role model the new standard; educators to reach as many people as possible in a target audience with a
relevant, practical message; and multiple media strategies for communicating and
increasing dialogue. To educate every staff member, we scheduled two sessions
for each shift: days, evenings, and during the night. Our first barrier was the difficulty in getting staff off the unit—together—for more than 20 minutes. In the
first session, we provided food and simply introduced ourselves and the study. In
the second session, all staff members (chaplains and nursing assistants included),
took a pretest questionnaire and were educated about the principles of good end-
of-life care and how the pathway would be used. We encouraged the nurses to
evaluate their caseload on a daily basis and ask the question, "Is this someone who
could die during this admission?" If a patient was identified as such, then the nurse
reported to the clinical specialist or nurse or case manager, who would then be
the liaison with the attending physician to consider the patient for PCAD.

It took us about one month to work out a routine schedule of when and how we would identify candidates for PCAD and for staff to process the principles of implementing the pathway. All housestaff (including physician assistants), nutritionists, dieticians, and even the nursing assistants were educated about the pathway and its goals.

During the in-service, staff members actually took a tool and demonstrated how to put a patient on PCAD and how to document their actions and observations. Every nurse was able to practice going through the steps. These activities were part of the one-month process of assessing skills and introducing the guidelines to staff on the unit. It took that long to reach all the day, evening, and night staff. We first did this on the oncology unit, then went through the same process on the geriatrics unit, and then followed one month later with the hospice unit. We gave specific in-services as per staff request, such as "the physiology of dying." We tried to meet educational needs weekly as they arose.

We also educated the large QI team by showing scenarios from the EPEC Series.[||] Drs. Portenoy and Wollner, both faculty for the national program, led the sessions and discussion groups.

IMPLEMENTATION OF THE PATHWAY

ALR: *How did you implement the pathway with real patients on the unit?*

MB: Following this intensive month of in-services to introduce the PCAD, we began implementation on each pilot unit. Someone from our study team was present frequently, sometimes every day and at least once a week. We worked with the staff, primarily nurses, as they reviewed patients for PCAD. We asked the following kinds of questions: "Are you asking the referral question?" "What difficulties are you having?" "Is this a patient for PCAD?"

The study nurse and I mentored the two pilot units as the staff began to implement the pathway. Each pilot unit had 32 beds, but only one or two patients on each unit were actively dying at any one time. We decided with each leadership team how we were going to evaluate patients for PCAD. We began discussing this on a daily basis and moved to a weekly schedule. We were invited to join the weekly discharge planning rounds on the geriatrics floor. During the early stages of implementation we found that the term "palliative care" needed clarification by the clinical nurse specialist and staff.

Another QI principle is to bootleg the new practice, or add it onto existing routine practices. Because nurses report on patients every morning, they chose to review patients for PCAD at this time. As they take or give report, they now ask, "Is this a patient for PCAD?" or "Is this a patient for comfort care? Let's consider PCAD."

[||]EPEC: Education for Physicians on End-of-Life Care is a curriculum and training project. For more information visit <www.epec.net>.

EVALUATING EFFORTS TO IMPLEMENT THE PCAD

ALR: *Can you describe the process audit?*

MB: The process audit tool is a variance tracking tool of sorts, similar to those used by case managers monitoring pathways.¶ Remember, the pathway is a set of guidelines, but since we are treating individual patients, we anticipate variation and wouldn't want people to implement the guidelines blindly. The concept of a pathway brings up questions of practice and variations in practice: "Did we do *x*? Did we do *y*?" This process audit tool helps to evaluate whether the guidelines are being followed or not and, if not, they provide an opportunity to learn how come. The study nurse who was monitoring the implementation of PCAD asked the nurses on the unit questions such as "When you spoke with the physician about putting the patient on PCAD, what was his or her response?" I would ask nurses about what they were doing: "I see you didn't chart *x*. Can you explain? I'm trying to make sure that the tool is really capturing what we want." It is best to learn what works and what does not from the nurse recording the practice, rather than trying to infer it from the chart itself. So, the process audit tool helps you to see whether the pathway is meeting the need of the patient and the need of the discipline to actually document care. This tool allows us to learn if the implementation is going as we planned and provides us with data about what needs to be fixed. It reveals some of the barriers to implementing the pathway.

BARRIERS TO IMPLEMENTATION

Added Paperwork

We identified one important barrier with the implementation of the MD Order Sheet. It is one of the three components of the pathway, which requires not only a physician's order, but it also requires them to rewrite all the orders. This adds

> *We want the clinical caregivers to think about what it makes sense to do or stop doing in terms of treatment. Patients who are dying may find it burdensome to be woken up to have a daily weight taken or have their vital signs checked, for example.*

a layer of paperwork that is a real barrier to implementation. This is another thing we hope to change in the future, with physician input. I would go back to the physicians, which we're going to do, and ask them to help us to redesign the intervention. "How can we make this easier for you, and at the same time make sure that all these areas are addressed?" The reason we asked physicians to rewrite the orders is because we are asking them to reassess the goals of care at the point the patient enters the pathway. We want the clinical

¶See Appendix B, p. 353, for a mini version of the process audit tool.

caregivers to think about what it makes sense to do or stop doing in terms of treatment. Patients who are dying may find it burdensome to be woken up to have a daily weight taken or have their vital signs checked, for example.

On the back of this new medical order sheet we posted guidelines of how to treat the 14 most prevalent symptoms experienced by people near the end of life. The physician housestaff appreciated the guidelines and used them to write orders on non-PCAD patients as well.

ALR: *What other kinds of problems and issues did you see?*

Lack of Readiness by Patient, Family, or Staff

MB: Initially, the 22-member team identified the areas that they suspected might present the biggest obstacles, and, in fact, the areas that they identified were the most difficult. The team predicted that we would encounter discomfort and a lack of readiness on the part of all disciplines to identify patients as imminently dying and then change their treatment plan to fit that trajectory. Readiness on the part of clinicians was less of a problem than for families. Clinicians and patients and families had to acknowledge that the patient was imminently dying in order to begin the pathway, so the physician had to have a conversation with the patient and family as part of the process.

We found that the biggest barrier was this readiness of patients and families. Most wanted "everything" done, not wanting to give up hope and chance for recovery and to go home one more time. While we may agree that having conversations at this late stage (two days before death) may be too late, this scenario is still the reality and we need to figure out how to make it better.

ALR: *Did you have to do special training with the physicians to teach them how to open up this conversation with families?*

MB: Our project did not directly address this issue. However, the hospital's ethics committee has an ongoing educational program to help housestaff (who rotate each month) to become more comfortable with discussing end-of-life issues with patients and families. The clinical nurse specialists and the nurse practitioners, the champions on the units, educated physicians about PCAD by having discussions about patients whom they thought were candidates. Within one year, all full-time physicians on the study units had placed at least one patient on PCAD. So I cannot say that they are totally resistant to this. We think that they choose patients sparingly, choosing only those patients who were clearly dying and whose families shared that view. Nine of 31 patients who died on oncology and geriatrics units during the six-month study period were placed on PCAD. Most patients were identified, but some died before we could get the process going, others wanted everything done, some we missed over a weekend or holiday, and some improved, which made them ineligible.

ALR: *Who has the discussion with the patient and/or family?*

MB: The attending physician or the housestaff is responsible for the discussion in concert with the nurse who's taking care of the patient and sometimes the social worker will be involved. It is usually interdisciplinary, meaning at least two of them were present. This is a conversation that goes on all the time. Did we educate them to do it better? I don't think we assumed that they needed help doing it.

ALR: *So you didn't see that as a barrier?*

MB: We didn't see it as a barrier to PCAD implementation, but this is not to say that we don't see communication as an issue. We did not target this area specifically, but I think we now know that communicating bad news is a skill that most clinicians can improve.

FINDINGS FROM PILOT STUDY

We showed several positive outcomes within this short pilot period. Symptom assessment improved on all the units involved in the study, namely, the experimental (including the inpatient unit of our department) and control units. In particular, assessment of pain, cognitive impairment, and breathlessness improved.

Practice moved in the direction that we wanted it to. The control units improved, but not as much as the experimental units, and the experimental units (geriatrics and oncology), moved closer to the level that we documented on the hospice and palliative care unit, in other words, the gold standard.

ALR: *Given these results, that is, improved symptom assessment on all units, how can you make claims about the specific utility of PCAD?*

MB: It is true that the control units also improved and the differences between the study units and the control units were modest. Remember, however, that simultaneously with this QI effort our new department was offering pain and palliative care consults throughout the hospital. We think that the combination of the department's broader efforts and diffusion from the study units combined to produce "contamination" of our efforts to measure the impact of the pilot implementation of the PCAD. Nonetheless, the finding of some differences between study units and control units at a time when this contamination was happening, and in a period of only a few months, makes us think that PCAD does indeed have real value as a means to produce change in the standard of care.

We believe that we initiated a cultural change in how people think about the care of imminently dying inpatients. This is a much broader mandate than showing statistically significant differences in symptom assessment. We walked onto the study units and tiptoed about until we could figure out where the openings were to begin to shape practice and educate staff. Our team didn't directly conduct in-services with physicians, but clearly a great deal of education occurred informally.

ENGENDERING CULTURAL CHANGE

ALR: *Can you say a bit more about what you mean by cultural change and how you documented this phenomenon?*

MB: First of all, the unit language related to end-of-life care has changed. Clinicians (nurses, physicians) now talk about goals of care. Focus groups with staff indicate that they are less afraid to use the "d" word, that is, death, and are more confident asking, "What are the goals of care for this patient?

The study team collected informal information every week about what changes were happening on that unit. We perceived that there was a social process going on. Data about behaviors need to be collected when you do this kind of research. Some of this information can never be obtained in the chart audit tool or the process audit tool.

> *. . . the unit language related to end-of-life care has changed. Clinicians (nurses, physicians) now talk about goals of care. Focus groups with staff indicate that they are less afraid to use the "d" word, that is, death, and are more confident asking, "What are the goals of care for this patient?"*

ALR: *How were you documenting what you saw as cultural changes?*

MB: We both observed and asked questions of the nurses on a weekly basis, when we did the review of all the patients and discussed who would be eligible for PCAD. We noted a change in the discussions about care. These began to include the comment "Refer to PCAD." We asked, "How have you seen change in behavior here?" Nurses told us, "We feel that there are more referrals to hospice. We are at least thinking more about patients who are eligible for hospice."

ALR: *Did you document increased referrals to hospice? Was that a goal of the implementation of the PCAD?*

MB: We did see an increase in referrals. But you have to understand some of the nuances here. If the staff is doing a great job on the oncology unit, maybe patients don't need to be admitted to hospice right at the end of life. So, just seeing improvement in referrals is only one measure of success and perhaps not the most important one.

Nurses told us that they feel that they assess patients sooner for hospice. But our numbers may not reflect the increase because (1) the patient may not have been eligible for hospice, or (2) the family chose to keep their loved one on the unit where he or she was receiving excellent care. Our sense was that there's more discussion about whether a particular patient is eligible for hospice or might be a candidate for PCAD.

DISTINGUISHING BETWEEN UNIT-LEVEL AND PATIENT-LEVEL OUTCOMES

The chart audit tool is used to assess how well we implemented the pathway; for instance, did staff members assess a greater range of symptoms with greater frequency? It does not tell us if someone had a good death or a peaceful death. The process assessment is really about implementing the PCAD and not about patient outcomes.

Our analyses thus far have been on the entire unit, not the patient. We did go into charts, but we aggregated the data, rather than looking at individuals. We did not compare pain scores of individual patients over time. We did not look at Mrs. Smith's last three days of life based on her chart, how the medications changed, how many she was on, what was withdrawn, what wasn't withdrawn, or if there was an interview with the family. We did not look at that kind of micro-level detail.

Instead, we sought to understand whether we could implement PCAD on a unit. Could we teach clinicians to treat patients using a new standard of care and access specific services that would be of benefit to dying patients? So, our data collection and analysis were conducted to assess how well we were implementing this pathway. One immediate goal was to begin to change the culture of a unit. Initiating the use of this standard of care is a step along the path to improving patients' outcomes and quality of care.

To get patient-level outcome data, you would have to do a concurrent QI study, in which you examine the death as close to the event as possible. Understanding individual patient outcomes is the next step. I think this needs to be done at the time it's happening. This is what I want to do next. You would look at the death of, say, Mrs. Smith and obtain data about the experience, perhaps from an after-death interview with the family or perhaps from assessment of outcomes directly from the patient immediately before death. Then the nurse looks at how well pain was assessed. The physician looks at the drugs that they used. Someone else looks at respiratory distress. Did we follow our guideline? Do we need a protocol? The chaplain determines if the patient had spiritual distress and whether a chaplain was involved or whether there was any indication that one was needed. One approach to improve overall practice on a unit in terms of patient-level outcomes would be to look more closely at the individual deaths on a unit with an interested team—at what they did and didn't do—using some guidelines for what is the ideal.

OTHER EVIDENCE OF IMPACT

We saw more consultations to the pain and palliative care team, because the unit staff and physicians realized how much we could offer families, especially once patients went home. They began to request continuity by the team for family support, symptom management, and titration of multiple drugs.

We learned early on in the project that our hospital needed to improve bereavement services. The hospice has excellent bereavement services, but then bereavement has always been integral to hospice. That is not the case for most hospital care of dying patients.

ALR: *How did you identify this deficit?*

MB: We conducted a debriefing session when a patient on PCAD died. The first part of our process was to debrief with nurses and nursing assistants about the patient's death. The debriefing was part of the PCAD educational process. Staff members loved it! The units have continued this practice on their own when they feel the need. For the benefit of the staff, the oncology unit, of its own initiative, is now doing a memorial service every six months for patients who died.

For families, we have created a condolence card from Beth Israel, which will be sent by the unit manager. The card is sent with an educational booklet, "Going Through Bereavement When a Loved One Dies." And on the back we list "Bereavement Resources" available in the community and a toll-free telephone number (Hospice Link 1-800-331-1620) for local bereavement groups sponsored by the Hospice Education Institute.

Limitations

ALR: *What do you think the limitations of PCAD are?*

Regarding implementation, I think the added paperwork of the MD Order Sheet, which required that they rewrite all orders, was a barrier and probably also a limitation. From a research perspective, the influence of the Consultation Service in the Department of Pain Medicine and Palliative Care could be seen as a limitation. Their presence and education of staff on all units (experimental and control) may have contributed to the increase in the standard of care (i.e., improved symptom assessment and treatment) on control units as well as on the experimental units. The influence could be viewed as contamination, or as diffusion of an innovation. Another limitation to generalizability to others is that we just tested this intervention in one hospital. PCAD is not a "magic bullet" to assure best practice in end-of-life care. It does, however, serve as an education and documentation tool, an interdisciplinary standard of care, and a catalyst to begin dialogue about the kind of care we all—clinicians, patients, and families—should expect when someone is imminently dying.

Advice

My suggestions for others, especially those working in a community hospital, who may wish to implement the pathway with little or no additional funding, are as follows:

1. **Start small.** Delineate the scope of your project: unit, service, and hospital.
2. **Work both "top down" and "bottom up."** What I mean by *top down* is gaining the buy-in and support from administration, unit physicians, and leaders who will pilot the intervention. The *bottom up* approach means getting the buy-in from staff who will be implementing the tool. The staff at the grassroots level gives you feedback and is crucial for working with you to make the intervention practical and relevant.
3. **Apply and adapt the PCAD tools to make them fit your own setting and disciplines.** For example, the MD order sheet—if doctors don't want to use it, come up with your own solution to getting goals of care addressed and treatments to reflect that patients are dying.
4. **Collect data to measure your current practice and to move the standard forward.** Go to the literature, find the best practice, seek to meet the benchmark. Keep yourself inspired by joining listservs or participating in Internet discussions, such as the one associated with *Innovations in End-of-Life Care*, or by reading other QI success stories.[#]
5. **Be patient.** Recognize that unit culture, like any change, takes time.
6. **Find and cultivate champions on the units targeted for change.** Champions are essential to this process. These are the people who find opportunities and strategies to increase dialogue and educate staff members and who keep the momentum going and role model the innovation. Leaders need to continue to mentor champions because it is easy for enthusiasm to wane after the initial trial period.

NEXT STEPS

I would like to develop a focused QI study with oncology and geriatrics unit teams (nurse, doctor, social worker, chaplain, dietician, ethicist) to examine individual patient deaths by asking the question "Was this a peaceful death, a good death?" In addition to learning about professionals' knowledge and attitudes about end-of-life care, I believe we would then learn a great deal about current practice, the systems impeding care, and the areas deserving accolades or needing improvement. I think we could develop a brief set of indicators to evaluate the salient factors that such teams believe characterize a good death. What are the criteria? Is

---

[#]For examples, see Lynn J, Lynch Schuster J, Kabcenell A. *Improving Care for the End of Life: A Sourcebook for Health Care Managers and Clinicians.* New York: Oxford University Press, 2000; and Solomon MZ, Romer AL, Heller KS, Weissman DE. *Innovations in End-of-Life Care: Practical Strategies & International Perspectives,* Volume 2. Larchmont, NY: Mary Ann Liebert, Inc., 2001.

the staff satisfied with how they cared for the patient and family? Is the family satisfied? Were symptoms well managed? Did we know what the patient's wishes were and did we meet them? Once the team can define what a good death would be on their unit, we can build the tool to help them to measure themselves against that benchmark, and the quest to reach a new standard begins. So that's what I will do next on these three units. We are still seeking funding to test PCAD at a larger level. Until then I'll start small and follow the steps I just laid out for others without funding. Get a team, get the dialogue going, develop a tool to track changes, give feedback, and be available with resources and ideas and support to make changes and raise the standard one more time.

ACKNOWLEDGMENTS

Marilyn Bookbinder, PhD, RN, would like to acknowledge the expertise and commitment of the QI Team, the pilot units, and the DPMPC Study Team: Russell K. Portenoy, MD; David Wollner, MD; Elizabeth Arney, RN, MS; Roseanne Indelicato, RN, NP; Marlene McHugh, RN, NP; Terry Altilio, ACSW; Joan Panke, RN, NP; Arthur Blank; and Pauline LeSage, MD.

REFERENCES

1. Bookbinder M, Coyle N, Kiss M, Layman Goldstein M, Holritz K, Thaler H, Gianella A, Derby S, Brown M, Racolin M, Nah Ho M, Portenoy RK. Implementing national standards for cancer pain management: Program model and evaluation. *Journal of Pain & Symptom Management.* 1996;12(6):334-347.
2. Bookbinder M, Kiss M, Coyle N, Brown M, Gianella A, Thaler H. Improving pain management practices. In *Cancer Pain Management*, 2d ed. D McGuire, C Yarbro, B Ferrell (eds.). Boston: Jones and Bartlett, 1995, 321-361.
3. Christakis NA, Lamont EB. Extent and determinants of error in physicians' prognoses in terminally ill patients: Prospective cohort study. *Western Journal of Medicine.* 2000;172:310-313.
4. Ross MM, McDonald B, McGuinness J. The palliative care quiz for nurses. *Journal of Advanced Nursing.* 1996;23:125-137.
5. Bookbinder M. Improving the quality of care across settings. In *Textbook of Palliative Nursing*, B Ferrell, N Coyle (eds.). Oxford, England: Oxford University Press, 2001, 503-530.

A Systematic Approach to Palliative Care in a Hospital and Community Setting

An Interview with STEIN KAASA, MD, PhD
Trondheim University Hospital
Trondheim, Norway

In the following interview with Anna L. Romer, EdD, Stein Kaasa, MD, PhD, chair of the palliative medicine unit at the Trondheim University Hospital and professor at the medical school in Trondheim, Norway, describes the evolution of that unit within the department of oncology as well as in the larger context of the provision of health care in Norway. The country is divided into health regions; the Trondheim University Hospital serves as the regional, tertiary-care specialty hospital for patients residing in the central part of Norway. Ten years ago the government decided to create the only palliative medicine professorial chair in the country at this medical school and to locate the first and still unique palliative care unit at the Trondheim University Hospital. This academic, university-based unit combines research, training, and clinical work and has served as a model for others in Scandinavia. Medical students have exposure to the palliative medicine unit during each year of their training; fellows and general practitioners also spend time on the unit to receive additional training in palliative medicine.

A REGIONAL PALLIATIVE MEDICINE PROGRAM

Anna L. Romer: *Describe the palliative medicine program at the Trondheim University Hospital.*

Stein Kaasa: The service includes a 12-bed acute palliative care unit, an outpatient unit, a hospital-based consultation service and a home care team, which consists of doctors, nurses, social workers, physical therapists, dieticians, and chaplains. The mean length of stay at the inpatient unit is 10 days, exactly the same as for the department of oncology.

ALR: *What population of patients does the unit serve?*

SK: Ninety-nine percent of our patients have cancer diagnoses. We should see patients with other diagnoses, but that's not the situation right now. We admit the majority of the patients from the hospital, either from the department of surgery, lung medicine, or from the department of oncology and other departments in the hospital. General practitioners in the community refer a smaller portion of our patients to the unit.

ALR: *Where do patients who leave the inpatient unit go?*

SK: We discharge 25 percent of our patients to home, another 20 percent go to a nursing home, and approximately 55 percent die on the unit.[1] Hospice is not a word we use so much. We use the term *hospice* quite differently in Norway. It refers primarily to a philosophy of care, but can also refer to a place, but it has no funding or regulatory implications. Nursing homes are the places where we offer inpatient, chronic, long-term care, including inpatient hospice care.

Recently, the palliative medicine unit established an agreement to collaborate with the city of Trondheim in the care of patients at two nursing homes. As a result, we now have four beds at one nursing home and three beds at the other. This new arrangement means that, when we discharge patients from the acute palliative care unit who cannot go home for various reasons, we can now send them to these beds in the nursing homes for longer-term inpatient palliative care. A doctor–nurse team visits the patients there once a week at least, and the long-term staff can request additional consults if they wish. The nurse also gives general support to the nursing staff. Recently, we have begun offering telemedicine teaching sessions to update their skills, and the staff of the nursing home participate in our teaching rounds and case discussions online with the staff of the palliative medicine program. In this way, other patients beyond the four in the designated palliative beds in each nursing home also benefit from this contact, as the nursing home staff can consult the palliative care team about their care as well.

ALR: *How is the staff of the palliative medicine service organized?*

SK: At first, we tried to have a floating organization with staff working in both inpatient and outpatient settings. But, after a couple of years, we realized that this was too complicated. We now have two doctors working on the inpatient unit and two doctors working at the outpatient clinic. The latter also consult at the nursing homes, in patients' homes, and in the rest of the hospital. Five nurses work on the outpatient team. The inpatient team includes 30 nurses. The doctors rotate annually across the units. The doctors who are visiting fellows spend the first half of the year on the inpatient unit and then the second half at the outpatient clinic. In addition, the palliative care staff that works with patients across all settings includes one and a half positions for physical therapists, one chaplain, one social worker, and one dietician.

ALR: *Can you perhaps take a typical patient, if there is such a thing, and describe how he or she enters your care, what you might do, and then where that patient might go?*

SK: A young patient with pancreatic cancer might have, for example, a family and a lot of internal resources and energy to live. The patient wants to be active for as long as possible, but has a lot of symptoms. He might have ascites. He might have a lot of pain because of the pancreatic tumor, but he wants to be at home. Most likely, this patient's oncologist will refer him to us as the care becomes complex, to offer support to the patient and family and to help manage the symptoms and home care. Quite a few of these younger patients don't want to be inpatients; they want to be outpatients. For these patients we try to establish a program tailored to their needs. We try to treat the patient in an outpatient setting and, if necessary, we go to the patient's home. Young patients with cancer often have children, so we spend quite a lot of time talking to the patient, the spouse, and the children. So, in this example, we would focus on the patient's symptoms and his family's needs. We would talk with him and his wife about how to inform the children, how to bring them into the process, and how they are going to actually prepare the children for living together while the father is dying and afterward. If the patient wants to die at home, we work in advance with the general practitioner and the home care nursing service so that this can happen.

Another example might be an 80-year-old man with prostate cancer, who is having lots of skeletal metastases and who has a wife who herself is not very fit. This patient decides he doesn't want to be in a nursing home; he wants either to be at home or in our inpatient palliative care unit. So, for this patient we try to establish as much support as possible at home. We try to treat him as an outpatient, because we have a limited number of beds in our palliative care unit. We also try to anticipate with him that he may get so sick that he can't be at home and then he would have to stay for a long time in a bed in an institution. We describe the beds we have at the nursing home and our close connection with these nursing homes, which might lead a patient to accept that option. Such a patient might, for example, come to our palliative care unit for several short inpatient visits, maybe to get radiotherapy or other types of tumor-directed treatment and/or to get his pain treatment monitored. Sometimes we might even take that patient in over the weekend or maybe for another three or four days to offer respite care so that his wife can relax.

In sum, we try to work flexibly with the primary health care team so that we can orient our care to the patient and family's needs across levels and settings as seamlessly as possible.

DEFINING PALLIATIVE MEDICINE: THE ROLE OF SPECIALISTS

ALR: *It sounds like your team plays a variety of roles with patients, from almost a primary care role to the consultant role. Can you elaborate?*

SK: We have a mixture of patients. All patients in Norway have a general practitioner. A recent change in the law has made that mandatory. In some cases there is a close existing relationship, in others less so. We are trying to classify our patients into three groups to help us best to monitor and respond to their needs. We call them A, B, and C patients, based on which health care professionals have primary responsibility for the patient's care. A patients are those for whom the palliative care team has primary responsibility—they are "our" patients. These cases are few, and the general practitioner has very little involvement. Then we have the B patients, for whom the general practitioner and the home care nurses have the primary responsibility, but our team still has substantial involvement. The C patients have been seen once or twice by us, but we don't have any regular follow-up with them. This system allows us to be clear with patients about whom to contact in an emergency.

Palliative care is more than just caring for the dying. We need to be preventive and we need to reach the patients before they are dying. Palliative treatment should not begin in the last couple of days of patients' lives. To implement this ideal, we need to be clear about which health care professionals are serving as the primary caregivers for the patient and family.

ALR: *What do you mean by preventive?*

SK: By preventive, I mean prevent symptoms, prevent suffering, and give psychosocial support to the family. You cannot just do that the last three or four or five days that the patient is alive. You have to know the family for a while. You have to know the patient in order to address his or her symptoms. You have to talk to the family. You may have to meet the children a couple of times and know the family before you can actually give them advice.

ALR: *Do you aim to make contact with these patients earlier in their disease trajectory, that is, doing* preventive *work and getting to know families?*

SK: It's a very good question, because it is also related to resources. When can you actually deliver your expertise best? Should we as specialists in palliative medicine have direct contact with more patients or only those with the most difficult problems? Should palliative medicine be in the mainstream so that most doctors have some expertise in it, or should it be a specialization? My answer is a little bit of both. In the Trondheim program, we want to see the problematic patients on our inpatient unit. We can admit them to our inpatient unit to get intractable symptoms under control. We can also design an individual home care program in collaboration with the primary health care system, if necessary. One of our strengths is that we have a great deal of flexibility in how we respond to patients' needs. We have skilled doctors, nurses, and other health care professionals who are working together as an interdisciplinary team.

However, we also see teaching and research as crucial to our mission. We want to consult to others, demonstrate what we know and do well, and disseminate our research findings to establish the evidence base for the field so that other physicians value and accept palliative medicine.

Ideally, I think oncologists and internists should deal with most of their patients themselves. Patients who are not suffering unduly could be managed by their primary health team or the specialists who have responsibility for their condition. But this is a two-edged sword. I do think that the palliative care specialists should be more heavily involved in symptom control and in planning care for the last months and weeks of patients' lives.

BARRIERS TO ACCESS TO PALLIATIVE CARE

ALR: *In the United States we have had regulatory barriers, as you know, in terms of the Medicare Hospice Benefit, which regulates who can gain access to hospice care. What kinds of barriers to accessing palliative care early in the disease trajectory exist in Norway?*

SK: The barriers are not regulatory, but we have barriers just the same. We have the same problem of patients being referred to palliative care too late in their disease trajectory. We have the same problems of denial, of physicians not wanting to give up on patients or transfer their care to other physicians.

We also have funding barriers to providing seamless care. I had to fight very hard from the beginning, when I established the palliative care unit, because doctors at the hospital do not traditionally leave the hospital. Doctors were not expected to go to patients' homes, and visiting nursing homes was unheard of, as care in that setting is reimbursed through a different budget. Three years ago, I was able to convince the politicians in the government that they should pay for doctors to go to patients' homes and to nursing homes. Now the hospital administration approves of these activities because they now get reimbursed for this time. At first, when we did this type of work, the hospital did not get any income from it. The doctors are on a fixed salary, so their reimbursement has not changed with these new activities.

ALR: *Did the nursing homes welcome you?*

SK: Yes. But there are also some economic barriers. Having patients who require more intensive care in the nursing homes costs more because we are asking for more expensive treatments.

The nursing homes have a certain amount of money each year, which they can use for medications. We may prescribe, for example, IV fluid, blood, bisphosphonates, and other kinds of drugs, such as antibiotics, which may be more expensive. Providing this more intensive care in the nursing home allows these patients, who would have been admitted to an intensive care hospital, to stay in the nursing home. So, for the patients themselves, it is probably better, less disruptive care, and for society as a whole this care conserves resources. This change creates savings on a grand scale, but the hospital and nursing home come out of different budgets. We might ruin the entire budget for a nursing home if we discharge a patient to them who is on some expensive drugs and getting blood transfusions and some other drugs for, let's say, two months. The nursing homes can lobby for more money, if they can prove that they have patients who are legitimately consuming more resources, but it's complicated.

INTEGRATION OF PAIN AND PALLIATIVE MEDICINE

ALR: *Integrating the pain service and a department of palliative medicine, as Dr. Portenoy has done at Beth Israel Medical Center in New York City,* is unique in the United States. Would that be novel for you in Norway?*

SK: It depends on what you define as pain and palliative care. In all palliative care programs, pain treatment is an essential component. You cannot separate them. But, from an organizational point of view, pain programs started much earlier in most hospitals than the palliative care programs.

I think during this development process it has often been very difficult to combine them, because the pain programs in Europe are very closely linked to anesthesiology. The pain programs are not only caring for palliative care patients, but also post-operative pain, chronic non-malignant pain, chronic back pain, and so on. We have a small pain clinic in Trondheim, and they are organized within the department of anesthesiology. We are having consults together with them. We look at patients together. If we feel that we need their expertise, then we consult with them, and we have meetings regularly. We have several joint research projects, and we are training doctoral students together. Yet we are not organized as one department. I've been thinking about this question, and there are actually both pros and cons.

ALR: *Philosophically, are there reasons that these departments do better when separate?*

SK: I don't think there is a philosophical reason. However, post-operative pain and non-malignant pain are somewhat different, and if you want to be really specialized, I think it is somewhat difficult to combine them. Physicians in each area go to different types of conferences and are reading different journals, and so on.

When I came to Trondheim, my idea was that there were so few experts in this field that pain and palliative medicine should really be combined. So, if I could make the decision in Trondheim, I think I would like to have one department including pain and palliative care. It's a little artificial to say "pain and palliative care" because pain treatment is so crucial within palliative care.

AVAILABILITY OF DIFFERING LEVELS OF CARE

ALR: *In some parts of the world, insufficient numbers of long-term care beds, insufficient financial resources on the part of patients and their families, or the absence of family members to provide "free" long-term care have all led to patients staying longer than is clinically necessary on acute care units. What is the situation in Norway?*

---

*See Developing an Integrated Department of Pain and Palliative Medicine: An Interview with Russell Portenoy, MD, pp. 53–67.

SK: Sometimes we have that problem. But since we have gained access to these seven beds at the nursing homes, it has been much easier. Earlier, we sometimes had patients staying for several weeks on our inpatient unit.

ALR: *Are seven beds in the long-term care settings sufficient to meet the more chronic palliative care needs of the population?*

SK: No. Trondheim is a city of more than 150,000 people. Currently, we have too few nursing home beds, and that's a big problem for the hospital in general, because there are too many patients staying in our acute hospital. For example, in the department of internal medicine, we have patients who should not be at an intensive university regional hospital. Patients' treatments are finalized, and the Trondheim University Hospital can no longer add to their care, beyond what a chronic setting can offer, but the patients are not discharged because there are no beds to go to. To take care of patients suffering from cancer in an adequate way, including the opportunity for optimal symptom control and optimal palliative care in general, we would need approximately 15 to 20 chronic, long-term beds.

ALR: *So it's not an expense problem, it's a beds problem?*

SK: Ultimately, it is an expense problem because the society has not built enough nursing home beds. To make changes within such a system takes time. Everything is paid for within the National Health Care System, including long-term inpatient care. But you cannot get that care if the beds do not exist. It is a governmental expense problem, not an individual family expense problem, except insofar as the family will have to care for the frail family member if sufficient long-term beds are not available.

STANDARDS OF CARE

ALR: *Would you say that the kinds of treatments that you offer and the general level of care in Trondheim are comparable to that offered in other parts of Europe or the United States? Or are there cultural differences in terms of what treatments are seen as appropriate palliative care?*

SK: There are not that many acute palliative care programs including inpatient beds specifically assigned for palliation in the United States. To my knowledge, there is one, as you mentioned, at the Beth Israel Medical Center in New York, one at the Cleveland Clinic in Ohio, and one at the Memorial Sloan–Kettering Cancer Center in New York. There is a regional program in Edmonton, Alberta, in Canada.

We were very much inspired by the program in Edmonton when we designed our program in Trondheim. Basically, the standard of care in these different units across the world is similar. We are all working in interdisciplinary teams, including experienced nursing staff. But I think that we who practice palliative medicine are still struggling with these questions: What is palliative medicine? What distinguishes palliative medicine?

I think that our answers are very much influenced by where different physicians are coming from. If a doctor is trained in neurology, he or she might be more interested in neurological problems; in anesthesiology, the doctor might be more traditionally pain oriented; if a doctor is trained in oncology, he or she might be more oncology oriented. One's focus depends on one's clinical training. This might explain the heterogeneity of palliative medicine, but we are quickly moving to a consensus on what palliative medicine is.

What I would like in the future is to really try to get an international curriculum for palliative medicine. It is needed, even though palliative medicine is developing all the time.

ALR: *One of the features of the Beth Israel program that has been highlighted is the Palliative Care for Advanced Disease (PCAD) pathway.[†] Do you have a similar type of pathway, either as a quality improvement effort to establish a clear standard of care or as a way to get people thinking about using palliative care or referring to palliative care in your hospital?*

SK: We are in the process of establishing standards for palliative care at our program, too. I believe standards are important, but we need to be flexible in our application of them. It is a great idea to have a clear pathway or set of standards and to be able to demonstrate what clinicians are actually doing. I think Dr. Portenoy has built a remarkably good program. All physicians in the United States who are interested in palliative care should know about his program, as well as the Edmonton program established by Dr. Eduardo Bruera.[‡]

TEACHING AND RESEARCH

I think teaching is very important—teaching in palliative care in general and also on specific themes, both of which we do. Teaching and doing rounds are ways to increase referrals and to spread knowledge of the principles of palliative care to physicians in other specialties. These activities improve the overall quality of care in the hospital outside the palliative medicine unit. I think they also build trust in our staff and increase requests for consultations.

It is also crucial to be on site within the different wards. As we go there regularly, we ask, "Are there any patients who could benefit from palliative care?" All these wards have their own routines. If we think that we can help them and that we can improve patient care, this is news to them. We have to be there regularly and actually show them what we can offer so that they can see how we might help.

[†]See Raising the Standard of Care for Imminently Dying Patients Using Quality Improvement: An Interview with Marilyn Bookbinder, PhD, RN, pp. 69–83.

[‡]For information on the Edmonton Palliative Care Program, see *Quality of Life*, Part Six of this volume.

We need the palliative medicine inpatient unit to teach medical students, fellows, nurses, nursing students, and other health care professionals. Having our own patients also enables us to do research and learn more about what the most effective treatments are and how to measure and attend to patients' quality of life. Research and teaching go hand in hand and reinforce each other in further establishing the field of palliative medicine.

Teaching medical students and teaching doctors is one worthy long-term investment. My main argument for investing a lot of my own resources in the medical school is that one has to have a long-term strategy to improve palliative care.

One problem with palliative care in general is that, in spite of a lot of enthusiastic individuals, we have not been able to incorporate palliative care into the system. When the enthusiastic individual champion disappears, the palliative care effort disappears. Our rationale for teaching in medical school is to change basic attitudes toward palliative care and to improve the knowledge base of doctors within the health care system.

> *When the enthusiastic individual champion disappears, the palliative care effort disappears. Our rationale for teaching in medical school is to change basic attitudes toward palliative care and to improve the knowledge base of doctors within the health care system.*

I think that medical doctors are extremely important as gatekeepers and role models for the health care team. When doctors accept palliative care nurses (who tend to be much more proactive), they are able to follow through more effectively with that care. If there is one doctor on the ward who is pro-palliative care and thinks differently about death and dying, then it's much easier for the nurses to work within this field.

INTERNATIONAL COMPARISONS: ACCESS TO CARE, CONTINUITY OF CARE, AND FUNDING

ALR: *Can you describe how the financing of care in Norway helps health care professionals provide what sounds like good continuity of care and perhaps make some comments about your experience in the United States?*

SK: First of all, hospitals in Norway are free. Patients pay a certain amount for outpatient care and for prescription drugs, but patients with cancer or other chronic, life-ending diseases don't pay for any medications. In the Norwegian system, everyone has an annual deductible of approximately $200 per year for prescription drugs.

I think the Norwegian system has many other strengths. First, we *have* a universal health care system and it is based on at least two levels: we have the hospital level with the doctors and nurses, and then we have the community level. All patients in Norway have to have a general practitioner. When a person has a life-threatening disease and wants to be at home during the end of life, this person will have access to some home care nursing. Another strength is that hospitals and other health care settings are not competing over patients, even though we do have budgetary conflicts, such as the one I described between the hospital and the nursing homes. The system works best when different health care institutions collaborate.

Limitations of the Norwegian System

There are limitations, because the health care system cannot provide round-the-clock care at home. Patients who are severely ill have to rely on family members for care in order to stay at home. Family members can be paid their full-time salary for four weeks in order to take care of a dying father, mother, husband, or wife. That's usually enough. If family members need more time, it is unpaid leave at the discretion of the employer.

One disadvantage with our system might be that patients in need of specialists, for example, palliative medicine care, might not have access to these specialists because the general practitioner thinks that he or she can do an adequate job. We have tried to address this problem by demonstrating to the general practitioners what skills we have. In Trondheim, we know the general practitioners, and they are training with us as fellows for half a year, so in our particular region this may not be such a problem.

Another problem lies in the professional skills at the nursing homes. We don't have enough experienced nurses working at the nursing homes. Quite a few of the nurses working are not registered nurses and have just one year of nursing education. Furthermore, up until now, work in nursing homes has had a very low status.

Our current collaboration with the nursing homes in Trondheim is helping to address this problem. We are asking staff at the nursing home for better documentation and more follow-up with patients. In the nursing home we are teaching for free. In this way we are increasing the general skills in medicine and in nursing for the doctors and nurses at the nursing homes. Increasing the general level of skill in palliative care has an impact on the care of other non-dying patients at nursing homes. We believe that this kind of collaboration can ultimately improve patient care.

Limitations of the US System

ALR: *Now that you are just completing a sabbatical year in the United States, what insights have you gleaned about how the differences in our two health care systems affect the provision of palliative care in our respective countries?*

SK: I think the system in the United States is problematic for palliative care. It should be a human right to get optimal care when you are dying, independent of your economic resources. To get optimal palliative care in the United States, either you have to be able to pay out of your own pocket or you have to have rather good private health insurance or be enrolled in the Medicare Hospice Benefit for care near the very end of life. That's my understanding of the system. I might be wrong.

I have also seen that the health care system could probably benefit, at least in palliative care, from more integration. To me, the US system is highly individualized and somewhat fragmented. As a doctor, a patient is *your* patient, and quite often I think the patient might benefit from being in a more integrated health care system, where quality and access to care depend less on access to one individual doctor who will save the day. I think patients would benefit from having a more trustworthy *system* of care.

For people with enough resources and the right health insurance, the United States probably offers the best specialized treatment in the world. No one can compete with that. But for those with a chronic disease, and dying is usually a chronic situation, I do not think the system is working optimally. Many successful interventions can be low tech; you don't need to do every sophisticated intervention. Patients do need access to doctors and nurses who actually want to provide quality palliative care, and you have to have a system that actually honors them for providing this type of care. Society needs the security that each individual will have access to this type of care through some kind of insurance, probably government insurance that adequately covers the costs of providing it. I know that this is a very difficult issue in the United States. But to an outsider who lives in a country where we have such a system, its absence in this rich and privileged country is startling.

> *Society needs the security that each individual will have access to this type of care through some kind of insurance, probably government insurance that adequately covers the costs of providing it. . . . to an outsider who lives in a country where we have such a system, its absence in this rich and privileged country is startling.*

REFERENCE

1. Jordhøy MS, Fayers P, Saltnes T, Ahlner-Elmqvist M, Jannert M, Kaasa S. A palliative-care intervention and death at home: A cluster randomised trial. *Lancet.* 2000; 356:888–893.

Selected Bibliography

Part Two

Selected references by contributors to this part:

Bookbinder M, Coyle N, Kiss M, Layman Goldstein M, Holritz K, Thaler H, Gianella A, Derby S, Brown M, Racolin M, Nah Ho M, Portenoy RK. Implementing national standards for cancer pain management: Program model and evaluation. *Journal of Pain & Symptom Management*. 1996;12(6):334-347.

Bruera E, Portenoy RK (eds.). *Topics in Palliative Care*, Volume 5. New York: Oxford University Press, 2001.

Bruera E, Portenoy RK (eds.). *Topics in Palliative Care*, Volume 4. New York: Oxford University Press, 2000.

Bruera E, Portenoy RK (eds.). *Topics in Palliative Care*, Volume 3. New York: Oxford University Press, 1998.

Bruera E, Portenoy RK (eds.). *Topics in Palliative Care*, Volume 2. New York: Oxford University Press, 1998.

Bruera E, Portenoy RK (eds.). *Topics in Palliative Care*, Volume 1. New York: Oxford University Press, 1997.

Ellershaw J, Smith C, Overill S, Walker SE, Aldridge. Care of the dying: Setting standards for symptom control in the last 48 hours of life. *Journal of Pain & Symptom Management*. 2001;21(1):12-17.

Ellershaw J, Foster A, Murphy D, et al. Developing an integrated pathway for the dying patient. *European Journal of Palliative Care*. 1997;4:203-207.

Ellershaw JE, Peat SJ, Boys LC. Assessing the effectiveness of a hospital palliative care team. *Palliative Medicine*. 1995;9(2):145-152.

Glajchen M, Bookbinder M. Knowledge and perceived competence of home care nurses in pain management: A national survey. *Journal of Pain & Symptom Management*. 2001;21(4):307-316.

Lloyd-Jones G, Ellershaw J, Wilkinson S, Bligh JG. The use of multidisciplinary consensus groups in the planning phase of an integrated problem-based curriculum. *Medical Education*. 1998;32(3):278-282.

Thorns AR, Ellershaw JE. A survey of nursing and medical staff views on the use of cardiopulmonary resuscitation in the hospice. *Palliative Medicine*. 1999;13(3):225-232.

Other selected references:

Berwick DM. A primer on leading the improvement of systems. *British Medical Journal*. 1996;312(7031):619-622.

Brenner P. The experience of Jacob Perlow Hospice: Hospice care of patients with Alzheimer's disease. In *Hospice Care for Patients with Advanced Progressive Dementia*, L Volicer, A Hurley (eds.). New York: Springer Publishing Co., 1998, 257-275.

Brooke RH, McGlynn E, Cleary PD. Quality of health care: Measuring quality of care. Part 2 of 6. *New England Journal of Medicine*. 1996;335(13):966-970.

Chassin MR. Quality of health care: Improving the quality of care. Part 3 of 6. *New England Journal of Medicine*. 1996;335(14):1060-1063.

Christakis NA, Lamont EB. Extent and determinants of error in physicians' prognoses in terminally ill patients: Prospective cohort study. *Western Journal of Medicine*. 2000;172:310-313.

Evangelista M. Transferable pathway benefits hospital, hospice. *Hospital Case Management*. 1995;3(5):75-78.

Gordon DB. Critical pathways: A road to institutionalizing pain management. *Journal of Pain & Symptom Management*. 1996;11(4):252-259.

Anonymous. Supportive care pathway comforts the terminally ill. *Hospital Case Management*. 1998;6(4):69-72.

Kitchiner D, Davidson C, Bundred P. Integrated care pathways: Effective tools for continuous evaluation of clinical practice. *Journal of Evaluation in Clinical Practice*. 1996;2(1):65-69.

Lafferty CL. Transformational leadership and the hospice RN case manager: A new critical pathway. *Hospice Journal*. 1998;13(3):35-48.

McClung LT. Clinical pathways for the terminally ill. *Caring*. 1997;16(11):26-28, 30, 32.

Ventafridda V, Ripamonti C, De Conno F, et al. Symptom prevalence and control during cancer patients' last days of life. *Journal of Palliative Care*. 1990;6(3): 7-11.

Wright PM. A critical pathway for interdisciplinary hospice care. *American Journal of Hospice and Palliative Care*. 2001;18(1):31-34.

Zander K. *Critical Pathways, Total Quality Management: The Health Care Pioneers*. Chicago: American Hospital Publishing, 1992, Chapter 9: 305-314.

Part Three

Supporting Family Caregivers

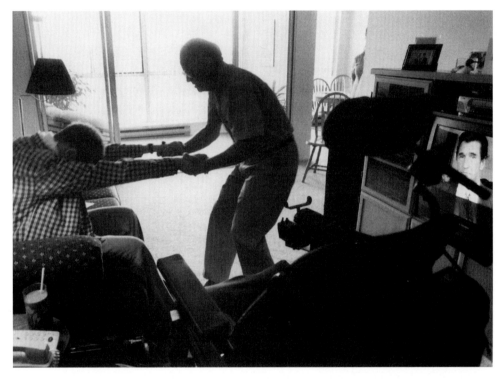

©1998 Roger Lemoyne and Living Lessons.

Hospital-Based Family Caregiver Programs: Building Institutional Resources and Community Ties

CAROL LEVINE

United Hospital Fund
New York, New York

Most family caregiving takes place at home, even for people at the end of life. But the long months and years of caregiving that precede the final stages are often punctuated by acute episodes of illness or trauma, when hospitalization is necessary. Whether these hospital stays are of a few days' duration or stretch out into weeks, they typically mark turning points in the patient's condition and in the caregiver's responsibilities. And for everyone involved the experience of hospitalization is usually full of anxiety, stress, and uncertainty. Ordinary life, even in the extraordinary conditions that characterize long-term caregiving, is suspended in the hospital environment.

In this part we focus on projects that are changing the culture and practices of hospitals to respond more creatively to the needs of family caregivers of people with dementia, who are often in the last stages of life. This group of caregivers, some of the 25 million Americans who take on this responsibility, has particularly acute needs. The United Hospital Fund's Family Caregiver Initiative, a $2 million effort that is making a difference in New York City hospitals and communities, funded the programs featured here.

Cabrini Medical Center in Manhattan has created two acute care dementia units called Windows to the Heart; one is at the medical center and the second is at the Cabrini Center for Nursing and Rehabilitation. These units provide a high level of empathic care to individuals with Alzheimer's disease and related dementias and their family caregivers. The Brooklyn Hospital has taken a different route toward its goal of improving care for a similar population of blacks of northern and central Brooklyn. With its community partner, Wartburg Lutheran Home for the Aging, the Brooklyn Hospital project has significantly reduced caregiver strain and improved follow-up care. In this project, a gerontologic nurse practitioner identifies families while the patient is hospitalized, teaches the family caregiving techniques, and follows up with them after discharge by making phone calls and home visits to ensure that the transition has gone smoothly. The Wartburg staff provides seminars available to all caregivers in the community.

WHY A HOSPITAL-BASED INITIATIVE?

If most caregiving takes place at home, why look to hospitals for help? This question arose early on in discussions within the Families and Health Care Project. Before determining a set of research activities, we held several meetings with providers from many different disciplines and types of affiliations, as well as with family caregivers. No matter what question the meeting formally addressed, again and again participants brought up the problems surrounding transitions or transfers from one care setting to another. Usually, the discussion centered around discharge from hospital to home or to another facility, but many people also mentioned the often chaotic admission process. Everyone was frustrated with abrupt discharge policies that shortchanged essential caregiver training and planning.

> *. . . one reason to look to hospitals for solutions is that they are part of the problem.*

Even more compelling was the sense that, whereas hospitalization may have improved the patient's physical condition by treating pneumonia or mending a broken hip, it had led to deterioration in the person's overall functioning and had been an anxiety-ridden experience for the caregiver. So, one reason to look to hospitals for solutions is that they are part of the problem.

A second reason was the conviction that hospitalization, while admittedly challenging, is an opportunity to reassess the caregiving situation and to provide family caregivers with referrals and resources to help them in the community. Various hospital professionals are involved with the patient's care and, if given time and incentives, can support the family through the hospital stay and help them to make whatever adjustments are necessary at home.

A final reason was pragmatic. While the extensive multidisciplinary research and analytic activities of the Families and Health Care Project are funded mainly through foundation grants, one of our goals has always been to determine how to use the fund's grantmaking to shape meaningful change in the health care delivery system. A major portion of the fund's philanthropic dollars, which are raised annually by the fund and United Way of New York City, is designated for hospital-based initiatives. "Hospital," after all, is our middle name. The Family Caregiver Initiative blends the fund's expertise in research and analysis with its philanthropic mission.

However, we knew that most hospitals had not done much for family caregivers, whose importance to the health care system in general was largely unrecognized. We wondered if we issued an RFP would anyone respond? In March 1998, we got our answer: 28 New York City hospitals responded to our Phase I RFP for six-month planning grants of $20,000. The applications were extraordinarily candid. They acknowledged the problems and promised a serious attempt to engage hospital staff and family caregivers in a process of determining where trouble spots existed and what programs might be instituted in response.

In May 1998, 16 of these hospitals were awarded grants to survey what was currently being done in their institutions specifically for family caregivers and to propose a programmatic response. At the end of the planning period, we issued an

RFP for program development. It specified that the program had to have high-level administrative support, multidisciplinary membership, participation of a community-based agency, and the involvement of family caregivers.

All 16 hospitals responded to the Phase II RFP for two-year implementation grants. The proposed projects were diverse, ranging from a hospital-wide program to educate staff and create resources for family caregivers (Mount Sinai Hospital) to the creation of a website (www.tbi-help.org) for caregivers of traumatic brain injury patients (Jamaica Medical Center). In February 1999, we awarded seven two-year implementation grants: six for $175,000 and one for $100,000. In February 2001, the board of directors approved third-year grants of $75,000 to each of the seven hospitals to enhance or modify their projects and to collaborate with us in a structured dissemination program.

All the hospitals have made important progress and have identified areas for improvement or modification. Interestingly, even before the project activities were underway, project staff reported to us that, because they had been awarded a grant and they now had identified staff concerned with family caregivers, they had new status within the institution and increased questions and referrals from their colleagues. Over the course of this initiative we have learned that, while hospitals cannot and should not provide all the services that caregivers need, they can be an important source of support and information at a critical point in the caregiving experience and can be good partners with other agencies in the community.

THE IMPACT OF THE CARE RECIPIENT'S HOSPITALIZATION ON THE CAREGIVER

As part of its research agenda, the Families and Health Care Project conducted a series of focus groups with experienced family caregivers, which gave us important insights into their problems with transitions in care settings. The findings of these focus groups are described in the United Hospital Fund Special Report, *Rough Crossings: Family Caregivers' Odysseys through the Health Care System.*[1] Briefly, caregivers told us that hospitalization led them to confront the deterioration in the patient's condition and intensified their sadness and sense of loss. They indignantly reported the difficulties that they encountered in getting information from hospital staff about the patient's condition and the results of tests or procedures. They reported that they felt invisible—or worse, unwelcome—in hospitals until the patient was ready to go home. They described the lack of training in complex medical equipment that they were responsible for operating at home. The training that was provided was perfunctory and dismissive of their fears. The staff did not appreciate, they told us, that caregivers were learning to do a task for the first time on someone that they love. On the other hand, small gestures of kindness or concern were gratefully remembered long after the event.

We learned more about the impact of hospitalization from a national and New York City random telephone survey of family caregivers conducted by the Families and Health Care Project in partnership with the Visiting Nurse Service of New

York and Harvard School of Public Health.[2] In this survey, New York City data did not differ in critical ways from the national data, suggesting that our focus groups' experiences are widespread. The respondents, a representative population-based sample, had all provided care for a family member or other person in the previous 12 months. About half were no longer providing care, and the most common reason was that the person had died.

Half of the care recipients had been hospitalized within the previous 12 months. After the hospitalization, caregivers' responsibilities increased in assisting with both Activities of Daily Living (ADLs) and Instrumental Activities of Daily Living (IADLs). (ADLs are personal care tasks, such as helping with bathing and toileting, while IADLs are household or management tasks, such as providing transportation and shopping.) This statistically significant finding confirmed our focus groups' reports that life was harder for them after the care recipient had been hospitalized.

It was not always so. In the past, people were kept in hospitals until they recovered, or at least until they had reached a stable condition. Now, even surgical patients are discharged with open wounds that need careful monitoring. Also, in the past, hospitalization was sometimes used to give family members a break from caregiving. While this was certainly an expensive and probably unjustified use of scarce resources, it at least reflected an appreciation of the difficulty of caring for a demented or dying person. However, hospitalization is now reserved for the most acute medical conditions, since almost everything else can be managed at home with the aid of technology. Although people who are admitted to hospitals are almost by definition very, very sick, hospital staffing patterns have changed so that there are fewer nurses and nurses' aides per patient. Tasks formerly performed by registered nurses are routinely assigned to less-trained staff.[3] Furthermore, publicity about hospital errors in medication and surgery has made family members concerned about patient safety.[4]

As a result, family members become hypervigilant, afraid to leave the patient alone, particularly if he or she is elderly, has cognitive problems, or has a complex medical regimen that must be followed exactly. Many family members organize shifts so that the patient is never left alone. Doctors often advise that if families can afford it they should hire private nurses or aides to provide essential care.[5,6] This kind of fear and constant vigilance plays havoc with caregivers' work schedules and other responsibilities, to say nothing of their emotional stamina.

Yet, as the Cabrini program shows, it need not be so. Trained staff and sensitive policies and practices can reduce caregiver stress and facilitate patient adjustment. Instead of seeing dementia patients as "crazy" or deliberately troublesome, staff members recognize that these patients are often reacting quite rationally to a totally disorienting experience. Imagine, if you will, being moved out of your hospital room in the middle of the night by strangers who do not say a word to you, take you on a circuitous route through the hospital, and then leave you in a cold, dark corridor—standard procedure for x-rays or CAT scans. Is screaming in fear under these circumstances irrational or understandable?

USING FAMILY CAREGIVERS AS A PATIENT RESOURCE

Family caregivers of dementia patients (and others as well) commonly complain that their intimate knowledge of the patient's behavior and medical condition is frequently disregarded by hospital staff, who assume that they have all the expertise that is necessary. As part of the Family Caregiver Initiative grant to the New York University Medical Center's Silberstein Aging and Dementia Research Center, the project staff created two tools for identifying and understanding patients with dementia as they are admitted to the hospital. The *Dementia Screen* flags patients with dementia at their initial entry point so that hospital staff can provide appropriate care and know that they need to interview family caregivers to obtain accurate information. The *Patient Profile* is designed to be completed by family caregivers identified as a result of the Dementia Screen. It provides assessment data that enable clinical staff to individualize and enhance care. Hospital information system (IS) staff developed and programmed data entry screens that facilitate data entry directly into the clinical record, which makes the information accessible to professional care providers.

WHAT NEXT?

Each of our grantees has plans to expand or enhance its projects. For example, Maimonides Medical Center in Brooklyn will expand its target caregiver population to all caregivers caring for elderly patients admitted to the hospital and will expand its staff education and postdischarge follow-up. Peninsula Hospital Center in Far Rockaway will revise its original assessment tool for caregivers of patients with traumatic brain injury to better understand their capabilities and future needs. It will also continue to track caregiver adjustment in the community and needs for further education.

Independently, several grantees have identified the same problem area: Most demented or seriously ill patients are admitted to the hospital through the emergency department (ED), where staff are not trained to distinguish dementia from other sources of anxiety. Television shows notwithstanding, most ED staff do not have time to spend interviewing family members or providing emotional support. Family members are shepherded away from the patient, who is left alone to be triaged for admission or treatment. The Cabrini project intends to focus on ED admission in the next year to facilitate the speedy assignment of dementia patients to the proper unit and to directly involve family caregivers in the intake process.

While the Families and Health Care Project dissemination plans are still in progress, we plan to spend the next year identifying the lessons learned from these projects and organizing ways to share this information with others. All the grantees have enthusiastically agreed to participate in this process.

To be sure, the barriers that existed at the start of this initiative have not been torn down and, in fact, may be higher in some institutions. Staff cuts, especially in nursing, are serious impediments to any program. Many institutions are under severe financial constraints and are not likely to assign resources for family caregivers unless they can see a direct economic benefit. Just as families have difficulties communicating with professionals, hospitals have internal communication problems. Information systems are not designed to collect important family data. Families who do not speak English and whose experience with the Western medical model is limited have special needs that few professionals are trained to address. Even more difficult to change are the professional and institutional cultures that frame families as "trouble," rather than as resources and allies.[7]

> *As more and more families are faced with the challenge of caring for a loved one at the end of life, medical institutions and health care providers, as well as other parts of society, will be moved to respond. It is up to us to shape this response in positive, compassionate, and humane ways.*

Still, compared to the situation just a few years ago, family caregiving has moved squarely onto the professional and public policy agenda. As more and more families are faced with the challenge of caring for a loved one at the end of life, medical institutions and health care providers, as well as other parts of society, will be moved to respond. It is up to us to shape this response in positive, compassionate, and humane ways.

REFERENCES

1. Levine C. *Rough Crossings: Family Caregivers' Odysseys through the Health Care System*. New York: United Hospital Fund, 1998.
2. Levine C, Kuerbis A, Gould DA, Navaie-Waliser M, Feldman PH, Donelan K. *A Survey of Family Caregivers in New York City: Findings and Implications for the Health Care System*. New York: United Hospital Fund, 2000.
3. Fagin CM. *When Care Becomes a Burden: Diminishing Access to Adequate Nursing*. New York: Milbank Memorial Fund, 2001.
4. Institute of Medicine. *To Err Is Human: Building a Safer Health System*. Washington, DC: National Academy Press, 1999.
5. Trafford A. When the hospital staff isn't enough. *Washington Post*, January 7, 2001, p. A1.
6. Parker-Pope T. How to lessen impact of nursing shortage on your hospital stay. *Wall Street Journal*, March 2, 2001, p. 19.
7. Levine C, Zuckerman C. The trouble with families: Toward an ethic of accommodation. *Annals of Internal Medicine*. 1999;130(2):148–152.

Windows to the Heart: Creating an Acute Care Dementia Unit

An Interview with JEFFREY N. NICHOLS, MD

Cabrini Medical Center
New York, New York

In 1999, Dr. Jeffrey Nichols, chief of geriatrics at Cabrini Medical Center (CMC) in New York City and medical director of the Cabrini Center for Nursing and Rehabilitation (CCNR), and his colleagues received a grant from the United Hospital Fund to develop an eight-bed, family-centered acute care unit for patients with dementia at CMC, a 500-bed hospital. Because of their location in Lower Manhattan, these institutions serve an ethnically diverse population, including many non-English-speaking people of Hispanic and Asian origin, and they have a high proportion of elderly patients, including patients with dementia.

This inpatient unit was created to address the widely recognized problem that, when dementia patients are hospitalized, the experience is frequently highly stressful for both patients and family or non-kin caregivers. Patients with advanced Alzheimer's disease and other dementias often suffer a precipitous decline in function during and following hospitalization, which places additional burdens on both the patients and their caregivers. Following some focus group research with family caregivers of dementia patients, Dr. Nichols and his colleagues realized that it was not sufficient to "tweak this, tweak that" in the traditional system of care in the hospital in order to meet the identified needs; rather, they had to take a comprehensive, carefully orchestrated, and holistic approach to change, encompassing the physical, operational, and cultural environment of the institution. In the following interview with Karen S. Heller, Dr. Nichols describes the challenges that he and his colleagues faced in starting this kind of unit in the acute care hospital setting and provides some preliminary evidence for its success.

GENESIS OF THE PROGRAM

Karen S. Heller: *How did this project begin?*

Jeffrey N. Nichols: This project, which we call Windows to the Heart, began three years ago, somewhat in response to the availability of a grant program launched by the United Hospital Fund to enable New York hospitals to look at ways that they could support family caregivers. Planning grants were given to more than twenty hospitals around the city to look at what they did and come back with a proposal. Because Cabrini Medical Center has an extremely high percentage of elderly patients, we decided that we would target the family caregivers of patients with dementia because they represent a large portion of our patient population. Although we were not sure exactly what proportion of patients in our acute care hospital had dementia, we were fairly sure that it was a significant number. Unfortunately, most hospitals don't do good screening, and hospital data systems don't capture the information because dementia is not usually the primary diagnosis. However, we have an affiliated nursing home where about 70 percent of the patients have dementia. This nursing home supplied a portion, at least, of admissions to the hospital. Plus, we knew that there were a lot of patients with dementia in the community. So we decided to pull together some focus groups of family caregivers who had had relatives at Cabrini. Remembering patients from the past few months, nursing staff identified patients whose care had involved family caregivers. We invited these family caregivers to come to some focus group meetings and share their experiences and suggestions with us.

HOSPITALIZATION IS "NOT GOOD" FOR PATIENTS

The focus groups were run by professional focus group coordinators. We were expecting the family caregivers to tell us that they needed support groups or more flexible visiting hours, perhaps better information about the disease, and better referrals for the time of discharge. We did hear these things. But even more loud and clear, people were saying that the hospital experience itself was *not* a good experience for the person that they loved or for themselves. They told us that they felt ignored when they came to the hospital and that they knew crucial things about what the patient needed, but that there was nobody to whom they could give this information. They told us that we were relatively insensitive to the emotional stress that they were undergoing. And they said that what they really would like is for us to take better care of the patients.

The family caregivers were very straightforward with us; they told us that Cabrini Medical Center wasn't *worse* than other hospitals, but that *every* hospital was bad. Many of them had had their family members at other hospitals, as well. In New York, we happen to be located in a cluster of hospitals in Lower Manhattan known in the community as "Bedpan Alley" because there are literally thousands of hospital beds here within a couple of square miles. Manhattan is terribly overbedded, and it is sometimes a matter of chance where an ambulance will take a patient.

In fact, when you look at the literature about hospitalization for patients with dementia, primarily with Alzheimer's disease, it tells you that patients suffer significant functional declines associated with acute hospital care.[1,2] This assumption of inevitable functional decline was the received wisdom in the field and has largely been taken for granted: this is simply something that has to happen because it is part of the disease. For many people with dementia, going into the hospital was always a disaster; they always wound up worse off than when they came in. Certainly, anyone who has worked in a nursing home will tell you that the patients always come back from the hospital in worse shape than when they left.

Now, in the focus groups, the families were telling us the exact same thing— that they brought patients in who were moderately functional, but had some acute problem. When they came out of the hospital, the acute problem was resolved, but their baseline functional status was dramatically worse. What's more, in the course of the hospitalization both the family caregivers and the person that they love went through some very humiliating experiences. Somewhat surprisingly, the hospital and its leadership were prepared to listen to this experience.

LEVERS FOR CHANGE

KSH: *What made your hospital administration receptive to this message?*

JNN: I think a combination of things made us responsive to this message. The United Hospital Fund's Family Caregiver Initiative was an encouragement to the hospital to choose family caregivers' needs as an area on which to try to focus in the short run. When foundations fund initiatives, they are able to bring attention to issues and to put these issues on an institution's agenda. For example, when The Robert Wood Johnson Foundation says that they are interested in adult day care or end-of-life care, it directs people to *think* about those domains. You may decide to do it or not, but it puts it on your list of something to consider.

A second factor that really made a difference is that there were individuals in senior hospital administration who were, in fact, caregivers themselves, some of whom have had their loved ones in the hospital. So, the stories that came out of the focus groups had a certain resonance for them, which they might not necessarily have had for someone else. That's really not so surprising, however; given the statistics on the percentage of middle-aged people who are family caregivers, it would be expected that at practically every hospital there are some senior staff who are, in fact, also serving as family caregivers. We were fortunate that the people that we invited to help us to think about the project had these experiences and, consequently, supported the project.

Third, our facility is sponsored by a religious order, the Missionary Sisters of the Sacred Heart of Jesus, known to most people as the Cabrini Sisters. As such, our hospital takes some mission issues rather seriously. It is part of our mission to provide family-centered care and to feel that we are involved in something slightly larger than just getting people in and out of a hospital. So, when we heard these difficult stories from family caregivers of our patients, we sat down and said, "How can all this be different?"

CHANGING THE CULTURE OF CARE

We pulled together a group of senior administrators from both the hospital and nursing home, and said, "If this is what's broken, how does one go about fixing all this?" The more we talked about it, the clearer it became that we could not change this in a piecemeal fashion—tweak this, tweak that, and we can make everything all right. In fact, we really needed to change the whole culture of care; by this I mean change the whole way we went about interacting with families, the whole way that we took care of patients suffering from dementia in the hospital setting. This change affected staff's job descriptions, the nature of their work, and what was considered important and not important. We realized that the whole culture of care had to involve the family caregiver directly. We *couldn't* just see the family caregiver as one more problem in a very busy day, which, to a large extent, is the way that they had been viewed. On a good day, you have some time to deal with *their* needs, too. But in the current hospital setting, it is a difficult process because there are six billion things to do, and the family caregivers' needs just seem like one more thing on top of everything else. So, we felt that care wouldn't change if we just put a patch on top of a bad situation—the patch being a little bit of extra time, especially if that extra time is being funded out of a grant.

> *. . . we really needed to change the whole culture of care; by this I mean change the whole way we went about interacting with families, the whole way that we took care of patients suffering from dementia in the hospital setting.*

Coincidentally, somewhat parallel to this effort in our institution, the Alzheimer's Association had a retreat in which they concluded that hospital care of Alzheimer's patients was a major, neglected area in which they wanted to try to become involved. When they had gone on their retreat, they had imagined all the different things that would need to be changed in the hospital to make it work. They envisioned that they would fund a hospital-based project that would try to do one of these things. Then they heard through their New York chapter that we already had started something, and they came here and discovered that we were trying to do *all* of the things that they were envisioning! We had naïvely launched ourselves to try to fix them all at the same time. But I think, in a way, that how we did it may be the only way that it actually could be done.

The intention was always to transform the care of the patients whom we already took care of, rather than seeking to increase referrals from outside the institution. When we went further along, attracting other patients became something that the unit staff identified as a potential index of our success. But this was never the hospital's original goal. Our goal was to do a better job of taking care of a group of patients and their family caregivers whom we were already seeing.

BARRIERS TO CHANGE AND STRATEGIES FOR OVERCOMING THEM

KSH: *In your own institution, what barriers did you encounter to making the kind of broad changes that you envisioned, given the preexisting culture and the way that things were set up? Did you anticipate them and were you able to address them?*

JNN: We thought that one barrier would certainly be the general belief that nothing could ever change, that the way things are is somehow inevitable. We knew that we were going to need major buy-in from senior administration in the hospital, because what we were doing was going to cut across many different boundaries and potentially, at least, was going to put people's noses out of joint. We wanted to make sure that everyone whose department was going to be affected had made a commitment in advance, had blessed the project, so to speak, that the project was *all right*, or else that we were prepared to deal with the reality that it *wasn't* all right. We didn't want to find out we couldn't implement the project because it was being secretly, or not so secretly, undermined by people who had different priorities or needs. So we tried very consciously to involve everybody in the senior administration relatively early on, to let them know what we were doing, to say openly, "These are things that are going to be different, is that all right with you? Is that going to present a problem? Tell us what the problem is in advance." We tried to prepare for a wide variety of different contingencies and for administrative opponents.

Our feeling was, first of all, that we *could* change the culture of the whole hospital; but even to change one piece of it was going to require a major investment of time and a willingness by all these other people. We thought that if we tried to create a unit that was separate and different, but not accepted by others, that ultimately it would be crushed. If it wasn't accepted, valued, and recognized from the beginning, then it couldn't possibly succeed. For this reason, we invested a great deal of time in planning and recruiting the interest, or at least the understanding, of other hospital personnel.

KSH: *What senior administrators did you involve?*

JNN: We involved the directors of medicine and nursing, excluding the director of surgery, because this was going to be a medical floor. In addition, we recruited the heads of food service, pharmacy, housekeeping, security, social work, discharge planning, chaplaincy, senior nursing administration, and senior medical personnel. For example, if we planned to change visiting hours, we knew it would be important to involve the admitting office and security. We tried to include all sorts of different people who, potentially, were going to be affected by our efforts to change the culture of care.

KSH: *Did these department leaders raise any concerns at the beginning?*

JNN: They did. I would say, initially, there was a lot of concern. For example, the human resources leaders were worried that there might be objections from union personnel about anything that appeared to change job descriptions and reporting. We were fairly careful about how we went about making changes, and it turned out to be *not* really an issue.

There were fewer problems than we anticipated. In any large bureaucracy (and this includes hospitals), people who have not been consulted are inevitably going to have concerns that they're going to want to have addressed later on. Very often, however, if they are involved in solving the problem or even framing the problem, they are going to be much more invested in the success of the project. So, we were very concerned that hospital staff and senior staff would feel, at least to some extent, invested in the project and willing to problem solve to make it happen. When they were asked to identify potential problems, in fact, they identified fewer problems. People were more flexible and more understanding of what the needs were going to be like than we had originally expected.

KSH: *How did you recruit the cooperation of these various departments?*

JNN: We knew, for example, that we were going to need extra time from social service. So, rather than scheduling the extra meetings we knew that we were going to have to conduct, and then hearing from the director of social service, "My staff doesn't have to come to all these meetings. We've got other things to do," we started with her and said, "How much time can you commit from your staff to attend the extra meetings that we know are going to be necessary? We are not going to schedule more time than you think that they reasonably can provide." With this approach, she actually gave us a larger number of hours than we probably would have asked for originally. At this point, it became an accepted part of the social work staff's responsibility to attend these meetings, and it was no longer a struggle to get that time.

KSH: *Did you involve quality assurance or risk management?*

JNN: Quality assurance was *not* involved. And I'm not totally sure why that's true. It didn't really exist as a separate department here. We didn't involve risk management, either, which might have reflected a lack of caution on our part because that's been a problematic area. Not that we've been sued, but, subsequently, risk management people came back with a series of concerns for which we had not really planned. So, we should have involved them at the beginning, too.

MINDFUL CHOICES CREATE COHERENT, PEACEFUL ATMOSPHERE

KSH: *Please describe what changes you made, briefly.*

JNN: We designed and opened one eight-bed unit on one medical floor of the acute care hospital. In designing the physical layout, we consulted with Lorraine Hiatt, probably the country's best known expert in dementia design. She is noted for her work in physical plant design and has collaborated on a large number of nursing home dementia units and adult day care programs. She spent a day with us and gave us some advice on how to make the space responsive to the needs of people with dementia, working within a limited budget.

We had what had been a stretch of rooms that went around the corner in a very large hospital unit. They were two-bed rooms and a corner four-bed room. We turned the corner four-bed room into a caregiver and patient lounge. So, we removed the beds and the wall equipment and put in couches, including a chair that turns into a day bed. We built a wheelchair-accessible bathroom and a family caregiver bathroom. We put in some shelves with patient education materials. We put in a lot of tables because dementia patients tend to eat better in a social setting. There are grab bars for the hallway. And we carpeted the lounge and the hallways and made sure that the infection control people signed off on this beforehand. These changes turned out to be no issue whatsoever, although everybody told us they would be.

The two-bedded rooms stayed almost exactly as they had been before. They were repainted to some more neutral colors, and we upgraded the lighting because shadows and odd lighting situations tend to induce paranoia and fear in patients suffering from Alzheimer's. One basic principle of Alzheimer's design is to make things *look* as much like what they're supposed to be as possible. You want doors to look like doors, so outlining the door in color helps people recognize that the door is, in fact, a door. Things that you *don't* want people to pay attention to should be the same color as the background so that they do not stick out. We tried to follow these design principles, so the stairwell that goes down to the street is done in the same color as its background wall with no outlining. But all the other areas that we want people to go into are as carefully outlined as possible. Some dementia patients will tend to wander—the general color and layout encourages people to wander in the direction of the caregiver room, which is where we want people to congregate.

We did something that seems like it's almost a violation of the patient's bill of rights—we took the TV sets out of the patient rooms. There is a TV in the lounge, but we can control what's seen on that, so you don't have the situation of people sitting around with TV sets blaring. Under normal circumstances, one watches what one wants. But here we were quite conscious that confusing, repetitive, loud, hostile presentations of sound are very difficult for patients. As a result, the unit is extraordinarily quiet. *And* we play music. It's not boring, necessarily, but it is extraordinarily quiet.

There's no traffic through the unit because it is laid out on the far corner of the floor. The only reason to come out to the unit is because you want to be on the unit. No one is wandering through with squeaky carts, nobody's yelling to the other end of the hall, "Get 17 out of bed. Have to go down to CAT scan." None of this goes on with a patient who may not know whether he or she is number 17 or not. There is no distracting overhead paging. So the only sounds that patients hear are sounds that are *intended*. In addition, we try as much as possible to bring them into the day room where they can interact with other patients and their families in a somewhat more spacious setting, because our two-bed rooms are not really that big.

STAFFING AND COST

KSH: *What is the staffing of your eight-bed unit?*

JNN: When we started the project, it was our intention that, with a sole exception, there would be no difference in staffing between this unit and any other unit in the hospital. Part of the reason for that was purely practical: there's no point in setting up a unit that requires special funding and then have it disappear after the grant money is gone. We had to come up with a plan that would be self-sustaining from the hospital's point of view. We are staffed primarily using our own in-house people reassigned from other units. The one difference in staffing between our unit and others in the hospital is that we have a pastoral care worker who is assigned almost exclusively to our unit. She is Latin American, bilingual, and has a lot of interaction with the Spanish-speaking patients and people from other ethnic groups who are Catholic.

> *We understand that dementia patients have special needs. Using a team approach has allowed us to meet these needs in an acute care hospital.*

We built an interdisciplinary team that looks at the patient and the caregiver as a unit, works with them, and responds to the patient's behavior as meaningful behavior that needs to be understood. We understand that dementia patients have special needs. Using a team approach has allowed us to meet these needs in an acute care hospital.

KSH: *Are staff exclusively assigned to this unit or do they rotate through it?*

JNN: Cabrini Medical Center is a voluntary hospital, and most patients have private attendings of their own. Any doctor in the medicine department can admit a patient to this unit. We have the regular house staff, that is, the interns and residents that any other unit in the hospital would have. Our unit has only eight beds, so it clearly doesn't have its own discrete house staff. In fact, it has been kind of a funny process, because the house staff recognizes that the care here is different from that in other hospital units and that they are expected to behave differently and to do different things. They observe that when patients in beds 6 through 21 get agitated they can order restraints. But if patients in beds 22 through 30 (our unit) become agitated, they are supposed to go see the patient and find out why he or she is upset. During teaching rounds we try to reinforce what some of the messages have been. The key message is twofold. First, the behavior of patients with dementia is meaningful. Second, caregivers can help us to understand what these meanings might be. But because of rotating coverage, not every doctor who is on the house staff has necessarily been educated about the unit and our approach to patient care.

From a nursing point of view, our unit has essentially the same staffing as any other unit in the hospital. One reason that we chose to have eight beds on the unit was that eight beds per nurse is the standard assignment for one registered nurse on the day shift. In general, seven of these beds are full at any given time. Family members had told us that one really difficult thing about the hospital was that they could never figure out who was taking care of their loved one. On most units, assignment sheets are not posted, nobody knows other people's names, and name tags are hard to read. So, family members would often spend long periods of time wandering through the floor trying to find somebody who knew whether their mother did or did not have breakfast this morning. Did Mom go for a particular test? And if Mom went for the test, was it completed? Or was it canceled because she was too upset?

We wanted it to be relatively transparent for families to figure out who was involved in the patient's care. So, if a family member walks onto the unit, which is physically separated through its design, and sees a member of the staff, that staff member is taking care of his or her loved one. The only dietician who comes onto the unit is our dietician. The only social worker present is this unit's social worker. One of the things that the team decided in the course of the planning was that our slogan would be "You can ask anybody because we're all involved in the care."

The worst that happens is that you ask somebody and they don't know the answer, but they know who *does* know the answer. If the person who's delivering the tray doesn't know what the patient had for breakfast, he or she at least knows who would know, so the family member can be directed appropriately. And this has been a really positive aspect of the unit. It allows staff to have much more meaningful interactions with family caregivers than the sort of milling around situation, which is unfortunately more common in acute care hospital settings.

KSH: *Tell me about the cost of the project.*

JNN: We had a Phase I grant of $30,000 from the United Hospital Fund and then a Phase II grant of $175,000 to implement our ideas. The hospital's capital contribution has been on the order of $90,000. The project had to be something that other people would see and say, "We can do that." We had worked with the Alzheimer's Association, and the New York City chapter wanted to be able to show that units like this could happen without a lot of extra funding. The grant covered the one additional pastoral care position and four consultants: an institutional change expert, the facilitator for the team planning meetings, the design consultant, and a research consultant who devised and implemented the satisfaction studies. The construction work was done at the hospital's expense. The only monies from the grant that went toward other staff costs, even during the training phase, were for overtime pay when we wanted to bring in staff from the other shifts so that we could have everybody together in the same room to plan together.

EXTENSIVE TRAINING AND PLANNING

Our goals required us to think both deeply and concretely about the needs of caregivers and of patients suffering from dementia. We really began with a very extended period of training, but training is almost the wrong word for it, because it really was a very extended period of *planning*. What we did was to ask every member of the team that was going to be on the unit, from myself as the director of geriatrics through the housekeeping staff, to sit down and think through how their jobs would be different if, in fact, they were responding to the needs of both the caregiver and the patient.

We did have some family caregivers involved in the project, and they participated in these planning meetings as well. We considered many of the different
tasks involved in daily care. For example, one task of an environmental aide is to
deliver the meal trays. We asked, "What was going to be different about delivering the meal trays in the new unit from the old unit? If we were going to involve
the caregiver and be supportive of the caregiver and the patient, what would we
do differently from the way we do things now?"

Our patients require a long time to be fed. A very large number of them need
to be assisted with eating in some way or another—either hand fed or reminded
to eat, cued, and so on. So our dietician made an arrangement with the kitchen
that our floor gets its food first, and the trays are picked up last. So, we actually
have about an extra half an hour between food delivery and pickup. This logistical change gives us extra time to feed these patients, and it accommodates for the
reality that we have limited staff at mealtimes.

IMPORTANCE OF FAMILY-CENTERED FOCUS

We spent relatively little time actually training people about dementia, as such. In
fact, over the course of almost a year of weekly meetings of an hour per week,
we devoted only two hours to Alzheimer's disease, just so people would feel that
they knew something. The point is that most people in the hospital do not need
to know much about the genetics of Alzheimer's disease unless they're going to
do genetic counseling. But what they really *do* need is to be able to look at a patient suffering from dementia and respond to him or her as an individual, and to
work with a caregiver who's telling them something and understand the importance
of what that caregiver is saying.

One reason we have had so much difficulty in taking care of dementia patients in
the hospital is that they can't tell us a huge
number of things about their daily care, and
we've just sent home the person who had
all the information! In fact, that person, the
caregiver, is usually at the bedside and
knows how this patient usually acts and
how to interpret what that person's non-
verbal behavior usually means. If the patient starts rubbing his stomach or pounding
the table it may mean "I need to go to the
bathroom" or "I'm bored, I want something
to do" or "I'm in pain" or "I'm only comfortable if I have a certain thing around." Be-
fore the patient came into the hospital, someone was feeding, dressing, and bathing
this person every day and, in most cases, responding to his or her needs remarkably well. Yet in many hospitals we completely ignore caregivers' vast experience

> *Before the patient came into
> the hospital, someone was
> feeding, dressing, and
> bathing this person every
> day and, in most cases,
> responding to his or her
> needs remarkably well. Yet in
> many hospitals we completely
> ignore caregivers' vast
> experience and sweep them
> aside, not realizing that we
> need them desperately to
> help us to provide the best
> quality care.*

and sweep them aside, not realizing that we need them desperately to help us to provide the best quality care.

KSH: *Did your history taking change as a result of attending to what caregivers tell you? Do you document what they say?*

JNN: Yes. That's one of the major differences in our unit. The first question that nurses ask when patients come to the unit is, "Who is the caregiver?" We ask, "Who knows what this person could do before so that we have some idea of what function it is that we are supposed to be preserving here? What seems reasonable to expect this patient to be able to do? And, if we have a problem, whom should we be calling to get more information?" These opening questions represent a completely new approach. Traditionally, nurses might be looking for the family member to ask, "Do you have the list of medications?"

In addition to approaching family members with new questions, when staff members get historical information from caregivers, they ask questions that show that they understand dementia and its effects. For example, if a family caregiver mentions a concern that the patient is someone who has a history of wandering or who sometimes calls out at night or things like that, it isn't treated as something bizarre. Rather, staff members are familiar with the kinds of things that people with dementia usually do at home. So they won't just be eliciting problems from the caregivers; they'll also be eliciting what have been solutions that worked at home and suggestions as to what should be done if a problem occurs in the hospital.

Over time, we've tried a number of different ways of getting information from family caregivers. We always ask about feeding, dressing, ambulation, and continence. We tend to ask more open-ended than directive questions. Family caregivers don't come in neat packages. Sometimes the caregiver is present at the time of admission, and you can get all this information. Sometimes, however, people are cared for by two or three different caregivers, or there's a family member who supervises, but there's really a paid caregiver who is with the patient most of the day. So you need to figure out what's actually happening with people.

We keep an independent, relatively informal log on all the patients in the unit, which is shared with the team. We preserve this log on the unit in case patients are readmitted so that we don't have to ask all these questions all over again. It doesn't become part of their hospital chart.

KSH: *What else is different for patients and their caregivers on your unit?*

JNN: There are unlimited visiting hours on the unit. So, if family members want to stay over or feel that they need to stay over because the patient needs them for whatever reason, they don't have to get the special permission of a nursing supervisor to okay it in order to have it happen. It's an automatically accepted situation.

We have a caregiver room, which has fold-down beds in it, for people who want to stay over, and we have fold-out cots if they need to stay in the room itself.

Because the units have two-bed rooms, we discourage staying in the room itself if it is not absolutely necessary because, obviously, this affects someone else's privacy.

At the very beginning, large numbers of family members said that they were going to want to stay, but once they are actually comfortable that staff members know what they are doing, very few family members wind up staying. We were prepared for three or four different caregivers staying on the unit the same night. We didn't know how much capacity we should build in. It turns out that most of the people had been staying the night, basically, because they didn't trust the hospital to take care of their loved one. Once family members recognize that we are both well-intentioned and moderately knowledgeable, very few of them stay overnight.

> *We professional care providers always tend to think it's all about* us. *The family members are coming to the hospital, they must want to see us. In fact, very often one of the benefits of being on the unit for family members is the opportunity to share experiences with other family caregivers.*

Interestingly, there have been a remarkable number of relationships that developed among family caregivers. We professional care providers always tend to think it's all about *us*. The family members are coming to the hospital, they must want to see us. In fact, very often one of the benefits of being on the unit for family members is the opportunity to share experiences with other family caregivers. Although we've attempted to provide some formal caregiver support, a lot of *in*formal interactions go on. For example, when people need assistance or reminders with feeding, families sometimes will make arrangements with each other: "If you're here this morning to help with my dad, I'll be here this evening to help with your mother."

END-OF-LIFE CARE

KSH: *What happens when a patient is seriously ill or dying? Do you provide palliative care to the patient and family caregiver?*

JNN: Most of the patients who have died on the unit have died unexpectedly. Because Cabrini has a very large and quite well-known hospice, when we have patients who are recognized to be terminally ill, we encourage families to become part of the hospice program. The hospice unit is right upstairs from ours, and so, normally, patients would be transferred up there, not so much because the clinical care is better or different there, but because hospice includes better bereavement services than we have, which is particularly important. Usually, end-stage dementia patients have very limited insight about what is happening to them. So, the biggest needs are usually the bereavement needs of the family. We have not done a lot with bereavement on the unit as such because we have had hospice here as a resource.

KSH: *How is pain managed on your unit?*

JNN: From my personal perspective, since I am board certified in palliative care as well as geriatrics, the biggest issue is getting staff to recognize that dementia patients have pain at all. Beyond that, very few end-stage or even moderate-stage dementia patients have pain that requires an anesthesiologist kind of pain team, which is pretty much what the standard has been. Instead, what these patients really need is pain medication. We worked to educate staff that symptoms such as agitation, restlessness, sleeplessness, and so on, are, in fact, common manifestations of pain among patients with dementia and that these symptoms need to be treated.

Another factor in this is that the attending physician or house officer who takes care of a patient on this unit is the same doctor who would take care of him or her on any other unit. This means that we have relatively little control over what they choose to do or not do. Although most house staff and attendings are reasonably open to suggestions, not everybody is equally open minded about this, so we don't have a guarantee that people will do what we suggest. We continue to do grand rounds, in-service training, and continuing education on topics such as pain management in dementia and caregiver issues.

KSH: *When you are considering moving a patient to the hospice unit, do family members ever feel concerned about a change in professional caregivers during the last phase of a patient's life?*

JNN: It hasn't come up much as an issue at all, probably because this is an acute inpatient unit, so most of the families really have not become that familiar with the staff. If it is obvious within a day or two of admission to the unit that the patient is dying, the family has only known the staff for a couple of days, so it isn't the same situation that you might face in a chronic care center. The second thing is that if the patient needs to transfer to hospice the patient is only going from one floor to another, to an in-hospital hospice unit, and the patient would not be expected to give up his or her usual physician. Even if some doctors don't really *want* to take care of patients on the hospice unit, they still would go up and visit. So, that piece of the common family abandonment concern really doesn't apply here.

MEASURING THE SUCCESS OF THE UNIT

KSH: *How have you measured your success?*

JNN: In the original grant proposal, we said that we were going to measure success based on, essentially, a *before* and *after* satisfaction study of caregivers and unit staff. One measure of success that was important to us was the satisfaction of both staff and caregivers. We used a before and after technique of questionnaires to determine satisfaction. Staff satisfaction has been extremely high, which is confirmed by minimal turnover in core staff over the nearly two years that we have been in operation. Caregiver satisfaction has also been very high.

In terms of other measures, we had involved the staff on the unit in identifying what they thought were the measures that would make *them* know that we were a success. These included a variety of different things, some which are very straightforward. Occupancy and length of stay are two such simple measures. Our sense is that quality care can shorten length of stay, and that if we were doing a good job our unit would be full or close to full most of the time. On average, our length of stay is 10 to 11 days and seven of the eight beds are occupied. I believe our length of stay is shorter than for comparable patients at other hospitals. Another measure of success that our staff thought would be telling is the hospital administration's commitment to the unit after the grant ends. For example, the administration might be inclined to keep the unit if they got a number of letters praising the unit or did not experience any new headaches from it. We weren't quite sure what administrators would be looking for. Since the project began, we have had a massive turnover in the hospital administration (including the CEO, assistant to the president, VP for nursing, and VP for medical care); however, we are gratified that the new administration has formally committed itself to maintaining the unit after the grant is completed, as part of how it sees the future of the hospital.

One measure that the staff on the unit believed would show whether we've accomplished something was if outside experts in the field came in and looked at the unit and said, "Yes, this looks like the kind of thing we think ought to happen." Certainly, on that measure we've been extremely successful. People from both the New York City chapter and the national Alzheimer's Association and from chapters around the country have visited the unit. Other visitors have included people from other hospitals and nursing homes and experts in dementia care, dementia design, and dementia clothing. It's hard to measure culture, but many people from the outside who have toured the unit have commented, "Yes, the culture of this unit *feels* like, *smells* like, *looks* like, therefore must *be* the kind of thing that we think is needed." So, this recognition has been a very gratifying thing for us. It is not the most objective measure, but still we felt and still do feel that it is quite significant.

Another measure was kind of a process measure; for example, do we use fewer restraints? We are also looking at patient outcomes; for instance, do our patients have less weight loss? Do we have, essentially, better outcomes than other units do with patients similar to ours? As of yet, I don't have the most solid data to support this, but it would *appear* that we have actually accomplished what we set out to do; there's a great deal less functional loss in our patients than occurs elsewhere in the hospital. For example, if they came into the hospital continent, our patients are much more likely to leave the hospital continent.

Although we have been tracking these kinds of indicators of functional outcome, the reason I'm saying it's not very scientific is that we have not compared our outcomes to a good set of matched controls. We keep track of what *we* do, but since the rest of the hospital isn't necessarily measuring things the same way and also isn't taking care of the same patients, we are not sure exactly how to compare our outcomes.

We would like to do a more careful job of measuring the impact of the unit on outcomes. Currently, we just have a sense of how things are going. We have what families tell us, which is certainly extremely favorable, but we don't yet have the formal data that would be useful for a better understanding of what units like this are about. We held preliminary discussions with the Samuels Foundation, in hopes of applying to do a much more formal outcome analysis with real case controls, real functional outcome data, and some better cost data to know, in fact, how much all this really costs. Despite considerable interest, they wanted a project even larger than what we were proposing, and there have been problems trying to get it all together. I am currently writing them a new proposal for a tiny planning grant to move this forward.

CHALLENGES AHEAD: CONTINUITY OF CARE AND APPROPRIATE REFERRAL

KSH: *What other challenges are you trying to address now?*

JNN: Ensuring continuity of care for these patients across our hospital units and appropriate referral to our unit from the emergency department remain unresolved problems. Sometimes the family will tell other hospital personnel, "My dad was on this dementia unit before, the staff there seemed to know how to deal with his behavior." But there's no formal mechanism to ensure that kind of continuity.

We had originally intended to involve the emergency department (ED) in our planning because we suspected, and families had told us, that emergency care for patients with dementia was a problem area in the hospital. This hunch was consistent with staff experience in other hospitals. So we were expecting that to be a major intervention area for us. Unfortunately, all the ED staff with whom we had originally intended to work on the project wound up leaving. For much of the planning period, they were without a director and were very short staffed administratively, and so they were unable to attend our meetings. Ultimately, their not being involved in the planning process hurt the project in a variety of different ways. For example, we have not been able to develop an effective communication system with the emergency room. Identifying patients who might be appropriate for admission to our unit is an area that still needs improvement.

So, we've applied to the United Hospital Fund for a Phase III grant specifically to work with our emergency department, because we still see that as a big, unresolved need. This has been something that has held us back all along; because dementia is not usually a patient's primary diagnosis, clinicians don't write it as a diagnosis on charts. When they are deciding where patients are going to go in the hospital, they don't think of admitting patients to our unit. When the patient ultimately *is* admitted, the admitting office clerks don't do mental status evaluations on patients, so they can't identify appropriate patients. As a consequence, the vast majority of our admissions have come because a family member specifically said, "I want that unit I read about in the paper." Other patients may have been admitted to a different floor and then, within some period of time, the patient was exhibiting problematic behavior, or sometimes staff simply recognized that this patient was appropriate for our unit and should be transferred to it.

One of our original ideas had been that we would be a source of reassurance and information for dementia patients and their caregivers from the moment of admission to the hospital. This piece has really not happened for a lot of patients. What happens is you have the first terrible day, when demented patients are agitated, pulling out their IVs, and tied down in restraints. And *then* somebody says, "This never happens with the patients who are down on the special unit for dementia patients, why don't we transfer this patient down there?" But it would have been nicer if the patient never had to go through that whole experience to begin with. We're still not doing the job that I'd like to be doing in this area. I don't think this problem is unique to us; most specialized units in hospitals revolve around the patient's primary diagnosis. Because dementia is so often really a co-morbidity, it's very difficult to get these patients into the system. Most hospitals don't have good mechanisms in place to identify these patients early on and so begin to provide them with the care that they're going to need at the time of admission.

BRINGING KNOWLEDGE OF BEST DEMENTIA CARE INTO THE HOSPITAL

KSH: *Overall, what do you feel is most innovative about your unit and approach to the care of patients with dementia and their caregivers?*

JNN: The unit brings into the acute hospital setting a lot of what's been known for some time about good dementia care in long-term care. It's hard to look at some of the individual things and see them as so remarkable if you are familiar with what good assisted-living programs, good adult day care programs, good Alzheimer's units, and skilled nursing facilities have been doing for years. We certainly didn't invent interdisciplinary care. Almost all the behavioral approaches that we use are things that were known to people in other contexts. But insofar as hospitals are at the top of the care system, hospitals have not previously been prepared to listen to what people in rehabilitation settings or long-term care know and to incorporate that knowledge into the hospital's culture and systems of care. One big advantage that we have here at Cabrini is that we are a connected hospital and nursing home: for example, I'm the chief of geriatrics in the hospital as well as medical director of the nursing home. This dual role means that I'm able to go back and forth between two different worlds and say, "These challenges can be tackled." And people believe me. A lot of what we've been talking about in terms of dementia care problem solving takes place on a daily basis in different settings. It just never has happened in hospitals before. In the long term, I think this is the most unique aspect about everything that we've done.

KSH: *Do you see a spillover into the wider hospital culture, from your unit?*

JNN: It certainly spread a little bit. We are, essentially, a subunit on a floor that also has other geriatrics patients and oncology on it. As I said, our unit is a standard assignment for nurses, but most of the other staff, in fact, go from one part of the floor to the other, or some nights and evenings one person might be assigned both to our unit and to some patients on the rest of the floor. The head nurse for the unit feels very strongly that there's been a lot of positive carryover with other patients on the floor, in terms of conveying a whole different approach to patients and families. That has been extremely positive.

PARTING THOUGHTS

KSH: *Do you have any advice for others seeking to start a similar unit at their hospital?*

JNN: One thing that we've struggled against is the notion that there are prefabricated solutions for problems. For one thing, we have tried to persuade people that you have to actually go and see the patient, that you cannot just "look it up" before prescribing or writing orders for care. You have to actually talk to the caregivers, rely on their expertise about the patient, and mutually find out how to solve a problem. So, our approach has been a problem-solving one, rather than coming up with a model that we would want people to follow.

> *One thing that we've struggled against is the notion that there are prefabricated solutions for problems. . . . You have to actually talk to the caregivers, rely on their expertise about the patient, and mutually find out how to solve a problem.*

From the very beginning, I never expected that this unit was going to be *the* model that everybody else would use. Rather, we have taken a stab at addressing the many challenges to show what *could* be accomplished. I could imagine this unit looking very differently, maybe even staffed differently and functioning differently. As proud as I am of everything we've done, I certainly recognize a lot of the limitations of what we've done and that most of it we made up along the way. I think that it's actually the process, and not necessarily the model, that is the really important thing. The really vital task is thinking through how to meet the needs of the patient within the context and culture of your institution, and not that the unit have eight beds or be set up a certain way. We made a lot of accommodations to the structure of the hospital. So, I'm not necessarily interested in persuading people to do it the way we did. I think that far more important than the solutions that we reached is the process of getting there, the careful needs assessment and planning, and people should not give up that process to mimic what we've done.

REFERENCES

1. Mace NL, Rabibs PV. *The 36 Hour Day*, 3d ed. Baltimore: Johns Hopkins Press, 1999.
2. Sager MA, Rudberg MA. Functional decline associated with hospitalization for acute illness. *Clinics in Geriatric Medicine*. 1998;14(4):669–679.

Supporting Family Caregivers of Neurologically Impaired Patients

An Interview with JOHN LARKIN, MD, ELLEN BARTOLDUS, MSW, CSW, and NEREIDA BORRERO, RN, MSN, GNP

The Brooklyn Hospital Center
Brooklyn, New York

The Brooklyn Hospital Center, in collaboration with the Wartburg Lutheran Home for the Aging, was awarded a grant from the United Hospital Fund to create a program to assist caregivers of neurologically impaired African American patients in northern and central Brooklyn during the acute and chronic phases of illness. They recognized this group as one that contains a long history of informal caregiving; often these caregivers do not seek assistance or tap into the available support services.

The Brooklyn Hospital Center Family Caregiving Initiative targeted these caregivers and created a program that merged the knowledge of day-to-day care from the Wartburg Lutheran Home for the Aging with the Brooklyn Hospital network of care. A geriatric nurse practitioner, working with two social workers, intervenes with caregivers when their loved one is admitted to the hospital. The geriatric nurse practitioner provides caregivers with a notebook, containing individualized information about the specific disease process, how to manage it, who to call in case of emergency, and how to access needed services. In addition, the nurse practitioner makes a home visit to follow up with the patient and family to provide additional caregiver training and assess the need for further assistance and support services. The program offers support groups for caregivers twice per month, as well as caregiver workshops bimonthly on such topics as advance care planning, navigating the emergency room, and how to speak with the doctor during a visit. A tip card for caregivers is one result of these workshops.

In the following interview with Samantha Libby Sodickson, the two principal investigators of the Caregiving Initiative, John Larkin, of Brooklyn Hospital, and Ellen Bartoldus, of Wartburg Lutheran Home for the Aging, together with geriatric nurse practitioner Nereida Borrero, discuss how the program came together, the community it serves, and what other hospitals can do to replicate this initiative.

PROGRAM BEGINNINGS AND DESIGN

Samantha Libby Sodickson: *What is the goal of the Family Caregiving Initiative, and when did it begin?*

Nereida Borrero: The goal of the program is to reduce caregiver burden by providing services to caregivers of neurologically impaired blacks in northern and central Brooklyn.

Ellen Bartoldus: The program was started in 1998 when Brooklyn Hospital and Wartburg received the initial grant from the United Hospital Fund (UHF). The first phase of the program focused on exploring the needs of caregivers of neurologically impaired blacks in our community. As a result, we were awarded a two-year implementation grant and the program has been flourishing.

SLS: *Can you tell me a bit about that population, and how you chose them?*

John Larkin: The population of northern and central Brooklyn, the community surrounding Brooklyn Hospital, is predominantly African American. The caregiving burdens of African Americans were described in a *New York Times* article,[1] which showed that the African American population was less likely to come forward for help and more likely to have a long tradition of informal family caregiving. There has been an observed reluctance in the African American community to place family members in nursing homes, and families often carry the burden of caregiving without formal assistance. So the needs of African American caregivers seemed like a logical focus for our efforts. We chose to focus on caregivers of neurologically impaired individuals because these individuals often exhibit particular cognitive and behavioral changes that are chronic and involve slow debilitation over time and so present unique challenges for caregiving.

EB: We began our project with a series of community focus groups. Caregivers were identified through Wartburg's Mobile Meals Program clients and Brooklyn Hospital's discharged patients. In these focus groups, caregivers were asked to identify specifically what their issues and frustrations were. There was a great deal of discussion about perceived and actual failures within the health care system, communication issues between physicians and caregivers, and family conflict and a sense of isolation among caregivers. Out of these focus sessions we formed a Community Advisory Board to guide us with program design and implementation.

SLS: *Can you describe what the disease process is in neurologically impaired individuals, and what the impact is on these caregivers?*

JL: The majority of our neurologically impaired patients are those with Alzheimer's disease, a long-standing, chronic disease that goes on for many years. We also see a lot of stroke victims. For patients with Alzheimer's disease, there's an increased caregiver burden, especially if it is a child who is caring for the parent. The role reversal between parent and child is quite stressful, as well as seeing the parent slowly debilitate.

EB: We also found that in the neurologically impaired population the ongoing behavioral issues, such as wandering, repetitive communication, incontinence, and so forth, create a type of constant stress, which is different from the physical stress of providing care. These changes are frightening to caregivers, who often have no experience in dealing with these behaviors. Caregivers sometimes perceive these behaviors as a "personality change," leaving the caregiver frustrated and uncertain as to how to relate to the patient.

INSTITUTIONAL COLLABORATION EASES CAREGIVER BURDEN

SLS: *Can you describe the collaboration that Brooklyn Hospital Center has with Wartburg Lutheran Home for the Aging?*

EB: Brooklyn Hospital and Wartburg had been discussing areas for collaboration in early 1997. When the UHF Family Caregiving grant became available, it was an area of mutual interest for both institutions. Dr. Eugenia Siegler initiated the program on behalf of the hospital. She and I began to speak about the ways in which the hospital and nursing home could offer complementary services for patients. Traditionally, there has not been good collaboration between our two institutions. It was important from the beginning to develop ongoing communication between the hospital and nursing home. The hospital's expertise lies in treating acute illness, whereas the nursing home provides the day-in and day-out caregiving, similar to what a caregiver at home would do. Through the collaboration of these two institutions, we are able to bring particular skills to the table that would help caregivers. For example, nursing homes are traditionally very good at healing and preventing bedsores. We're also good at managing behaviors, and we are *very* good at managing behaviors without restraints. The hospital has a lot to offer in the realm of up-to-date medical treatment and care. Therefore, this joint Family Caregiving Initiative makes perfect sense.

SLS: *How is the collaboration implemented in terms of staffing the program?*

EB: Dr. Larkin and I jointly oversee the operations of the program. Program staffing consists of representatives from both facilities. Nereida Borrero is a member of the Brooklyn Hospital staff. Lisette Sosa, CSW, one of our social work consultants, is the director of social work at Wartburg. Caregivers were recruited both from the hospital and from Wartburg's community-based programs. Nereida did a lot of active recruiting among the hospital staff in order to establish linkages for referrals. We have learned a lot from one another, which has greatly contributed to our success.

SLS: *What kind of response did you have from hospital staff?*

JL: The hospital as a whole has responded very well to this. It has been a team effort. A lot of our workshops have been conducted by different disciplines in the hospital, such as nursing, the emergency department, our geriatrician, and our hospital ethicist. Our discharge planning nurses, who are usually responsible for the initial referrals, also have been quite receptive to this collaborative effort.

EB: Hospital staff also has responded favorably to the collaboration with the nursing home on specific care skills and workshops.

IMPLEMENTATION OF THE FAMILY CAREGIVING INITIATIVE

SLS: *Could you walk me through the process of identifying the patients and admitting them into the program, all the way through the home visit?*

JL: The discharge planning nurses, who have been made aware of this program, refer the patient to Nereida, who would then contact the patient in the hospital for an initial interview. We also encourage all our physicians to refer families from their practice.

NB: I usually see the patient and the caregiver before the patient is discharged from the hospital. At this time, I explain the program and assess the needs of the individual. I offer support and facilitate the transition from the hospital into the community by identifying equipment or supplies needed in the home before the patient is discharged. When the patient goes home, I follow up with a scheduled visit to assess the home for safety, and I offer education and ongoing support. If the patient goes into acute rehab, I keep in touch with the caregiver by phone and mail. When the patient goes home from rehab, I follow the same process as when the patient was discharged from the hospital.

In my follow-up home visits, I do assessments to identify the home safety issues, as well as to determine if there is any additional need for equipment or supplies. I also identify whether there are any family dynamics problems that I can help with. Sometimes, family members complain about other family members not cooperating enough or not helping out with the patient. They may be having problems communicating with one another. On a few occasions, we've had family group discussions together with the social worker and myself. Other times, referrals are made for individual, short-term counseling. I also teach skills necessary to reduce caregiver burden.

SLS: *What kind of skills are those, generally?*

NB: I teach the family caregiver how to provide skin care, wound care, tracheal care, how to do tube feedings, and any other skilled care needs that apply. For example, let's say that the patient is going home with a new PEG (percutaneous endoscopic gastrotomy) tube. This could be very stressful to the caregiver because, most likely, this is totally new to them. The family caregivers are usually instructed in the hospital before the patient is discharged, but often during this time period caregivers feel frightened and overwhelmed. It takes time to get used to doing certain treatments—they need more than a quick lesson. It's a positive experience for caregivers when I'm able to follow up with training at home. Even if the patient leaves with home care services, in the state of New York, home attendants and home health aides are not permitted to perform any skilled nursing functions, such as wound care, tracheal care, or tube feedings. The family has to be able to do that themselves.

> *. . . in the state of New York, home attendants and home health aides are not permitted to perform any skilled nursing functions, such as wound care, tracheal care, or tube feedings. The family has to be able to do that themselves.*

SLS: *Do they have access to you after you make a home visit, if they have other questions?*

NB: Yes, they do. I have voice mail, so they call me and leave a message, and then I call them back if I'm not in the office. They know that they have access to me almost 24 hours a day because I also retrieve my messages from home. If there's an acute situation, I call them. Many a time I have called someone from my own home.

SLS: *How many patients and caregivers do you have enrolled in your program at any one time? Do you handle all these families yourself?*

NB: Seventy-eight families have been enrolled as program members since we began in 1998. Five members have been placed in a nursing home. Thirteen program members have died. One member didn't return my calls, and two were discharged from the program because they no longer wanted to participate. Another family moved out of the area. So, the total number of active families right now is 56.

With regard to collaboration and assistance running the program, I work very closely with two social workers. One social worker helps me a lot with the family's practical needs. For example, she helps if a family needs assistance getting entitlements, or increasing hours for home care, or accessing other resources in the community that they might need, but don't know how to go about getting. Another social worker helps me with the counseling and the support groups.

ALLEVIATING ISOLATION AND SHARING THE BURDEN

SLS: *How do you help caregivers to deal with their emotional needs?*

JL: One complaint often made by the caregivers is that they feel isolated and lonely. The support groups, which are run by a trained therapist, Beth-Ann Gillery,

CSW, have worked quite well in getting individual caregivers together. This part of the program is essential in that it provides caregivers with an opportunity to air their collective concerns about family caregiving and allows individuals to share their personal coping skills with their peers. The workshops also have helped by reinforcing and teaching caregiver techniques to family members. We also have a video library set up at the Brooklyn Hospital for which Nereida is responsible. In addition, Nereida compiles a loose-leaf notebook for each caregiver that is basically tailored to the patient's individual illness and can help to educate the caregiver.

SLS: *Please describe the caregiver notebook that you provide for each family.*

NB: Because we deal mostly with Alzheimer's patients, I have a separate notebook for people with Alzheimer's disease, as well as one for patients with stroke. A couple of our patients have multiple sclerosis, and some have Parkinson's disease. So each caregiver notebook is tailored to the needs of the individual. Each notebook is divided into different sections: Disease Process (signs and symptoms, management, complications); Caregiver Needs; Resources; Home Safety Issues; Skin Care; Legal Issues (advance directives, living will, power of attorney, and so forth) and, if needed, information on tube feeding.

SLS: *Can you tell me about some of the issues that are addressed in the support groups?*

JL: Beth-Ann Gillery, the therapist who runs these support groups has done a wonderful job of getting the caregiver to realize that, in many cases, there is a need to acknowledge the anger and guilt involved in being a caregiver and that these are natural reactions. We know that caregivers do an incredible job and a noble job, but there is still a reaction to a loved one who can no longer care for him or herself. Part of the support is getting caregivers to recognize this and to vent their anger in more positive ways, as opposed to neglecting themselves and therefore, inadvertently, not being able to take care of their loved ones.

> *. . . in many cases, there is a need to acknowledge the anger and guilt involved in being a caregiver and that these are natural reactions.*

EB: We also found that caregivers often have health concerns of their own. For example, one caregiver was a diabetic and had not been seen by a physician for quite a while. We were able to convince her that she needed to take care of her own diabetes in order to function as a caregiver. So we've been trying to make caregivers aware of the importance of self care.

Also, the social workers have found that the release of emotion is very helpful—that people need to cry and laugh. They need to be touched, to be hugged by somebody. They benefit from knowing that they are not the only ones struggling with these issues; that they are not crazy, and it's not that they just can't cope. The support groups have helped caregivers to realize that "I'm not the only one who feels that way." Then they can make a shift from having the disease run their lives to knowing that they do have some power and control. It has been interesting to see natural leadership develop within this group. We really encourage folks to say, "You know what, I am not the victim here. I can be in control." This has been *really* positive.

JL: Basically, we encourage them to think about *self*. A lot of times they get so caught up in the caregiving that they often neglect themselves, which is a factor in the increased mortality associated with family caregiving.

SLS: *How are caregivers able to attend support groups and workshops? Do you have any arrangements for respite care for their loved ones?*

NB: There are a few places that I usually recommend for respite care. I make the initial phone call to get in touch with the respite care service. Then I give the information to the caregiver and assist in any way that I can for the placement. The caregivers seem to be able to come to the workshops because we hold them right in the hospital, and most of the caregivers and patients live nearby.

JL: One thing that we stress in the support group is sharing some of the burden. We know that the caregiver most likely will be the eldest child, usually the eldest female child. Beth-Ann Gillery has been working with the caregiver to learn when they need to ask for help and when the other family members, for example, the other brothers and sisters, must share some of this burden.

EB: One other thing that we found was the *need for education*. When we started this project, we were amazed by the caregiver's lack of concrete information. One of the first workshops we did, based on the first recommendation from our Advisory Council, was instruction on how to communicate with a doctor. In this workshop, we were able to get the doctor's perspective and the family member's perspective. We, as a team, learned an awful lot about the process of communication between physicians and family members.

After each workshop, which are primarily educational in nature, although they do take on an element of support, we create what we are calling *Quick Tips*. These are cards developed from the educational workshops. We take notes during the program and then incorporate the questions that the caregivers ask and suggestions for action. Ms. Gillery designs them, and caregivers can carry them in a pocket or purse and pull them out for reference when information is needed to handle a certain situation.

The tip card on making a visit to the doctor* includes suggestions for making a list of the questions that you want to ask, focusing on the critical questions and writing down the physician's answers and comments. A new *Quick Tips* card that

---

*See Appendix B, p. 357, for the tip card, Quick Tips for Working with the Doctors.

we are working on relates to navigating the hospital emergency department. These cards give folks a lot of information right at hand when they are feeling overwhelmed and confused, and offers concrete steps to follow.

JL: The emergency department workshop probably deserves some special mention, because it was one of the more successful workshops. The chairman of the emergency department here at the Brooklyn Hospital facilitated it. He went through the hierarchy of the emergency department and broke it down for the caregivers and patients so that it wouldn't be as confusing for them when they arrived in the emergency room. We then conducted a tour of the emergency room and explained all the different aspects of the emergency room from the initial triage, to the emergency department's evaluation, to the admissions process. Feedback we gathered from our Community Advisory Board had suggested that this admissions process was especially stressful. We had an excellent response to this workshop, and it reinforces the hospital as an ally in the community.

EB: It also relieves some anxiety for the caregivers. They were able to see what the emergency room looks like and were told, "When *this* happens, *this* is whom you call. This is the title of the person in charge." It was very helpful. I, personally, learned a lot, and I think it was very reassuring to the families.

MEASURING CAREGIVER BURDEN

SLS: *How are you assessing the caregiver burden?*

JL: We're using the Robinson Caregiver Strain Index Questionnaire.[2] At baseline zero, 6 months, and 12 months, caregivers fill out the questionnaire, and we compare the data at these times.

SLS: *Have you been able to measure any change in caregiver health, satisfaction, or ability to cope as a result of the program?*

JL: Although the results are still being analyzed, preliminary data show a decrease in caregiver stress, particularly as it relates to the item "a sense of feeling completely overwhelmed." We believe this to be significant and look forward to finalization of the data. I think that we will have some pretty good numbers reflecting decreased caregiver stress.

NB: I experienced something wonderful yesterday, which I think speaks to this topic. I was visiting a family in which the caregiver is a 35-year-old male who is taking care of his mother. I know it is overwhelming for him because one of the things he said is, "I feel very uncomfortable and very embarrassed to wash my mom." That's so real for many caregivers. But while visiting this person, he said to me, "I can't believe how much help I've been getting from this program. I wish

I could tell more people because before I started with this program I didn't know what to do. I was so overwhelmed!" He's still overwhelmed, I'm not saying that everything is perfect, but he says, "I know that I can call you anytime." He can call the doctor. He also knows that there are a lot of resources available that I'm working to connect him with.

SLS: *Are there other kinds of measures that you're hoping to start using as the program continues?*

EB: We would like to see if our program has had any effect on reducing the number of "non-emergency" visits to the emergency room. Since this was not part of our original project design, we have no baseline data, but we do know that emergency room visits are stressful to both the patient and caregiver. This was clear in both our initial focus groups and caregivers' request for a workshop in the emergency room. If education and support can decrease unnecessary use of the emergency room, it would be beneficial to both patients and the hospital.

JL: We have had an overwhelming response to this program in the community; there is a great need for it. This is actually a limited program right now, so you can imagine what would happen if it were open to greater numbers of patients.

SLS: *Do you feel that given the current scope of your program, there are populations that you'd like to be able to reach, but cannot as yet?*

JL: Yes. Cancer patients would be very interesting to work with. Many patients could benefit from this, not just neurological patients.

SLS: *Is anyone ever turned away from your program?*

JL: We try not to do that. We have already gone over our target number of enrolled families, but we've definitely continued to provide information to all the people who are referred to Nereida. All patients and caregivers are given invitations to the support group and the workshop, but they don't all get the benefits of the home visit. Instead, we give them an open invitation to use the tools that we have.

SUSTAINING THE INITIATIVE

SLS: *Have you considered how you will keep the program going if grant funding were to stop?*

JL: Of course, we'd love for this program to continue. We'd even love to expand it for the hospital. I believe we've secured funding for at least another year, but after that time we are going to explore other possibilities for getting some additional funding.

EB: It is important to note that both Brooklyn Hospital and Wartburg Lutheran have supported the program with in-kind services. Most of the workshops have been given by Wartburg and Brooklyn Hospital staff without reimbursement. This collaboration has been an important experience for all of us and we believe in its value to caregivers. We really do want to see it continue. Although special grant funding has been invaluable to this project, I believe that strong collaboration and cost sharing between health care institutions can keep this program going. There are significant benefits to both institutions, which, it could be argued, are worth the financial investment. For the nursing home, which is often seen in isolation from the community, it provides an opportunity to be seen as a resource for education and support, as well as a source for available residential care when care at home is no longer an option. For the hospital, it demystifies the institution and encourages caregivers to see the hospital as an ally. The Family Caregiving Initiative can help to improve the public perception of the hospital as a vital part of the community and can benefit individual physicians through better coordination of services to their patients. A relatively small investment can reap substantial rewards.

BARRIERS TO IMPLEMENTATION

SLS: *Have you had any barriers to implementing your program?*

NB: One barrier I have found lies in gaining the trust of family caregivers. They might be reluctant to take advantage of our service due to fear of an undisclosed financial burden. This is not something that we have talked about a lot, but I'm usually the first person with whom they make contact after they are referred to the program. Often, when I interview the caregiver and offer this service, they can't believe that they will not be charged.

SLS: *How are you able to get them to make that leap of faith? How do you get them to really come to trust you?*

NB: I'm very honest. I explain about the program—how it started, how it's funded, and how they will never receive a bill. Making the home visit also reinforces their trust. The key is consistency and follow-up. In the very beginning they might have some reservations, but when I follow up with the phone call, as well as with the home visit, and when they call me and I respond, they know that I'm really there for them. That's very important.

EB: I think one other barrier is the caregiver's need to be relieved of his or her caregiving duties in order to get to the workshops and the support groups. We try to be extremely flexible in terms of time, but I think that not having respite care available has been a barrier for some caregivers. I would love to be in a position whereby this program could send in substitute caregivers for two hours. Another piece, too, is that caregivers tend to see the hospital and the nursing home as these big institutions. Nereida has been able, through the force of her personality and skill, to break down that barrier to some degree.

JL: We feel that the hospital is truly an ally for the community, and the caregiver is an ally for the physicians in the hospital. Without them, physicians would have a much harder time meeting these patients' needs and the burden to the hospital would be that much greater.

ISSUES TO CONSIDER IN REPLICATING THIS PROGRAM

SLS: *If other hospitals were to try to replicate your program, what kinds of things would they need to have in place, and what kind of advice would you like to offer?*

JL: The discharge planners would need to be fully aware of the program and then assist in identifying who the caregivers are in order to refer them to the nurse practitioner before discharge.

EB: We have been working with the Brooklyn Hospital Home Care Program, which has been quite helpful. Through this collaboration, we can offer better coordination of services to our caregivers. For example, we can utilize home care social workers and nurses in conjunction with the services offered through our program. Our nurse practitioner often collaborates with the rehab team from the Home Care Program to ensure that the patient receives proper treatment and necessary equipment. This takes some of the burden of coordinating services off the caregiver.

NB: I also go to the hospital's weekly length-of-stay meeting, so I'm able to identify patients who are really in need of this program. Although we receive referrals from the discharge planning nurses or the utilization review nurses, doctors also call me and identify some of the patients who are in need of our services.

EB: One piece of advice would be this: Do not confine your vision to the medical model. It is important to see that caregiver strain and stress involve more than just the medical and physical aspects of care. The full partnership between the hospital and nursing home has helped us to focus on psychosocial, spiritual, and emotional issues, in addition to medical and physical care. I think the success of our program lies in the fact that we have done this in a coordinated and holistic way.

> *Do not confine your vision to the medical model. It is important to see that caregiver strain and stress involve more than just the medical and physical aspects of care.*

NB: Integrating all the pieces that Ellen just mentioned is very, very important. The population that we deal with here in Brooklyn is a very spiritual population, very religious. The professionals who are involved with this program have to be able to understand and *respect* these beliefs.

SLS: *Is faith or religion directly addressed in your workshops or your support groups?*

NB: I think it's woven into the program in general, starting with the first interview, and it goes on with the visits and support groups and interaction with the caregivers, and also with the patients.

EB: We've encouraged the caregivers and patients to make use of the resources within their own communities of faith. In Brooklyn, particularly in the African American community, churches play a central role. So we've talked to people about really accessing the services available in their spiritual communities.

DECISION MAKING, ADVANCE CARE PLANNING, AND END-OF-LIFE ISSUES

NB: I want to mention that, beginning with my first visit in the hospital, we assist families with decision making, nursing home placement, and sometimes the placement of a patient in an acute rehabilitation center. Some families are very skeptical about sending their loved ones to a nursing home, and when they think about acute rehab, I have to explain that the placement is temporary and for their own benefit. I also have written letters of support to employers, especially when the caregiver can't go to work in the beginning. Caregivers have a great need for people to understand what they are going through. I also assist them with DNR orders and advance directives.

SLS: *When you raise the end-of-life discussions with caregivers, what responses do you get?*

NB: In the very beginning, sometimes it's denial. Then, as we discuss it more, they come to understand that it's important to talk about these issues.

EB: The social worker focused a support group session on how to begin to raise these difficult questions. The workshop focused on advance care planning and end-of-life decisions. It was conducted by the hospital's ethicist, Alice Herb, JD, who covered specific issues in end-of-life care. Caregivers find it hard to talk about these things. Few of us want to admit that we will have to face these decisions. But I think it's helpful for the caregivers to begin to think about and realize the importance of understanding the values and desires of the person for whom they're caring so that they know what that person really wants. Then they are working much more in tandem, particularly when it comes to some of the difficult end-of-life decisions.

IN CONCLUSION

SLS: *Is there anything more that you think would be important for our readers to know?*

EB: I would like to say that lately a great deal of emphasis, and rightly so, has been placed on end-of-life care, which is a critical issue. But there is a time *before* end-of-life care, which stands between wellness and functioning and death. This is chronic illness, the issue that we are trying to address. It's one thing to take care of someone for three weeks. It's another thing to take care of them for three years or longer. That is the place where the Family Caregiving Initiative really tries to step in and meet the caregiver's needs.

REFERENCES

1. Rimer S. Blacks carry load of care for their elderly. *New York Times*, March 15, 1998, p. 1.
2. Robinson BC. Validation of a caregiver strain index. *Journal of Gerontology*. 1983;38:344–348.

Extending the Family in an Era of No Growth: A Rumination on Family Caregiving

JAMES A. THORSON

University of Nebraska, Department of Gerontology
Omaha, Nebraska

I

I took a group of nurses and physicians to China some years ago. Our purpose was to see how our counterparts cared for the elderly, given the vaunted Confucian reverence for the aged. We visited colleagues in hospitals in cities and on communes, medical colleges, representatives of medical societies, and so on, and we found it all very interesting. But, other than observing what we would call step-down care within acute-care hospitals, we didn't accumulate much in the way of things we could take home and use.

Several times, we asked our guides from the government tourist organization where their long-term care institutions were. We wanted to see a Chinese nursing home. Met with blank looks, we persisted: Where, we asked, were the old people cared for who could not take care of themselves, the demented, for example, or those with degenerative illnesses who were nearing the end of life? The guides responded that people in those situations were cared for by their families. But what, we asked, became of people who had no family or were being cared for by family members when their son or daughter unaccountably predeceased the elder? Light bulbs went on: "Oh, you wish to see an institution for people whose children were *martyred*." Older people in China have lived through the Japanese invasion in 1936, World War II from 1940 to 1945, the Revolution that ended in 1949, and the Cultural Revolution of the late 1960s and early 1970s. Many have lost adult children in one of these upheavals.

We were taken to the First Peoples' Social Welfare Institution for the Aged, a three-story concrete building that housed 150 older people (an addition that would handle 120 more beds was being built at the time). We were told that it was one of four such institutions in Shanghai, a city of 12 million people. I reflected that the city where I live has about half a million people and has 37 nursing homes.

Our first experience upon entering the place was to be met by patients and staff who were applauding vigorously. Being visited by a busload of foreigners was a big deal, and no one who could get out of bed wanted to miss any of the action. After greetings, the residents hurried back to their own rooms in anticipation of individual visits. Like most delegations visiting Chinese institutions, factories, schools, or communes, our first task was to have the orientation. In a large conference room we were served green tea and listened to speeches from the staff. We were told that almost all of the residents were without any family and that they had been bereaved of their child or children too late in life to then form a *kai* relationship with a younger person.

A *kai* bond is a form of sworn kinship not unlike a blood brotherhood or sisterhood. In the case of older people without children, it was often a kind of foster parent relationship:

> The common theme of *kai* relationships was that of need on the part of one and nurturance on the part of the other. The *kai* relationship of greatest significance to the elderly was that in which an older person *kai*ed a young adult, preferably one without parents of his own. The two would exchange gifts publicly with the senior providing services to the junior in the early years of the partnerships and the latter providing services to the senior in the later years. Supernatural sanctions and the force of public opinion encouraged the participants to fulfill their obligations.[1]

In other words, the childless adult could acquire a young person to sponsor, guide, and nurture, expecting that an obligation would be created that would be reciprocated later. One could see how it would be difficult to form such a bond if an individual, say, in her eighties were to lose an only child. It would probably be too late for her to then seek a *kai* relationship. We were told that such bonds were breaking down with the urban migration that had been taking place in China. Community pressures present in village life were absent in the anonymity of the city.

After the orientation conference we were loosed upon the residents, and we spent quite some time going around in small groups to visit. The first floor was made up of women residents who were ambulatory, the second had men who were ambulatory, and the third floor was what Westerners would recognize as a nursing home for both men and women. So the institution was really a kind of continuing care retirement community with care at multiple levels.

One thing we found most remarkable was the enthusiasm of the greeting we received, whether the people we stopped in on were bedfast or not. Later, in an exit interview, this was remarked on. The administrator said, "Remember, these are people who have *no* visitors." Our few hours there was a very special occasion, for us as well as the residents. One of the ladies there had received her BA in 1929 from Macalester College in St. Paul, Minnesota, having been sent there by missionaries.

On the bus ride back to the hotel, some of us noticed a billboard along the highway showing a bright young couple holding a bouncing baby girl. We asked our guide to interpret the legend that was printed on the side of the happy picture:

"It is best to have just one child, even if it's only a girl." The message was a reminder of government-sponsored (or government-imposed) birth control. And it was understandable that people would want to continue trying to have a male child in a Chinese culture where it is the son's filial obligation to care for his parents. If a couple has just one child and she is a girl, then later she'll marry some young man and go off and care for *his* parents. With social institutions and community values in China in flux, many are wondering if they can form a *kai* relationship that can be depended on. Thus, the willingness of many Chinese to risk sanctions by having more than one child. They'll need a family caregiver in later life.

> *If a couple has just one child and she is a girl, then later she'll marry some young man and go off and care for* **his** *parents. . . . Thus, the willingness of many Chinese to risk sanctions by having more than one child. They'll need a family caregiver in later life.*

II

I was the adult child in charge of orchestrating my mother's dying. That I believe I may also have accidentally killed her will be explained in due time.

I had not been present at my father's death in 1970. He was in an Illinois nursing home, demented and failing rapidly; I was off in graduate school at Chapel Hill with a wife and a newly born son. For a variety of reasons, my father didn't get visited very often while he was institutionalized. While I have no reason to suspect that he received poor care, his death had to have been a lonely one. I vowed that when the time came this would not be the case for my mother.

She was hospitalized four times during 1997, the final year of her life. At 84 she was frail but lucid, living in a senior apartment. I joked with friends that keeping my mother independent was running me ragged. My wife, our sons, and I provided almost every service my mother received. Since the boys lived in other cities and my wife had a job where regular hours were required, I did most of the shopping, hauling, sitting in doctors' waiting rooms, scrubbing of carpets when she'd had diarrhea, and delivering of meals and laundry. I recall being told by my graduate students that adult daughters are the nurturant ones who deliver all the care to elders and responding, "Yes, I was reflecting on that very thought the other night while cutting my mother's toenails." Visiting nurses served as family extenders and eased the load during the final months.

At her last hospitalization when she was admitted for a touch of pneumonia, it was clear that my mother's kidneys were failing and it was just a matter of time. It turned out to be six weeks, although we had expected a bit less, I suppose. After acute care hospitalization, she was sent to a geriatrics unit where she received subacute care. Fortunately, about half of the staff on that unit are former students of mine. As a keen observer of the influence of staff perceptions of social value when working among the terminally ill, I made sure that my mother wore her mink coat when she was transferred. It worked. Not only was she *Doctor* Thorson's mother, but she was a *real lady*. She was treated like a queen.

As the weeks went by, the docs were open to my suggestions that the heart and blood pressure meds my mother was on were in fact an echo of a previous time when we were hoping to extend her life. They agreed to withdraw everything now that our intention was simply to keep her comfortable. Our goal had changed, and it seemed necessary to articulate that fact. Had I not brought it up, I'm sure everyone would have continued to pretend that she would get better.

My role was to be in charge of the visitors, as my mother held court until the final two days of her life. I was literally like an orchestra conductor, now bringing in the woodwinds, now the strings. I was also in charge of keeping *out* the large and boisterous family friend who made a pest of herself by visiting *too* often. Out-of-town relatives came and went, but it was the regulars who really pitched in and helped. It was an astonishing parade, an extended community of church ladies, and getting their schedule together meant that I could go back to the university and teach my seminar as well as my morning undergraduate class. I'd go to the hospital and eat lunch with Mom and then come back and spend the late evenings with her. One of the things she enjoyed most was being read to. I recall that the last book was a thick biography of the Windsors (Mother was a Royalist); near the end, she asked me what page I was on, and when I told her it was 86, she said, "Read faster."

At the very end, she was not in much pain, but was restless and semiconscious. A morphine drip with a patient-controlled analgesic (PCA) pump was installed; it had a hand-held clicker that would allow a predetermined dose once every 15 minutes. I, of course, was on it like a telegrapher, and it helped Mom a lot. However, when I was summoned to come in at 4:30 the final morning, the morphine pump didn't seem to be doing much good. Hugging my mother and mopping her brow seemed like the best I could do in terms of comfort measures, until at 8:30 I noticed that the wheel of the steel cart holding the IV bag was sitting on the IV's plastic tube. It was a natural reaction to roll the cart off the tube. All the morphine that had accumulated in the tube during the previous three hours then seeped into my mother's arm, and she slipped into the next world.

III

Jerry, an old friend from a dozen years of singing together in the church choir, called one evening to let me know of his frustration with the hospital care that his 85-year-old father was receiving. His dad had emphysema and congestive heart failure. He'd been in a nursing home for three months. When he had a respiratory arrest there, they pumped him up and sent him to the hospital. He was now in the ICU, there was a tube down his throat, and he was barely clinging to life. The docs wanted to do a tracheostomy and put the old man on a ventilator.

I asked Jerry if he knew that once his father was on the ventilator there would be little chance of ever getting him off of it. He did. I also asked him why they wanted to do that procedure on a man who was so apparently near the end of his life. Jerry said that when Dad had entered the nursing home they'd had him fill out advance directives. Asked if he wanted to be resuscitated if the situation arose, he checked off "yes" on the form. Now, the people at the hospital had seen this in the file and had taken it as a directive that he wanted all available means taken to keep him alive. I asked Jerry if that was what he thought his father, in fact, wanted, and he said no, he didn't think so. He was, in fact, sure that Dad specifically did *not* want to spend his last weeks or months on a machine breathing for him. Several times already his father had tried to pull out the tubes that were in his nose and mouth.

So I advised Jerry to meet with the surgeon immediately. "Tell him or her that you are the person responsible for your father, the situation has changed since he was admitted to the nursing home three months ago, that you do not authorize them to go ahead with the surgery, and that you want only comfort measures for your father."

That was on a Sunday evening. On Thursday I got a call from Jerry's wife. She said the staff had been only too willing to go along with his request. They'd actually been waiting to hear something from the family to prevent what they thought would probably be a useless procedure. Dad was now out of intensive care, in a regular hospital room, his daughters were in from California, and everyone was reconciled to the fact that this was the end of his life. There was just one thing: their youngest son Jeremy would be playing the trumpet solo at the last high school program of the year that evening, and since all the aunts were in from out of town. . . .

I picked up on where that was going: "And you don't want Dad to die alone. What time do you want me to be there?" So I took a stack of term papers with me to grade while I sat in the hospital and watched an old man die.

He was lying there on his back with his mouth open, obviously close to the end. His breathing was labored, short little puffs that weren't doing him any good. He wasn't conscious, but he wasn't comatose, either. When I went over and took his hand to tell him who I was, hoping he'd remember me from the many times we'd met, one eye did flutter for a moment. It didn't focus on me, but it did open. And he squeezed my hand.

As I sat there reading my papers, it was clear that the old man wouldn't be able to keep breathing like that for much longer; he would die of exhaustion. I clocked him. At 7:00 he was taking 23 breaths per minute; at 8:00 it was up to 30; by 9:00 he was taking 43 breaths per minute. I shouldn't say breaths, they were pants. Try taking 43 breaths per minute.

There was a monitor hooked up. The top LED (light-emitting diode) gave his blood oxygen levels, the bottom his pulse. He had an oxygen tube in his nose and an intravenous line giving him saline or glucose. Respiratory therapists came in twice while I was there to suction the gunk out of his trachea. When the light on the monitor indicated that his heartbeat had slipped below 50, it would turn from green to red and a beeping noise would sound. I asked a nurse to turn down the volume, as the noise agitated him. She said, "But if I turned off the sound, we couldn't hear it."

"That's right. It's okay if you don't hear it." It seemed necessary to come to an agreement. She understood, and she turned off the sound; she acknowledged that he was a "do not resuscitate" patient and there was no need for the alarm. We were then in an open awareness: the man was dying and it was all right. On the other hand, he was still hooked up to an antibiotic drip. Damned if I know what good *that* was going to do.

> *The first time both monitors went flat and read zero I figured that was it. The old man continued to pant along, though, and I began to have less faith in electronic monitors and more in the basic instinct to cling to life.*

The readings on both monitors gradually slipped down and down. The light on the pulse monitor was now blinking red much of the time, reading mostly in the forties. His breathing became even more labored. The first time both monitors went flat and read zero I figured that was it. The old man continued to pant along, though, and I began to have less faith in electronic monitors and more in the basic instinct to cling to life. The monitors went down to zero several more times while I was still on shift.

Jerry and his sister came in to relieve me late that evening. They'd enjoyed the program at the high school and were most appreciative. Dad died at 1:00 that morning. He wanted a Dixieland band at his funeral. He got it.

IV

By far the greatest amount of the care that is given to older people is delivered by family members. There is no greater illustration of this than what we see around us every day with example after example of older wives caring for their husbands, husbands caring for their wives, sons and daughters caring for their parents and grandparents, and so on. Whether it is a service so simple as stopping by the store for someone or as all-encompassing as caring for an Alzheimer's patient for the rest of his or her life, family members and friends perform countless acts of service for old people. This care goes in both directions; in many instances the primary beneficiary of extended households is the adult child.[2] In other words, there is a mutuality to family caregiving as well as an expectation that older adults will help their adult children when possible and adult children will be expected to help their parents when the time comes.

Some adult children may perform the services that they do out of an anticipation of some type of reward or repayment, a clear example of the exchange theory of aging. Actually getting payment or expecting an inheritance may happen less frequently than getting some kind of psychic reward, feeling good for satisfying a filial obligation, getting praise or positive reinforcement from others, or "building up credits" in the expectation that in the broad scheme of things they will eventually be repaid. Most people, though, have little expectation of any tangible reward for the services that they provide for family members and friends. Rather, they help their loved ones because of a sense of filial obligation, the notion that they are *supposed* to help them merely because that is the way members of a family behave.

This family feeling is the cement that holds civilizations together. Call it support for the group, tribal loyalty, family obligation, or norms and values of a culture; the interpersonal regard and care provided within families are among the most important factors in human relationships. As a general rule, in the field of gerontology we say that people in late life who have families seem to do better in many ways than those who are without families. When family systems break down, there is a potential for depression and burnout among family caregivers.[3]

In the cases presented, we have seen the need for extending family resources. The Chinese are richly aware of their own demographic problem. The nation is bursting at the seams with too many people, and the result is a Draconian birth control policy that has been enforced for the past 20 years. Where will the family caregivers come from for the next generation of Chinese elders? Many more old people will be like the residents of the Shanghai nursing home we described: childless and without visitors.

In my own case, the family extenders consisted of visiting nurses to my mother's home during the last few months of her life as well as a parade of helpful church ladies during her final weeks. In Jerry's case, I was the family extender. And in both of our cases an important point should be recognized: the extension of help was both exceedingly welcome and only temporary. For Jerry, the help of a friend was of great relief to the family and it was only for three and a half hours. In the case of my mother, the visits were spread out over a longer time, but they were relatively brief in terms of duration. These small but important services are what friends do for one another. One wonders what our own brave new world will look like. The birth rate has declined steadily for two generations.[4] It is no secret that the fastest-growing proportion of the population is elderly. Many people are remaining childless.

We must conclude that they had better have lots of friends. And this may be the conundrum of the twenty-first century. Many of us no longer know our neighbors, or we move so often as to sever neighborhood bonds. Fraternal organizations are literally dying off. In my mother's case, the helpful friends came from congregations, but we have seen a steady decline in church and synagogue participation since the mid-1950s.[5] It would seem that the group activity of choice among many young urban professionals is going to a fitness center to engage in solitary exercise with others who are also thus engaged. Although some colleagues point to the community strength among older African Americans, which is centered on the church, in fact, African Americans are no more likely to be churchgoers than anyone else.[4]

This is not to say that all hope is lost. Plenty of people are making plenty of friends all the time, despite our stereotype that most people are becoming urban hermits. Neighbors are helping neighbors. Hochschild found old ladies caring for each other in San Francisco single-room walk-ups.[6] Kastenbaum observed older people caring for one another in Arizona retirement communities.[7] Many a person with AIDS has been cared for by a non-kin caregiver. The American equivalents of *kai* relationships are no doubt being formed even as we lament our collective loneliness. People wise enough to plan for their financial future in old age may surprise us by planning for their social futures as well. Unexpected communities spring up unaware like weeds growing through sidewalks.

The point of extending families when we're running out of family members is that a little help goes a long way. We need to remember, too, that there is a mutuality to help, so we need to be open to opportunities, to be eager to form relationships, to go to places where friendships are likely to be formed. We need to care for one another.

REFERENCES

1. Ikels C. The coming of age in Chinese society: Traditional patterns and contemporary Hong Kong. In *Aging in Culture and Society*, C Fry (ed.). New York: JF Bergin, 1980, 84.
2. Speare A, Avery R. Who helps whom in older parent–child families. *Journal of Gerontology: Social Sciences*. 1993;48, S64–73.
3. Kosloski K, Young R, Montgomery R. A new direction for intervention with depressed caregivers to Alzheimer's patients. *Family Relations*. 1999;48(4):373–379.
4. U.S. Census Bureau, *Statistical Abstract of the United States*, 119th ed. Washington, DC: US Government Printing Office, 1999.
5. Thorson, JA. Spiritual well-being in the secular society. *Generation*. 1983;8(1):10–11.
6. Hochschild AR. *The Unexpected Community*. Upper Saddle River, NJ: Prentice-Hall, 1973.
7. Kastenbaum RJ. Encrusted elders: Arizona and the political spirit of postmodern aging. In *Voices and Visions of Aging: Toward a Critical Gerontology*, TR Cole (ed.). New York: Springer, 1993, 160–183.

Apple Tree

DOUGLAS BISHOP

Brookline, Massachusetts

The year my father died was the year the apple tree finally fruited.

Planting it, almost ten years before, was an example of my father's role as peace-maker in our family. I was always seen as the radical tree-hugger, leading to interminable arguments whenever someone decided to cut down a tree, so when the old white pine fell over on its own and I suggested planting an apple tree in its place, he was quick to endorse the idea. He took me to the local nursery and we picked out a dwarf apple tree, which the nurseryman said should fruit in three to five years.

The long gestation of his cancer began at about the same time, even as he was retiring from his profession of thirty-seven years. Immediately, he started to travel and play tennis more regularly. He bought a new computer and learned to do his taxes and finances there, as well as eventually hooking into the Internet and e-mail. He also began to study Spanish, and I took up the language with him. We went to Mexico together for a short vacation—just the two of us. On that trip and in the time afterward, I began to get to know my father in a way I never had before. The night after the day we planted the apple tree together, I was lying in bed, feeling satisfied with the work we had done, and I began to think back to my childhood, trying to remember times with my father. It was difficult to remember any specific incidents with him, even through all the years we had lived together. I made a decision then to reach out to him, and the trip to Mexico was part of that. I wanted to get to know him in a new way, but the years of distance were still strong. The trip to Mexico was like opening a window through which I could call to him. He would sometimes show his face at the window, but often he was more comfortable with talking into the air, in a dreamlike way, where we could hear, but not see each other. Then it became easier to talk about the little things that were passing in each of our lives.

Each year, I came back in the winter to prune, watching it grow to a mid-sized tree. But it never had blossoms, never bore fruit. After six years, seven years, eight years, I was starting to think that something was wrong. I suggested to my father that we go back to the nursery and ask the owner about the tree. Maybe there was something that we could do for it—or not do to it. My father was interested; he thought it was a good idea.

©2001 Apple Tree by Douglas Bishop. Published here with permission.

But by then the cancer had spread to his lymph system and he was having trouble walking. I remember the last time I went with him on his morning constitutional up the steep dirt road to the crest of the hill. He was clearly struggling, even with his cane in one hand and me on the other arm. I asked him if he wanted to stop to rest or even turn around and go back, but he insisted on completing the walk. He made it to the top of the hill, but on the way back down, on the curve by the white garage, his legs began to go out from under him, and I had to half carry him the rest of the way. Even then, he didn't want to stop. I suggested sitting down, but he wouldn't hear of it. We got back to the house with my arm around his waist, him walking bow-legged forward. We made enough of a scene that my mother came out of the house to see what was wrong. His answer was the usual: "I'm OK." My mother and I half carried him into the house and got him sitting, puffing at the breakfast table. In that context, we never got around to doing anything about the apple tree.

By the time the blossoms came on the tree, we knew that he wasn't going to last very long. He went through another round of radiation treatments to try to ease the stiffness in his leg, but it didn't really show any result. The summer the first green apples appeared on the tree was when the doctor stopped all chemotherapy because everything had been tried. When he finally left the family property in Vermont for his retirement home in Florida, with both my brothers serving as nurses and a bed set up in a rented van for the journey, there were about twenty apples on the tree. The apples were sweet, but a little soft, rose and gold streaking across the skin, but we were all too busy to harvest them as we rushed around to get him ready for the long trip south, which everyone knew would be his last, even though no one could really say it. In the end, the apples fell on the ground, maybe left for a nervous deer in the late November gray.

Sometimes it takes that long for a life to find fruition. It's not only the great ones that struggle with their posterity—sometimes simpler lives struggle for an ending—like my father, who fought in a world war and emigrated from one country to another, who wrote one book and fathered three sons, who enjoyed a rural childhood and a prosperous old age, but never really felt accomplished. Maybe that's why he fought the cancer for so long. He must have been waiting for something tangible, like a final piece of new fruit falling on frosted grass.

International Perspective

A National Network of Support for Carers in the United Kingdom

An Interview with ALISON RYAN

Princess Royal Trust for Carers
London, England

The Princess Royal Trust for Carers (PRTC) was founded in 1991 by Princess Anne to provide and coordinate comprehensive services to family caregivers, known as "carers" in the United Kingdom. This organization now sponsors a network of 102 carer centers across the country. These centers provide direct services to carers, as well as networking with statutory health and social service organizations to meet the needs of carers. Of the roughly six million carers in the United Kingdom, the carer centers make a particular effort to reach out to children and teens under the age of 18 who care for another family member. These young carers are variously estimated to number between 50,000[1] to half a million.[2]

Alison Ryan, the chief executive of this not-for-profit charity and a carer herself, describes the mission and work of the Princess Royal Trust, the challenge of defining and identifying carers, and the 1999 National Strategy for Carers, which is the new official British policy on carers.[3] In this interview with Anna L. Romer, EdD, Ms. Ryan details some of the new activities at PRTC that spring from this new national policy, as well as the ongoing challenges of financing and evaluation of services.

Anna L. Romer: *What is the mission of the Princess Royal Trust for Carers (PRTC)?*

Alison Ryan: Our mission is to support carers practically. Initially, the approach was through providing information to the carer; if carers had any kind of problem, they could get information from us. But as we've evolved we have realized that actually what the carers need, before they get information, is emotional support. Carers need to feel valued for the people that they are and the experience that they're having. If a carer comes into a carer center and says, "I can't stand it any longer," we would say, "We understand that it's a very difficult thing you're doing. We're here for you to provide emotional support." So first we provide emotional support, then we provide information and other services.

ALR: *What does it mean when you say that PRTC sponsors a carer center?*

AR: For us, it means that we provide a third of the money for the first three years. We also negotiate with the local health or government authorities located in the area that the care center is going to cover to get the remaining two-thirds of the funding for the center. Beyond that, we support the carer centers so that they are able to do their work. We keep them in touch with policy and good practice and offer training and consultancy. The Princess Royal Trust provides training and materials to the centers. We facilitate communication across the network so that staff members are always learning and improving good practice. We have published a number of resource booklets and reports.*

ALR: *Are the carer centers totally independent financially after the first three years?*

AR: They are. They are meant to be independent organizations, which are led by carers but run by professionals. This means that the strategy for each carer center will be determined by a group of voluntary carers. The center is structured to respond to the needs articulated by local carers. The trustee board running the center is designed to be dominated by carers, and the centers also have a duty to run carer consultation events and forums. Each center is run, however, by a cadre of paid professionals.

ACTIVITIES AND STAFFING OF CARER CENTERS

ALR: *Can you describe the staffing at a typical carer center?*

AR: Most centers have about six to eight paid staff and a lot of volunteers, as well. The paid staff are usually social workers or nurses, with about half working full time and half working part time. Most centers have no fewer than 3 paid staff members nor more than 12.

ALR: *What kinds of things do the paid staff do?*

AR: One important thing that staff members do is to make links to the other organizations in their communities. Carers are getting support from many other organizations, such as health services, social services, and schools. We have a huge commitment to young carers—children and teens who are providing care for other family members—so that is why we work with schools. Staff also work with local employers so that local employment practice acknowledges that there are carers in the workforce.

In addition, staff members provide information on the benefits to which the

---

*For a list of selected references from the Princess Royal Trust for Carers see p. 167.

carer is entitled and ensure that the carer is accessing these benefits. In the United Kingdom, carers are entitled to benefits, and people who are disabled and suffer from long-term illness are entitled to social security benefits. Yet the uptake is very low. We have found that, on average, each carer center brings in £0.5 million [approx. $717,600] of benefits per year to the carers that they serve. It's a staggering amount of money and the input to each local economy is enormous.

For the actual carers themselves, staff members provide direct counseling and emotional support. In addition, staff members advocate for individual carers. For example, if a carer is having a problem with a doctor and wants the carer center to take up the issue, they will do that.

ALR: *What is the role of volunteers for the PRTC?*

AR: There is some variety in what volunteers choose to do. Often former carers run some of the hobby groups. If a former carer is a talented artist and some of the carers want to get together and paint pictures, then that volunteer might run such a group. Another popular activity is to provide transport to carers who get stuck. Carers also just help doing all types of office work: e-mails, bulletins, newsletters, or whatever needs doing.

ALR: *What other activities do the carer centers engage in?*

AR: The carer center is also responsible for consulting with local carers so that they can inform the development of services in the community. For instance, if the local community wants to close a hospital and replace it with a day service, then it's up to the carer center to make sure that the carers have been consulted properly about this change. And if carers are opposed to the idea, the carer center will make their voices heard.

The carer center sponsors a range of fun activities. They set up times for hobbies and networks so that people can get together and enjoy some good times. A center might offer sessions on aromatherapy or reflexology, for example. Young carers get taken out for weekends off so that they can socialize. The center sponsors social and physical activities for young carers, such as skating or playing football. Arranging respite care is an integral part of running all these activities.

Our mission includes attending to the needs of former carers, those people who stop being carers because the person that they were caring for died. Most carer centers will usually keep up contact with former carers for a couple of years.

ALR: *How do they interact with former carers?*

AR: The staff at the center actively seek to help the person on the road to rediscovering his or her identity. They often help former carers to get back into employment or education. Or if these choices are not appropriate, then they may actually help the person to find some other meaningful role. Some former carers become volunteers; some support current carers.

There is a particular role for counseling at this time, because if someone's been a carer for a long period of time he or she probably dropped out of employment and might well have become socially isolated. Then when the person who was being cared for dies, the carer can lose all focus. Suddenly, the carer has nothing to do with his or her time and has no sense of role or identity. This is often when carers really do hit big-time trouble. Some carers may be at risk for suicide after the loved one being cared for dies.

> *. . . when the person who was being cared for dies, the carer can lose all focus. Suddenly, the carer has nothing to do with his or her time and has no sense of role or identity. This is often when carers really do hit big-time trouble.*

ALR: *Is employment counseling one of the activities of each carer center?*

AR: Yes. We have a national program. We've been working on carer-friendly policies and working with major employers, so we can provide lots of advice nationally on that. Our work includes educating employers to the idea that they have carers on their staff already. Often workers who are tired, seem unmotivated, and have poor attendance records are carers. Our work is to encourage employers to manage this problem with family-friendly policies so that carers can continue to take on both sets of tasks. Such policies include allowing carers flexible hours or the right to take private phone calls at work. We also provide financial assistance to carers to help them to retake vocational training to help them back into employment, if they have had to drop out.

ALR: *How much continuity is there across centers in terms of what they offer?*

AR: They are similar in that they all have to do the key work of emotional support, advocacy, information, and providing a voice for carers in their community. How they accomplish these tasks may differ. Most carer centers have a shop front on the main street so that people can just drop in. We're very clearly brand managed, so they see our gold and blue colors and our name, "Princess Royal Trust for Carers," and people can go in off the street.

Most centers are a real drop-in center five days a week, and then usually there's a phone answering service. At most centers, someone who phones in with a crisis will receive a reply within 24 hours. Nearly all the centers also have hotlines.

In urban centers, the shop front space is where the meetings happen and the offices are located. But in rural areas like the north of Scotland, this wouldn't be appropriate because the population is very scattered and the nearest town is often 100 miles of poor roads away. In these settings, the center would have a tiny office with a number of outreach workers who travel to community centers for an afternoon every week, for example. They'll work through other agencies far more. Some of the centers work by getting bigger and bigger and seem to take over all welfare services in their community, and some work primarily through partnerships with other organizations.

In Bristol, which has a large Chinese community, instead of having a Chinese worker, they have trained members of the Bristol Chinese women's group, and every week for one afternoon a Mandarin-speaking Chinese woman will answer the carers' hotline in Bristol. They advertise this service around the city: "If you speak Mandarin and you want to speak to a Chinese person about your caring, phone Wednesday afternoons." Other centers do similar kinds of outreach with other minority groups. These partnerships are essential.

IDENTIFICATION OF CARERS

ALR: *How do you find these carers? How do they know about these services?*

AR: Well, that is a really important question. It is not easy because, traditionally, carers have been defined by the number of tasks that they do or the number of hours that they spend doing it. We find that this "task and time spent" approach is not a very helpful way to describe this often invisible population that we are aiming to serve.

My approach is that the carer gets identified when the carer has problems. Carers can have problems doing 10 minutes of work if the relationship starts to become distorted. The person wakes up one morning, and she no longer feels like a wife, she feels like a carer. Or the carer might be a child, but this child is now the one who is responsible for and protecting his or her parent, not the other way around.

It seems to me that it is at this point when the stresses and strains of caring get serious. When the relationship, as it was before, can no longer be sustained, the carer may find him or herself in crisis. Sometimes it happens because the disease that a person has is a personality changer, such as with dementia or multiple sclerosis. I think hours and tasks are important, but it is often not what makes a difference between a carer who is coping and a carer who isn't coping. The breakdown of the caregiving systems seems to be due to this relationship distortion. Change in the basic nature of the relationship is not dependent at all on hours or tasks.

There's quite a lot of general publicity now in the United Kingdom to raise public awareness about the existence and needs of carers. But what we have to do is send out messages saying, "If you find it hard to be a carer, it's not because you're a lousy, inadequate human being. It is because the task of caring for someone nowadays is much more difficult." People

> *But what we have to do is send out messages saying, "If you find it hard to be a carer, it's not because you're a lousy, inadequate human being. It is because the task of caring for someone nowadays is much more difficult."*

are much more ill at home than they were when long hospital stays were common. In the United Kingdom it is judged that people are discharged sicker now than they were 10 years ago. People also survive with more serious conditions for longer, leading carers to face more challenging caring tasks at home. The current economic circumstances mean the carer has to juggle the caring with all kinds of other activities, and the nuclear family may be less supportive than in the past.

NETWORKING WITH GPS AND COMMUNITY PHARMACISTS

Locally, we are trying to link with all the professionals with whom carers naturally interact, even if they don't identify themselves as carers. That's where our work with primary health care and community pharmacists comes in.

Here in the United Kingdom, everyone is registered with their general practitioner (GP). Under the National Strategy for Carers, the British government said that GPs were to identify all the carers on their books, but doctors have found that really hard to do. At the Princess Royal Trust, we've placed a clearly identified member of staff from the carer centers in GP waiting rooms across the United Kingdom. These staff invite people to identify themselves. This self-identification then leads to referrals to carer services. We did a good bit of publicity about the effort in the surgery and the local press, so patients weren't surprised by this presence. We began this effort in Scotland and are now rolling it out across the rest of the United Kingdom. Corporate sponsors in the United Kingdom have supported this effort.

The GPs were very worried that this activity was going to produce more demands on their time. For this reason, they resisted this intervention, initially. In fact, identifying previously "invisible" carers has meant that the doctors get better and more appropriate referrals for their services. The carers who have got stress problems arising from their caring responsibilities now go to a carer service and are getting help. So, in fact, making the needs visible hasn't increased physicians' burdens because the carer center staff members are doing the case management to meet these people's needs. In the absence of this carer center effort, this case management burden might have fallen on the primary care health team.

We have also developed a project with community pharmacists. In contrast to GPs, community pharmacists have been much more interested in working with us. These pharmacists recognize who the carers are because they see them coming constantly into the chemist's shop to get medication or to ask for advice. Many carers do actually get advice from their pharmacists, not from their doctor, because they find the pharmacist more approachable. In the United Kingdom, where GPs are free (and grossly overworked), we are all very worried about troubling them unnecessarily and thus seek help elsewhere if we can. Pharmacists are very anxious to use their considerable expertise and are often easy to chat with while you are waiting for a prescription to be made up.

ALR: *What do you actually do with the community pharmacists? Tell me a little more about this outreach effort.*

AR: We are giving each community pharmacist a resource packet about carers, and we're making sure that all their local primary health care teams know about this intervention so that the GP primary care team is ready to pick up on anything that the center refers to them. Included in this packet are a set of simple one-ply leaflets that offer some descriptions of the kinds of carers, and the common problems encountered by carers, and where carers can access help. The goal here is to empower carers to seek help, to help them to identify themselves, and to make clear how many carers there are and how much of a contribution they are making. If the pharmacists suspect that the customer is a carer, they can pop this leaflet into the same bag in which they give the medication. There is a law in this country that says all medication has to be given in a bag, so logistically it is a very easy intervention. We hope to have a message about carers printed on the pharmacists' bags sometime later this year.

> *The goal here is to empower carers to seek help, to help them to identify themselves, and to make clear how many carers there are and how much of a contribution they are making.*

We are not asking pharmacists to say, "You are a carer, you may need help." That would not be helpful. Instead, we harness pharmacists' existing local knowledge and intuitive hunches about their clients, without being intrusive. When pharmacists put the informative leaflet in the bag, they offer the carer the opportunity to identify him or herself as a carer, a first step to accessing services.

ALR: *Can you speak a little more about young carers?*

AR: We are actively attempting to address the needs of carers under the age of 18. I've been working with Gail Hunt of the National Alliance for Caregiving (NAC) in the United States and from what I understand young carers have not yet been recognized by carer organizations in that country. Gail came over to a young carers conference we had in January 2001. I think the NAC had difficulty trying to find even one project that works with young carers in the United States.

ALR: *How did you come to recognize and consider this group?*

AR: About seven or eight years ago, people suddenly realized that there are children who are primary carers. It is a problem that has been hidden because families conspire to hide it, they collude, because they are worried that if the authorities hear that a youngster is looking after Mom, who has got multiple sclerosis, and Dad's not around, the child will be taken away. That's a knee–jerk reaction. People say, "That's a terrible situation, we must take the child into care." In fact, all the child wants to do is to be with Mom, who loves him and has a good relationship with him. So both parents and children tend to hide what's going on.

We now know what signs to look out for. We look out for bad behavior in school—someone who was doing well, but now is doing badly. We encourage teachers and administrators to look out for someone who has been bullied, is having problems keeping up, is turning up dirty, late, or not at all. We encourage the school teachers and administrators to start wondering if there's something going on at home. If there is an illness at home, we'd like them to start thinking about this child in a new way. Perhaps this child doesn't need disciplining. Perhaps this is a child who is trying to juggle an impossible number of responsibilities. In those places where we have a carer center, schools nearly always refer the child to the carer center. Sometimes a child will identify himself or herself. We put posters in schools saying things like, "Do you look after someone? Is this you? Call the Carer Center."

ALR: *How have the schools reacted to this?*

AR: Many school people can't believe it's happening until they actually identify a young carer in their midst. If we approach school personnel carefully and in a reasoned way, then we find it rings a bell and they are responsive. We hope that our approach allows them to see what is happening. For many school people, it is really the first time that they have thought about children in this role. Schools can do an awful lot to support young carers even in the absence of a carer center.

If the caregiving burden is not recognized, children who are carers can get into terrible trouble. These children can lose out on education and, particularly, on social skills. They don't tend to play with other kids because they are always hurrying home. They can't have someone for tea, and they're not wearing fashionable clothes. They might get abused on the playground, the other kids saying, "Oh, your mommy's in a wheelchair." Kids are not always kind. So these children who are caring for other family members can become very isolated. Missing out on childhood and adolescence can lead to suffering and difficulties in becoming responsible, well-adjusted adults.

ALR: *Was the PRTC the first group to address this issue?*

AR: No. An organization called National Carers Association,[†] which is a lobbying group and the carers' membership organization, was the first to pick it up. We work with them in a sisterly kind of way. They appointed a research worker to investigate about four or five years ago and it was thought that there were 50,000 young carers; we now think that there are probably more like half a million young carers in the United Kingdom.

ALR: *How did they come up with those numbers?*

AR: By going through census reports, social service reports, and the local authority records.

ALR: *Let's take an example. What happens if a teen who is taking care of his*

[†]See <www.carersonline.org.uk/> for more information.

dad has a problem and calls the carer center on a Saturday afternoon? Would that teen get a real person or a recording?

AR: A child who is already known to the center will have someone available 24 hours a day, someone whom the child trusts and knows. If it's a new child, we pick it up almost as quickly, actually. On weekends the call is usually taken by a telephone answering machine. But the answering machine gets monitored, so a person will get back to the caller pretty fast. The staff member would find out what the problem was and, if medical intervention were needed, would help the child to get that care.

ALR: *What's the process when a young carer contacts a center? How do you connect with them and what kinds of resources does the center make available to this young person?*

AR: Referrals for children and adults are much the same and there is no set pattern. People self-refer or are sent on by friends or professionals. If it is a child, however, the young carers specialist will pick up the referral. The first step of any referral is always the same: a welcome, and then an assessment of the carer's perceived needs. The center will match the young carer with a worker whom the center knows and trusts. The young carer will have personal contact numbers for this person and so will know how to get hold of the contact person if he or she needs to. This contact person must be an adult who is extremely well equipped to deal with whatever the problem is. With the young carer, it is a professional— a social worker or someone trained and vetted to work with young people. Volunteers who work with children have to be police-checked to make sure that they have not been lawfully registered as child abusers, and they must be trained very carefully. But on the whole, for control reasons, you would normally choose someone on the staff to be the contact person for a young carer.

Working with vulnerable people is something you have to do very carefully. There are a lot of issues about child protection that we have to be extremely careful about. It is the law, but it also has to do with quality standards. When providing direct care to vulnerable people, services should not employ persons who are not specially trained and able to respond appropriately.

FINANCING

ALR: *How are all these services paid for?*

AR: Financially, it's a total nightmare, or rather a challenge! The centers do provide a great many services. Centrally, we raise £1.5 million a year. We have restrictions on what kinds of fundraising we are allowed to do, because we are a Royal Trust. The good thing about being a Royal Trust is that many people quite like meeting princesses, so they are willing to come to fundraising events where they can do so.

ALR: *How do you raise the money to support these centers?*

AR: The money for the central work that we do, which is basically the training and consultancy and providing our third of the start-up funding for the centers, comes on the whole from big companies and wealthy individuals, and it comes through the influence that we can have, simply because we are very well connected. The entire social establishment in the United Kingdom is on our board or we know them or can get to them. So we are privileged in that way, and we use that privilege all the time.

The carer centers don't have that kind of clout. However, they now seem to be occupying such a core part of the provision of social services and health service in their communities that they are funded largely from local statutory funding. Perhaps now is the time to talk about the political context and the new National Strategy for Carers.

THE NATIONAL STRATEGY FOR CARERS

The National Strategy for Carers became the national policy not because the Labor government is full of kind people, even though they'd like you to think so, but because it made financial sense. I have to say that Tony Blair, the prime minister, was a young carer. When he was a teenager, his mother had a stroke and his father had a bit of a nervous breakdown. Tony did most of the caring for a time, so he has some sympathy for this plight.

However, it was the research on the actual monetary contribution carers are making to the welfare economy that spawned this new policy. Now, as you know, in the United Kingdom health and social services are largely provided free of charge and we don't have health insurance. On average, a carer in the United Kingdom cares for someone for five years; clearly, some people provide care for many more years than that average, some people for fewer. A recent report estimated that the six million carers providing these five years of voluntary care save the government £34 billion per annum.[4] If the government could increase the duration of this voluntary caregiving by 10 percent, to five and a half years, it could save an additional 10 percent on the replacement costs of the carer, or an additional £3.4 billion per year. [Carol Levine and her colleagues have calculated the comparable "savings" generated by voluntary caregiving in the United States.[‡]]

These statistics had an impact on the British government. If these people were put off being carers, then paying for what is now "free" care, from the government's point of view, would be a phenomenal drain on national resources.

[‡]Carol Levine offered a "midrange national economic value of informal caregiving" estimate of $196 billion in 1997, citing Arno PS, Levine C, Memmott MM. The economic value of informal caregiving. *Health Affairs.* 1999;18(2):182–188 in Levine C. *Always on Call.* New York: United Hospital Fund, 2000, 5.

Additional costs can emerge from this kind of caring. Carers can become patients themselves because of the problems of being a carer. Another risk to carers is that as they drop out of the paid work economy they are no longer accruing retirement pensions. Without a pension, they run the risk of becoming a burden to the state in later life.

In 1999, the government took a proactive approach and designed a holistic National Strategy for Carers. Within this new national policy are some obligations that were then translated into law in various pieces of legislation. The strategy looks at the kind of information, training, and consultation that carers need. But, more importantly, it addresses key underlying issues: How can the community work to keep carers in school? What allows carers to remain employed? How can we as a society keep carers connected to their communities and so avoid social isolation? Carers need support to remain whole people. And it is to everyone's advantage that carers retain access to their whole world. The National Strategy for Carers is a powerful document that advocates strongly for the rights and needs of carers. However, the impetus for this policy came from the financial and economic statistics on what these people save for the nation. Investing in carers benefits us all.

The National Strategy for Carers works through the agency of the National Health Service (NHS) and the local government. The strategy lays a requirement on both the NHS and the local government to do certain things for carers, and if they don't do those things, they don't get central government money. There is also real money behind this strategy. The first thing that was centrally funded was a project for carers to get short-term breaks.[§] This new policy also inspired the creation of new Quality Standards for Local Carer Support Services.[‖]

The King's Fund, another independent health care charity in the United Kingdom, set up a working group to establish the Quality Standards for Local Carer Support Services in response to recommendations laid out in the National Strategy for Carers. The working group included a representative from the Princess Royal Trust, as well as someone from the Carers National Association and representatives from the NHS, the Department of Health, and other government and charity organizations involved in this field.

Poor-quality services have been a real problem for carers, so these new standards should help support carers in very concrete ways. We are now working on how to implement these standards.

ALR: *Are there other pieces coming out of this new national strategy?*

AR: The work we are doing with primary care GPs to identify hidden carers, which I mentioned earlier, is very much part of the National Strategy for Carers.

[§]See <www.kingsfund.org.uk> for more information on the King's Fund. Click on the link to the Health and Social Care Support page for an analysis of local authority plans and progress reports on the use of the Carers Special Grant (Year 2) written by Penny Banks and Emilie Roberts.
[‖]See Carers—Government Information for Carers at <www.carers.gov.uk> for a link to these standards.

Another major national effort is that the 2001 census of the population is going to have a question in it about carers. As a result, we will be able to quantify the numbers of carers a bit more accurately, as well as their distribution by region.

BUILDING PARTNERSHIPS TO ACHIEVE MISSION

ALR: *Can you say more about partnerships that you have built with other organizations to achieve your goal of providing comprehensive care to carers in the United Kingdom?*

AR: Currently, the Princess Royal Trust for Carers reaches about 100,000 carers in the United Kingdom. We want to get to a million. We cannot expand our network tenfold, it is just financially impossible. So the way we hope to get support to the million carers is by forming strategic alliances with people who may already be working with carers, but may not recognize these individuals as carers. We would like to share the kind of carer insights that we have gained through our carer center network with these other individuals and organizations.

The usual trajectory of a carer seeking help is that the carer does not go first to a carers service. I know this from my own experience caring for my husband and my mother-in-law. Carers go first to the organization that deals with the disease afflicting their loved one. So, in my case, I used to go to the Hemophilia Society and the Liver Trust. These disease-specific organizations can be wonderful. They provide fantastic information, but often they are not "carer-alert." What I mean is that they are not oriented to the experience of being a carer. They don't know the added little bits that I would need as a carer. They offer the technical information necessary to do the caring. We believe that we can help these organizations to become more "carer aware" and provide more carer-focused support. In this way, they would increase the effectiveness of their information.

If we at the Princess Royal Trust can form alliances with the people who the carers actually go to for information, especially in the first days of caring, then I think we can start making a difference in the lives of more carers without actually having to expand our own network. So we will make an alliance with anyone that we can. We have made a very strong alliance with Crossroads,¶ which provides short-term breaks and respite care. In fact, we're getting together with Crossroads to train our staff jointly. We have a very good alliance with the National Carers Association and with a lot of other national organizations. Locally, our carer centers will make strong links with whoever is available in their own communities.

EVALUATION

ALR: *How do you evaluate the work that the carer centers do?*

¶See Crossroads—Caring for Carers at <www.crossroads.org.uk/>.

AR: We are working on that at the moment. We are trying to make sure that the carer's experience of the work is at the core, because we believe that the carer's experience is the prime determinant of success or failure. We are working on all kinds of feedback. Virtually every carer center has developed its own system of getting feedback. Now we're trying to work out which system represents best practice. It is very lively work, right at the moment.

ALR: *What is the range of ways that centers are currently using to obtain feedback on the carers' experience of the services that the centers provide?*

AR: Some centers recontact carers who have not accessed the service for six months, with the goal of finding out what's going on and whether the service met their needs. Staff members from the center inquire by phone or send a questionnaire to these carers.

> *One problem in eliciting feedback is that carers tend to be so grateful that anybody did anything for them that they tend to be a bit uncritical.*

One problem in eliciting feedback is that carers tend to be so grateful that anybody did anything for them that they tend to be a bit uncritical. So it is very hard to get real feedback and actually determine what's being done really well and what's being done less well.

In some areas, we will have consultation days. We'll bring in 14 or 15 carers to participate in a focus group. We ask them to explore the issues that they are facing and then we inquire how the carer center is addressing these issues. The goal is not just to find out what the carer center is up to, but also to learn how the local services provided by statutory bodies are working. Getting these focus groups together is terribly hard because, in order to get a group of carers together, we always have to provide respite care for each person being cared for.

Another mechanism we're using to develop good practice is to use action learning sets. We bring together the more highly trained specialist workers, like those who work with young carers' or center managers, to look at the common problems that they face. Based on their cumulative experience and knowledge, they develop a standard of good practice.

An additional challenge that we face is to understand why hidden carers are staying hidden. One might consider their not accessing the center as evidence that the center is doing something wrong or that the center is missing something. So I wouldn't say that we've got that one right, but we're working on it.

ALR: *Do you conduct any kind of anonymous surveys of carers?*

AR: We haven't conducted a national survey. I think we may get some of that kind of information from our website. All the carer centers are on the Web, and one benefit that they offer carers who don't have Internet access in their own homes is access from the center.

ALR: *Have you learned anything about carers' experience and the quality of services from the carers' chat and discussion on the PRTC site?*

AR: The chat and discussion venues are developing quite slowly. The discussion hasn't taken off yet, but we think it will.

The other thing we've learned comes directly out of my experience as a carer. I have extensive experience speaking to carer groups, as a carer. When I speak publicly and am willing to say that I've always found caring pretty difficult, this honesty helps to provide an atmosphere in which people are less afraid to talk about their own real problems. This makes a real difference, especially with men, who are perpetually weeping on my shoulder. That's no good, because I just weep back.

The whole question about quality and evaluation is huge in the not-for-profit sector in the United Kingdom. We use a number of models, which are broadly used in this sector. Our problem is that they tend to be process oriented and geared toward assessing the organizations' activities. We can tick off all the boxes and have all the meetings, but these measures do not assure that we are hearing real carers' voices about their own experience. Accessing their experience is not in the model. Yet that's what you have to do.

REFERENCES

1. Young carers research group. *Young Carers in the UK.* Leicestershire: Loughborough University, 1998.
2. Pettitt G, Kenny D. *Carers Count: A Research Report on Carers in London.* London: The Princess Royal Trust for Carers, 2000.
3. HM Government. *Caring about Carers: A National Strategy for Carers.* HM Government, February, 1999. Available at <www.carers.gov.uk> in PDF format.
4. Warner L, Wexler S. *Eight Hours a Day and Taken for Granted?* London: The Princess Royal Trust for Carers, 1998:2, citing General Household Survey (GHS) 1995.

Book Review

Caregiving and Loss: Family Needs, Professional Responses edited by Kenneth J. Doka and Joyce D. Davidson*

SAMANTHA LIBBY SODICKSON

Education Development Center
Newton, Massachusetts

An assumption underlying the movement to improve end-of-life care in the United States is that somehow, in the process of providing help to families through better delivery of medical care, the redesign of systems, and extending access to hospice and social services, we will be able to alleviate the physical and emotional burdens that go hand in hand with caring for the dying. *Caregiving and Loss* provides us with many voices and perspectives with which to consider how far that assumption takes us and how we fall short. In her piece "Voices: Hoping This Could be Somebody Else's Life," Elizabeth Halling shows us that with a dying child nothing may ever seem to be enough. "Finally, I thought, we're going to be surrounded by people who know what to do and how to help. Finally, we won't have to be the experts anymore. We'll have someone to share the burden, someone to show us the way. The big step we've taken of putting ourselves in their hands meant that somebody else could take some big steps now, and big soft wings would enfold us, and we wouldn't have any more pain. Turns out the hospice people are just people, not angels" (p. 35).

The burden of caregiving grows ever larger as an increasing proportion of our population enters the Third Age. In her introduction, Carol Levine notes that 23.5 million adult caregivers in the United States contribute an estimated $196 billion per year in free labor (in 1997), with an average of 20.3 unpaid hours per week (p. 5). The implications of this burden are staggering. Caregivers repeatedly report the loss of promotions at work, financial resources, and the emotional support of friends and family who cannot relieve the heavy burden of the caregiver and thus turn away. At the same time, the caregiver is experiencing the ongoing deterioration and impending loss of a loved one—lifelong partner, parent, child. Who is responsible for providing this care, and what can we, as a society, do to understand, appreciate, and ease this heavy duty of service?

These are the questions that are raised in this multifaceted book, which provides a collection of resources, personal stories, examples of programs that work

---

*Doka KJ, Davidson JD. *Caregiving and Loss: Family Neeeds and Professional Responses*. Washington, DC: Hospice Foundation of America, 2001.

to support caregivers, and the current thinking on grief, bereavement, and the physical and psychosocial complications of caregiving. Connection between people remains at the heart of caregiving. There are many players in this complex and fragmented health system: the professionals who repeatedly step into the homes and lives of those for whom they care; the health care professionals who diagnose disease, manage symptoms, and are relied on to support patients, caregivers, and their families; the professionals who counsel families in turmoil; the family and community members who give of themselves to assist loved ones and neighbors. There are intricate family dynamics, awkward and stressed systems that are not easily navigated, complex and often illogical financial constraints, and the often overwhelming burden of grief. Kenneth J. Doka and Joyce D. Davidson have created a compilation that gives voice to the experiences of the professional and family caregivers who are caught up in the streams of assistance that slowly trickle in to them, as well as those professionals who are working to open the rivers of care that caregivers of the dying need so desperately to flow to their doors.

Doka and Davidson define caregivers as the persons who are caring for a dying patient. This could mean members of the immediate family; members of the community who are non-kin, but considered to be a part of the family network; and the professional caregiver who provides care in a nursing home or long-term care facility or who enters the home of a family in need and provides care. All caregivers—professional, family, and non-kin—are essential in providing quality care to those who need it.

Part I of *Caregiving and Loss*, "Caregiving as an Issue: Policies and Programs," addresses the size and scope of the role of caregiving, while highlighting several programs within the community and the workplace that try to assist family caregivers. For example, AT&T provides a service to its employees called Life Tracks, which is housed on its intranet and provides referral resources to employees for life transitions, including caregiving and end-of-life care. AT&T also offers flexible scheduling options, such as compressed work weeks, telecommuting, and part-time work for up to 24 months, as well as family care leave benefits for a period of up to 12 months. The company has found that many people who would otherwise have had to leave their jobs were able to remain employed as a result of this program. In New Jersey, the Grotta Foundation bound together local synagogues, funders, and the local aging service groups into a network of support called the Grotta Synagogue HOPE (Help, Opportunities, and Programs for Elders). They created opportunities for Jewish congregants to aid the elderly community and provide care and assistance at the end of life.

Part II of *Caregiving and Loss*, "The Caregiving Experience: Implications for Professionals," focuses on the ongoing challenges faced by professional caregivers and the many medical and support professionals who interact with the patient, family, and caregivers. Effective caregiving happens when professionals can fully engage with their patients and families. The ongoing cycle of grief and the low-wage work of caring for the dying place many of the most essential personnel in this field at risk. Caregivers working through home care agencies and some nursing homes are often unable to grieve for the loss of their patients, largely due to the fact that they cannot afford even one day off from work to attend the funeral or visit the family. Eileen Chichin, Orah Burack, and John Carter describe how some nursing homes and long-term care facilities, such as Jewish Home and Hospital in New York City, are trying to acknowledge these caregivers' attachments to their patients. The administration honors their grief in the form of leaving a rose on the bed after a patient has died and allows the certified nursing assistant the opportunity of a short break to write the family a note on company time.

The very real need for professionals to have sensitivity in dealing with many ethnic and cultural groups is discussed in "Cultural Differences: Sensitivities Required for Effective Caregiving" by Bernice Catherine Harper, Michon Lartigue, and Kenneth J. Doka. Their recommendations begin with knowing oneself and then move on to suggest that caregivers and professionals ask direct questions so as to determine what is meaningful to each patient and family. William Lamers discusses the need for doctors to be willing and able to provide caregivers with reassurance and clear expectations about the symptoms and disease trajectory of a dying patient, what constitutes an emergency, and whom to call if and when assistance is needed. Susan Reinhard writes about the role of nursing in supporting family caregivers. She advocates for social policy changes that address financial reform for services on a sliding scale basis, collaboration among health care leaders, consumer-driven home care programs that have public support, insurance benefits for family caregivers, and better intervention research.

Also included in this part of the book are the personal voices of psychological and spiritual counselors who work with caregivers toward the goal of helping to ease their burdens. Barry Jacobs tenderly details working with a caregiver who would only agree to help herself if he could convince her that, by participating in therapy as part of an education program for medical students, she would be helping him. "I invited Carla because selfless caregivers are among the most difficult patients for any health care professional to know how to help. . . . In my clinical career, I'd seen several caregivers eventually crash and burn because they steadfastly neglected to take care of themselves" (p. 161). In "Self-Care: The Path to Wholeness," Beth Witrogen McLeod poetically addresses the spiritual context of the family caregiver in a youth-obsessed society. Where does the family caregiver fit in society at this critical turning point, and how can he or she protect the fragile sense of self that exists separately from the caregiving role in a day and age where we are expected to be everything to everyone at all times? "The fear of admitting that we are not supermen and superwomen carries such power over us that we neglect ourselves in order to measure up to an outside, disempowering ideal. . . . In molding ourselves to what is socially acceptable, we have become untrue to our whole selves, and thus invite dis-ease" (p. 197).

> *Inevitably, all caregivers face the final moment when their loved one dies. In supporting caregivers up to the time of death, we are only doing part of the job.*

Inevitably, all caregivers face the final moment when their loved one dies. In supporting caregivers up to the time of death, we are only doing part of the job. Part III of *Caregiving and Loss* addresses the more existential questions of grief, loss, and moving forward. Often overlooked are the torment and questions caregivers face about the sequence of events leading up to the death. "Did I do the right thing? Did I make the right decision?" These are questions that continue long after a loved one has died. Reverend George Blackwell and Rabbi Harold Stern write of the spiritual practice of connecting and being present, often helping people through the experience of a crisis of faith in "Providing Spiritual Support to Family Caregivers." Deborah Sherman speaks to the importance of addressing the memories and experiences of grieving families. How they feel about what they remember, rather than actual fact checking, is the focus of grieving, and she notes "the importance of hearing 'I am sorry' from their family member's physician and caregivers following the death of a patient" (p. 262). The value judgments contained in ethical decision making during prolonged illness and the need for patients and families to be supported while making such decisions, especially under the weight of grief that families experience at this time, are the topics of David M. Price's piece, "Hard Decisions in Hard Times: Helping Families Make Ethical Choices During Prolonged Illness." Families often feel limited by either/or choices about care. Price advocates for families to have a clear understanding of their choices and acknowledges the need for professionals to recognize the influence of grief and guilt during this critical time. He provides a guide to many common turning points faced by families at the end of life, for example, should we have a DNR order? Should we put in a feeding tube? Should we discontinue aggressive curative approaches?

Under the best of circumstances, these questions have no easy answers. *Caregiving and Loss: Family Needs, Professional Responses* provides a wealth of information for all persons involved in answering these questions. The breadth of topics covered and the honesty of the individual stories and professional compassion contained in these pages are a tribute to how deeply the importance of caregiving is felt. As Joyce D. Davidson concludes, "Somehow, no matter what we humans are going through, nothing gives us more comfort than the presence of someone with whom to share our journey" (p. 299). The heart of this book lies in the hope that caregivers will not have to travel this road alone; that professionals and members of the community alike will hold torches aloft to light the way and tread gently, steadfastly alongside.

Selected Bibliography

Part Three

Selected references by contributors to this part:

Arno PS, Levine C, Memmott MM. The economic value of informal caregiving. *Health Affairs.* 1999;18(2):182-188.

Crabtree H, Warner L. *Too Much to Take On: A Report on Young Carers and Bullying.* London: The Princess Royal Trust for Carers, 1999.

Levine C (ed.). *Always on Call: When Illness Turns Families into Caregivers.* New York: United Hospital Fund of New York, 2000.

Levine C. Family caregivers: Hospitals' most vulnerable partners. *Trustee.* 1999;52(2):24-25.

Levine C. Home sweet hospital: The nature and limits of private responsibilities for home health care. *Journal of Aging and Health.* 1999;11(3):341-359.

Levine C, Zuckerman C. Hands on/hands off: Why health care professionals depend on families but keep them at arm's length. *Journal of Law, Medicine & Ethics.* 2000;28(1):5-18.

Levine C, Zuckerman C. The trouble with families: Toward an ethic of accommodation. *Annals of Internal Medicine.* 1999;130(2):148-152.

Pettitt G, Kenny D. *Carers Count: A Research Report on Carers in London.* London: The Princess Royal Trust for Carers, 2000.

Warner L. *Seven and a Half Minutes is Not Enough: A Good Practice Guide for Carers, Support Workers, and GP Practices.* London: The Princess Royal Trust for Carers, 1999.

Warner L, Wexler S. *Eight Hours a Day and Taken for Granted?* London: The Princess Royal Trust for Carers, 1998.

Wexler S, and The Carers in Employment Group. *Carers in Employment: A Report on the Development of Policies to Support Carers at Work.* London: The Princess Royal Trust for Carers, 1995.

Other selected references:

Annerstedt L, Elmstahl S, Ingvad B, Samuelssen SM. Family caregiving in dementia—An analysis of the caregiver's burden and "breaking point" when home care becomes inadequate. *Scandanavian Journal of Public Health.* 2000;28(1): 23-31.

Ayres L. Narratives of family caregiving: The process of meaning making. *Research in Nursing & Health.* 2000;23(6):424-434.

Brown D. *The Caregiving Years: Six Stages to a Meaningful Journey.* Park Ridge, IL: Tad Publishing Co., 2000.

Canam D, Acorn S. Quality of life for family caregivers of people with chronic health problems. *Rehabilitation Nursing.* 1999;5:192-196.

Carlisle C. The search for meaning in HIV and AIDS: The carer's experience. *Qualitative Health Research.* 2000;10(6):750-765.

Chou KR. Caregiver burden: A concept analysis. *Journal of Pediatric Nursing*. 2000;15(6):398-407.

Corcoran M, Gitlin LN. Managing eating difficulties related to dementia: A case comparison. *Topics in Geriatric Rehabilitation*. 1996;12(2):63-69.

Dilworth-Anderson P. The structure and outcomes of caregiving to elderly blacks: A research agenda. *African American Research Perspectives*. Spring 1997.

Doka KJ. *Living with Life-Threatening Illness: A Guide for Patients, Their Families, & Caregivers*. San Francisco: Jossey-Bass Publishers, Inc., 1993.

Doka KJ, Davidson JD (eds.). *Caregiving and Loss: Family Needs, Professional Responses*. Washington, DC: Hospice Foundation of America, 2001.

Fourteen Friends LLC. *Fourteen Friends Guide to Eldercaring*. New York: Broadway Books, 1999.

Glajchen M, Fraidin L. Caring for the caregivers. *Pain Medicine and Palliative Care Newsletter*. Vol. 2, No. 3. <www.StopPain.org/for_professionals/newsletter/newsletter/no3/caregivers.html> (accessed 26 Jul. 2002).

Haley WE, LaMonde LA, Han B, Narramore S, Schonwetter R. Family caregiving in hospice: Effects on psychological and health functioning among spousal caregivers of hospice patients with lung cancer or dementia. *Hospice Journal*. 2001;15(4):1-18.

Karpinski M. *Quick Tips for Caregivers*. Medford, OR: Healing Arts Communications, 2000.

Koch T. *Mirrored Lives: Aging Children and Elderly Parents*. New York: Praeger Books, 1990.

Lynn J, Harrold J, Center to Improve Care for the Dying. *Handbook for Mortals: Guidance for People Facing Serious Illness*. New York: Oxford University Press, 1999.

McGadney BF. Family and church support among African American family caregivers of frail elders. *African American Research Perspectives*. Spring 1995.

McLeod B. *Caregiving: The Spiritual Journey of Love, Loss and Renewal*. New York: John Wiley & Sons, 1999.

MetLife Mature Market Group and National Alliance for Caregiving. *The Metlife Study of Employer Costs for Working Caregivers*. Based on data from *Family Caregiving in the US: Findings from a National Survey*. Wesport, CT: Metropolitan Life Insurance Company, 1997.

Nijboer C, Triemstra M, Tempelaar R, Mulder M, Sanderman R, van den Bos GA. Patterns of caregiver experiences among partners of cancer patients. *Gerontologist*. 2000;40(6):738-746.

Parks SM, Novielli KD. A practical guide to caring for caregivers. *American Family Physician*. 2000;62(12):2613-2622.

Pickett M, Barg FK, Lynch MP. Development of a home-based family caregiver cancer education program. *Hospice Journal*. 2001;15(4):19-40.

Ramirez A, Addington-Hall J, Richards M. ABC of palliative care: The carers. *British Medical Journal*. 1998;316(7126):208-211.

Sachs GA. Sometimes dying still stings. *Journal of the American Medical Association*. 2000;284(19):2423.

Sankar A. *Dying at Home: A Family Guide for Caregiving*. Baltimore, MD: Johns Hopkins University Press, 1999.

Sarnoff Schiff H. *How Did I Become My Parent's Parent?* New York: Penguin Putnam, Inc., 1997.

Sokolovsky J (ed.). *The Cultural Context of Aging: Worldwide Perspectives*, 2d ed. Westport, CT: Greenwood Press, 1997.

Van Staa AL, Visser A, van der Zouwe N. Caring for caregivers: Experiences and evaluation of interventions for a palliative care team. *Patient Education and Counseling*. 2000;41(1):93–105.

White TM, Townsend AL, Stephens MA. Comparisons of African American and white women in the parent care role. *Gerontologist*. 2000;40(6):718–728.

Part Four

On Grief and Bereavement

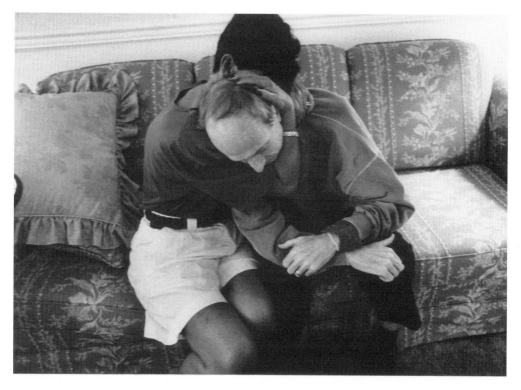

©1998 Roger Lemoyne and Living Lessons.

Living with Grief, Rebuilding a World

PHYLLIS R. SILVERMAN, PhD

Massachusetts General Hospital
Institute of Health Professions
Boston, Massachusetts

In this part, we look broadly at the experience of bereavement and at how health care professionals might respond. In doing so, this framework implicitly expands the population that professionals working in end-of-life care have typically considered to be the focus of their care. When we talk of bereavement and what happens to survivors after people die, we must include not only those who are grieving losses from long-term illnesses, such as cancer, but also those who are grieving sudden, unanticipated deaths caused by disease, suicide, accidents, murder, and war. We also need to keep in mind that even when a death is anticipated, the grieving that occurs before the death differs from what happens once someone has died. Another process is set in motion as mourners learn to live with the fact of death, and all that this means for their ongoing lives.

> *... even when a death is anticipated, the grieving that occurs before the death differs from what happens once someone has died.*

Grief touches people socially, emotionally, physically, and spiritually and can have far-reaching and unanticipated consequences. Rarely is there is a single mourner; many lives are changed by most deaths. It is the family, and sometimes the larger social network into which they extend, that becomes the unit of care. Ultimately, I see living through grief as a process that involves not only coping with a range of intense and painful feelings, but of finding a new sense of self and a new place for oneself in the world. I also view the nature of grief within a developmental and relational framework. Applying this framework to the clinical practice of providing bereavement support calls some current models of care into question and gives more robust support for others.

In this part, "On Grief and Bereavement," two hospital-based efforts are spotlighted. Both represent an attempt to respond to the families' needs for bereavement care in a proactive manner. The Featured Innovation spotlights the University of California at San Francisco (UCSF) Children's Medical Center's Family Bereavement Retreat, held for the first time in 1994. This effort is grounded in the philosophy that the health care professionals who care for a dying child are in a position to offer support to families after the child dies, due to the ongoing relationship that has developed over the course of the child's illness. By pairing the health care professionals with outside bereavement experts to co-lead groups that support grieving parents and siblings, this intensive weekend-long retreat can be "healing" for all involved.

The Promising Practice, St. Vincent's Hospital and Health Care System in Indianapolis, has taken a proactive approach in its recently developed bereavement care track. There are three elements to its program: (1) They capture all deaths that occur in the hospital system and reach out to all bereaved families, regardless of whether the death was anticipated or not. (2) Staff and volunteers reach out to bereaved next of kin by initiating phone calls at one month, three months, and six months after the death, in addition to mailing brochures and written materials to the families. (3) The volunteer network is made up of staff, often those who were involved in the care of the dying person before that person's death, allowing staff, who are interested and able, the opportunity to follow up with these families.

THEORETICAL MODELS OF DEVELOPMENT AND GRIEF

For much of the twentieth century, theories of grief and the research associated with it focused on the mourner's intrapsychic or emotional reactions to the loss, with the major focus on identifying problem behaviors that might result.[1] Following a model attributed to Freud, the bereaved were encouraged to "decathect" from the "object," that is, to let go of their attachment to the deceased, as if by remaining attached to the deceased they would not be free to develop other relationships.[2] During this same time, the field of human development focused on how people achieved separation and individuation.[3] This perspective sought causes for maladaptive behavior in the events of the individual's early life, ignoring the fact that human experience rarely unfolds in such a simple manner.[4]

This theoretical stance has led to what can be described as an illness or a deficit model of grief and bereavement. Bereavement counselors often describe grief as something that mourners will "get over," such as an illness from which one recovers with the appropriate treatment. This approach is reflected in the vocabulary available for describing the direction that grieving should take. Clergy, health care professionals, friends, and now the media—especially when they report on survivors of disaster—talk of "a time of healing," of "getting over it," "working it through," and "finding closure." Yet, for many who grieve, this vocabulary does not match their experience. It is important to recognize that, while the pain of loss may be tempered by time, time does not heal. The bereaved do not recover, in the sense of returning to life as it was before the loss. Rather, they make an accommodation to their new situation, and this accommodation does not have an end product, but changes as the bereaved change over time. People visit and revisit the loss so that, in time, they "run the pain, it no longer runs them."[3] In his Personal Reflection, David Browning, a social worker specializing in bereavement work, shares his 35-year sojourn through grief resulting from the death of his mother when he was just 13. When the bereaved are unable to achieve the sense of closure expected by those around them who believe that their grief should "resolve" and be completed, the bereaved can feel defective and stigmatized, as if something must be wrong with them. David Browning so ably describes this process.

The focus on the resolution of grief is often accompanied by a message that a lack of resolution could lead to dire emotional problems or psychiatric illness. Currently, there is a serious movement to develop a new category for DSM IV, called Traumatic Grief.[5] A small minority of people who have experienced a loss may, in fact, suffer from such a syndrome.[4] However, if this initiative succeeds, it will have repercussions for how we consider the bereaved. They become persons who are suffering from a psychiatric diagnosis or a condition eligible for reimbursed services from mental health professionals. There may be a benefit here for some in making services thereby available, but I believe we need to consider what it means when predictable, expected aspects of the life cycle experience are called disorders that require expert care. We need to consider how to promote care and concern for and with the bereaved in the community in which they live and in the helping networks in which they participate.

The approach that I am proposing here is grounded in an understanding that our values, attitudes, and beliefs about death and bereavement are not fixed in stone, but are responsive to and modified by dynamic historic, economic, and social forces.[6] French cultural historian Philippe Ariès described how significant changes in attitudes and values have led to new understandings of death and of grief over time.[7] His work offers evidence of the socially constructed nature of attitudes about death. Practically, this means that what is expected of us as mourners and what we expect of others who mourn with us varies across time, place, and culture.

A relational and developmental lens focuses both on the relationship that is lost and the changes that ensue from this loss. It assumes that the mourning individual's sense of self is integrally linked to the relationship with the deceased. One's experience as the parent of a particular child, for example, continues to shape one's sense of self, even if this child dies. Relationships with others frame our sense of self and how we live our lives. To understand the ripples set off by an individual death, we need to ask who the deceased was and what role he or she played in the lives of those who are mourning this death.[8] Emphasis on relationship as central to individual development is consistent with earlier sociological and psychiatric theory[9] and has gained new importance in light of research focused on women's experience.[10,11] Recent work has focused on the importance of relationships in girls' and women's lives and has contributed to the articulation of a new goal of human development—one that values mutuality and interdependence rather than autonomy and independence. This perspective now informs our understanding of all human experience, not just that of women, and provides new insights into the meaning of loss in the life of the individual mourner, the family, and the community in which they live. It helps us to understand that when a death occurs more than a life is lost; a relationship is broken, yet this relationship does not end with death. The relationship may end in one sense, but in another it goes on as we find new ways of remaining connected. As David Browning notes, "It was the notion of saying goodbye that I had trouble with." Similarly, in another Personal Reflection, Christian Busch, a Danish chaplain, describes his work with a grieving mother and how she found a way to express her feelings about the loss of her son. This mother does not use the language of letting go or closure, but rather speaks of creating a healing story, which allows her to hold on to her memories of her child and her love for him. In looking at programs for the bereaved, we need to ask how they help the bereaved change their relationship to the deceased so that they can find ways of remaining connected that are appropriate to who they are and to their relationship to the deceased. The process changes and grows as those mourning the death do.[8]

LOSS ENTAILS DISRUPTION AND ACQUISITION OF NEW ROLES

Some losses require the bereaved to assume new, often unwelcome, roles, such as "widow," "orphan," or "single parent." In these new roles, the bereaved must not only grapple with grief, but also find new ways of living in the world given this changed situation. Habits of daily living are irrevocably changed and cannot be reconstituted as before.

Facing new challenges can be the impetus for development that involves new ways of understanding one's self and the world.[12] Change takes place on many levels. On one level, the bereaved find new ways of relating to themselves and to others. They may see themselves as more sensitive or appreciate life differently. Values and attitudes often change. They begin to develop new stories about themselves, new ways of living in the world, of making meaning, of listening and of feeling heard. One way of describing this is that the bereaved develop a new capacity to be audience to their own performance and to their relationships with others.[13] David Slavitt, a poet and novelist whose mother was murdered in 1982, has written about the ways inconsolable grief can lead to a new identity. He wants health care professionals to resist the temptation to intervene and attempt to cure grief. He suggests that they work collaboratively to "ask each patient who he is and what he wants and what is acceptable to him."[14] Over time, bereaved people often speak of being empowered by the loss: they find themselves developing new voices, whereas before they were silent.

NO FORMULAS

There are no easy formulas for dealing with grief and bereavement and no real alternative to living with it and through it. As health care professionals and compassionate caregivers, we need to be sure that the readings that we suggest to the bereaved do not suggest otherwise. To cope effectively involves learning to live with the fact that people die and that the kind of change that comes with death is part of living. Yet how many of us live our lives with this as part of our awareness?

> *There are no easy formulas for dealing with grief and bereavement and no real alternative to living with it and through it.*

When death occurs, it is invariably accompanied by uncertainty and a bit of chaos. Yet, in the face of loss, we may look for structure and certainty, which often evade us. Coping styles differ, as do our understandings of death. These differences will influence our social and emotional resources. Some of these resources are consistent or compatible with our needs; others are not.

We need to find a language for recognizing that the processes that we have been talking about extend over many years and typically become part of the remainder of a mourner's life. In spite of my skepticism about a lock-step stage theory, we can look at bereavement as a developmental transition that unfolds with some sense of direction (not linear, but more of a spiral), with no set times when particular insights or understandings should occur. I see the process of bereavement as unfolding in various phases that reflect mourners' experiences. People are numb at the beginning, even when death was expected. There is an honest sense of disbelief that this could happen. It is difficult to take death in all at once, and often years later the unreality of the loss still lingers. Most people realize that the person is indeed dead, but only gradually are they able to allow themselves the fullness of their feelings. While they may move toward their pain, they may use distraction to move away from it, and this in part is the nature of the spiral to which I am referring.

WHAT HELPS? THE IMPORTANCE OF COMMUNITY AND FRIENDS

Bereaved people need different kinds of help over time. Initially, they need friends to help with the concrete tasks of living and managing their family from the time before the funeral and immediately afterward as they try to simply keep on living with the pain and the stress. As time goes on, if existing friendship groups and community ties are not sufficient, sometimes new friends and communities can emerge from places that provide opportunities to explore ways of coping with the loss and expand the bereaved's repertoire of coping skills. Sometimes these opportunities come from formal helping programs, sometimes from meeting others through friends and in the community.[10]

Many people find that religion can be very important in trying to find a way of living with the fact that people die. Religious groups can rally to form a helping network at the time of death. Funeral directors may offer after care programs, as well. People need help in establishing a lifestyle appropriate to their new situation. This sense of need may be felt one or two years after the death or even longer. Resources for help still need to be there whenever the bereaved feel ready to access them.

Not everyone is a talker. We know that some men find talking in support groups less helpful than being involved in activities that distract or require physical energy. Most bereavement workers note that women are more likely to want to process and talk about what they are experiencing. Some question whether these qualities in men and women are really gender specific or relate more to coping styles.[15] Whatever the gender or coping style, help must be responsive to the needs of the bereaved. Help must legitimate their feelings and provide them with the opportunity, information, and support they need to learn how to live in their new role in the world.

How support is provided at the time of death and how mourners respond tell us something about the way that relationships are valued in a community, how care and concern are expressed, and how much a community recognizes the interdependence of its members. A strong mission to serve families and the larger community may be an important element in what fosters innovative approaches to bereavement care, such as at St. Vincent's and the UCSF program. It is noteworthy that both of these institutional efforts depend on staff donating their time in order for the program to succeed. In fact, many bereavement programs involve volunteers who come to this work from their personal experience with grief, which informs their interest in helping. The Widowed Person's Service of the AARP and the Dougy Center for Bereaved Children in Portland, Oregon, have developed in exquisite detail programs for training volunteers to use their personal experience well.

INTERVENTIONS: REBUILDING A LIFE

If we think of bereavement as a time of transition, what do people need to know in order to make this kind of shift? The work of Irwin Sandler, Tim Ayers, and their colleagues at the Prevention Research Center at Arizona State University exemplifies how a psychological and educational program can provide concrete ways to help both bereaved parents and children to adapt to the new family constellation and its shifting roles. These researchers have designed two dovetailed courses for surviving spouses and bereaved children, respectively, to teach skills that help the family to invent new ways of living in the face of the loss of a parent or spouse.* Pathfinders, another skills development program, emerged from the observation of the need among the elderly widowed for more information about how to care for their own health and how to live alone. Michael Caserta, Dale Lund, and Sarah Rice found that the widows and widowers who participated in this course improved their perceived competencies in a variety of self-care skills.[16] Specifically, enduring physical activities, identifying and using community resources, organizing and using sources of help, and simple yet important life skills, such as keeping a household organized and keeping tax information, were all domains in which the participants reported improvements.

HEALING STORIES

There are many ways in which people integrate their loss into who they are and will become. The bereaved themselves are often quite creative in terms of coping

---

*See Vol. 3, No. 6 (November–December 2001) of the online journal *Innovations in End-of-Life Care* at <www.edc.org/lastacts/> to read more about the Family Bereavement Program at Arizona State University.

with loss. As caring professionals, we need to be sure to hear their voices and let ourselves learn from them. One family I know goes to the cemetery on their father's birthday with a bunch of balloons that they release, and then they go to his favorite ice cream parlor. Many use the arts and literature to not only connect to the deceased in meaningful ways, but to find a way of talking about their experience. Literature can help the bereaved make some sense of their changing life story, as demonstrated in Christian Busch's Personal Reflection, in which he uses the Danish writer Isak Dinesen's piece, "The Roads of Life" from *Out of Africa,* to catalyze new ways of making meaning of loss. Writing poetry, keeping a journal, or expressing oneself through painting or sculpture can also be therapeutic.[17,18]

SUPPORT GROUPS

Support groups provide people with an opportunity to learn from each other. Peer support is needed throughout the life cycle; at each new stage or phase, people seek to learn from others who have gone before. Learning is easier when the helper is one step ahead of the person in need and has experience with the problem to use as a guide. In addition, dealing with a peer is a way of normalizing the experience. With time, this kind of experience provides the opportunity for mourners to "repeople" their lives with new friends, new activities, and new foci for some of their energies.[19]

Many benefits can ensue from participation in a well-run support group. These include feeling cared about and understood, discovering a common language, developing a sense of mutual obligation, gaining new information, and learning new skills, as we see in the examples provided by Pathfinders and the Family Bereavement Program at Arizona State University. Additionally, in her contribution, Yvette Colón offers a concise review of some Internet bereavement support groups and raises issues to consider when using this new medium to create community and support for this longstanding need.

JOINING A CAUSE, CREATING A MOVEMENT

The impetus for some powerful advocacy, educational, and support groups comes from the bereaved themselves, which exemplifies the creative transformation of grief. Compassionate Friends, Mothers Against Drunk Driving, and the Louis Brown Peace Institute are examples of what bereaved parents and friends can accomplish out of their pain.[†] In my experience, we learn from these organizations that the bereaved themselves are the most effective "helpers" of the bereaved. They can really listen, as well as allow others to listen and hear one another, thus en-

---

[†]Visit the websites of these organizations at <www.compassionatefriends.org>, <www.madd.org>, and <www.institute4peace.org>.

hancing the lives of the bereaved and creating a sense of community as people learn to be there for one another over time in both recipient and helper roles.

IN SUM

Those of us who work in this area are always faced with our own humanity. We will all know death and grief in our lives. In a sense, we are each our own laboratory, using our own experiences to test out theory and practice.

REFERENCES

1. Lindemann E. Symptomatology and management of acute grief. *American Journal of Psychiatry*. 1944;101:141-148.
2. Silverman PR, Klass D. Introduction: What's the Problem? In *Continuing Bonds: New Understandings of Grief*, D Klass, PR Silverman, SL Nickman (eds.). Washington DC: Taylor & Francis, 1996 3-27.
3. Silverman PR, Nickman SL. Children's Construction of Their Dead Parent. In *Continuing Bonds: New Understandings of Grief*, D Klass, PR Silverman, SL Nickman (eds.). Washington, DC: Taylor & Francis, 1996, 73-86.
4. Stroebe MS, Hansson RO, Stroebe W, Schut H. Concepts and Issues in Contemporary Research on Bereavement. In *Handbook of Bereavement Research: Consequence, Coping and Care*, MS Stroebe, RO Hansson, W Stroebe, H Schut (eds.). Washington, DC: American Psychological Association, 2001, 3-22.
5. Prigerson HG, Jacobs S. Traumatic Grief as Distinct Disorder: A Rationale, Consensus Criteria and a Preliminary Empirical Test. In *Handbook of Bereavement Research: Consequence, Coping and Care*, MS Stroebe, RO Hansson, W Stroebe, H Schut (eds.). Washington, DC: American Psychological Association, 2001, 613-645.
6. Fulton R, Owen G. Death in Contemporary American Society. In *Death and Identity*, 3d ed., R Fulton, R Bendickson (eds.). Philadelphia: Charles Press, 1994, 12-27.
7. Ariès P. *The Hour of Our Death*. New York: Alfred A. Knopf, 1981.
8. Silverman PR. *Never Too Young to Know: Death in Children's Lives*. New York: Oxford University Press, 2000.
9. Sullivan HS. *Personal Psychopathology, Early Formulations*. New York: W.W. Norton, 1972.
10. Gilligan C. *In a Different Voice: Psychological Theory and Women's Development*, 2d ed. Cambridge, MA: Harvard University Press, 1993.
11. Brown LM, Gilligan C. *Meeting at the Crossroads: Women's Psychology and Girls' Development*. Cambridge, MA: Harvard University Press, 1992.
12. Kegan R. *The Evolving Self: Problem and Process in Human Development*. Cambridge, MA: Harvard University Press, 1982.
13. White RW, Epston D. *Narrative Means to Therapeutic Ends*. New York: W.W. Norton, 1990.
14. Slavitt DR. The treasures of grief. *Journal of Pain and Symptom Management*. 2000;20(5):357.
15. Martin TL, Doka K. *Men Don't Cry: Transcending Gender Stereotypes of Grief*. Philadelphia: Bruner/Mazel, 1999.

16. Caserta MS, Lund DA, Rice SJ. Pathfinders: A self-care and health education program for older widows and widowers. *Gerontologist*. 1999;39(5):615–620.
17. Hotch P. *No Longer Time*. Albuquerque, NM: La Alameda Press, 2001.
18. Henderson C. *Losing Malcolm: A Mother's Journey through Grief.* Jackson: University Press of Mississippi, 2001.
19. Silverman PR. The widow as a caregiver in a program of preventive intervention with other widows. *Mental Hygiene*. 1970;54(4):540–547.

A Weekend Retreat for Parents and Siblings of Children Who Have Died

An Interview with ROBIN KRAMER, MS, RN, PNP

University of California San Francisco Children's Hospital
San Francisco, California

Many families who experience the loss of a child also lose the supportive relationships that they have had with the health care providers who cared for their child throughout the course of his or her illness. The creation of the University of California at San Francisco (UCSF) Children's Hospital Bereavement Weekend Retreat was fueled by Robin Kramer's conviction that bereavement care for families is a responsibility of the health care professionals who treated the child and with whom the child's family has already developed a relationship. The retreat, which occurs in an outdoor setting over the course of a weekend, creates an opportunity for families of pediatric oncology and bone marrow transplant patients who died to reconnect with staff members who cared for the deceased child and to join with other bereaved families in remembering these children. The weekend contains a series of grief and bereavement workshops for parents and siblings, presentations by experts, and a memorial service. A unique feature of this program is the pairing of outside bereavement counselors with UCSF staff to co-lead support groups for parents and groups for siblings of the deceased children. The first retreat was held in 1994 and the fifth in June 2002. In the following interview, Robin Kramer MS, RN, PNP, speaks with Samantha Libby Sodickson about how the model for the retreat has changed over time and how she feels health care professionals can better serve the needs of families who have lost a child.

IMPETUS FOR THE BEREAVEMENT RETREAT

Samantha Libby Sodickson: *Can you describe the work that you do in your daily practice, and how you came to start the bereavement retreat?*

Robin Kramer: I have worked at UCSF Children's Hospital since 1983 as a pediatric oncology clinical nurse specialist and pediatric nurse practitioner. I function mostly in the advanced practice role of a clinical nurse specialist, although I do periodic, limited histories and physicals as they relate to handling problems, such as the management of side effects.

When I started at UCSF Children's Hospital as a new master's-prepared nurse, I was impressed with the home death program established by the division of pediatric oncology. Families were acculturated to the practice of family-centered care, which supported and even encouraged the choice of having their child die at home. The majority of children had planned home deaths. This was novel in 1983. It was, by and large, because of Arthur Ablin, MD, professor emeritus, who was the division chief of pediatric oncology at that time. Dr. Ablin had very strong feelings about end-of-life care for children and their families. His approach was based on the premise that one *always* provides treatment for children—treatment is never stopped. Dr. Ablin emphasized that the goals for treatment may change from cure to palliation, but that pediatric palliative care focuses on extending the child's life as long as possible while promoting comfort measures and quality of life. Dr. Ablin believed that children with incurable disease should, if possible, help to establish the goals for treatment with their families before choosing what this treatment should be. The goals for treatment determine the appropriateness of various treatment options. I was quite impressed with this philosophy and really embraced it—it felt like the right way to help children at the end of life and their families.

About seven years ago, we had an excellent conference at UCSF on grief and bereavement. Linda Silver, RN, MFT, a psychotherapist facilitator, presented core didactic content and conducted interactive group work with the staff. The group was multidisciplinary, with nurses, social workers, and child life specialists primarily in attendance. The conference helped us to identify and better understand the complex needs of families and staff with regard to grief and bereavement. At the end of the day, we participated in a brainstorming session to develop strategies that would address these needs. It became very apparent to me that we really had no formal bereavement follow-up. All of a sudden I saw how these relationships between families and staff, which often span several years and become very meaningful and supportive, come to an abrupt end when the child dies. I don't think we fully appreciate how important the support that families receive from us can be. What parents experience as helpful is not always obvious, sometimes it is just being there and listening—it isn't always about handling a crisis situation. But after the child dies, all that shared history and all that support seem to disappear.

> *It became very apparent to me that we really had no formal bereavement follow-up. All of a sudden I saw how these relationships between families and staff, which often span several years and become very meaningful and supportive, come to an abrupt end when the child dies. . . . But after the child dies, all that shared history and all that support seem to disappear.*

I think that the separation is also hard for the nursing staff. At the conference, there was some discussion about feeling guilty after a child dies—many times we never know if the families recover from their loss. Because we have primary nursing, the nurses on the floor often keep in touch with the families, but by and large it's on their own time; it's very informal and sporadic. Our social workers also provide bereavement follow-up, but, realistically, the needs of children and families at the medical center take precedence. It is often hard to find the time and energy to call bereaved families. It was clear that what we had in place was not an ideal bereavement follow-up program.

During this conference, we talked about how isolated families often feel after the death of their child. The feedback we had received from families indicated that there was a reluctance on their part to depend solely on friends for continued support. They found it difficult to talk to most people about their feelings, because they sensed that such discussion makes others feel uneasy. Often, bereaved families perceive that other people have an expectation that they should be getting on with their lives.

At that point, I realized that we were probably in the best position to offer support to families because we had experienced the child's illness and, ultimately, the child's death with them. Many of these families lived several hours from San Francisco, so I knew that we couldn't be responsible for *all* their bereavement support. Every community differs in how much support is available. If the child had died at home, families would have been connected with a hospice, which provides bereavement services. It occurred to me that we could try to augment what was already available in their communities. Families benefit from having different types and sources of support. I felt a strong sense of obligation and responsibility to these families for providing a piece of their bereavement care.

SLS: *Some grief and bereavement professionals believe that bereaved families find it too painful to reconnect with the people or place associated with their child's death. Can you speak to this concern?*

RK: My experience has been that, even though parents do find it difficult to return to the medical center, they seem to want to stay in touch with the people who cared about and cared for their child. It is the physical structure, not the health care professionals, that they associate with the child's death. This is not to say that families do not experience ambivalent feelings when they reconnect with hospital staff. Talking with or seeing people associated with their hospital experiences can bring back painful memories. I suspect this is the reason why we have had several families cancel their plans to attend the retreat at the last minute or just not show up.

GERMINATION OF THE RETREAT MODEL AND INITIAL FUNDING

SLS: *How did you come to see the weekend retreat as a solution?*

RK: When you call families periodically, as many follow-up bereavement programs do, it can be very limiting in terms of how much you can help them. There is only so much counseling or assessment that you can do on the telephone. I really felt that in order to provide something of significance to these families it would be helpful to have a face-to-face intervention that occurred over a longer period of time. At an intensive weekend retreat we can address difficult issues in more depth, and families can choose to engage at the level that is most meaningful to them. As staff, we have the opportunity to follow up with families and then to check in with them informally over the course of the weekend to see how they are doing.

SLS: *How did you make the jump from having the idea of an intensive weekend to implementing the steps to put the retreat together?*

RK: One of the things that made it possible was the availability of funds. In 1990, Patrick Thomson died from relapsed leukemia after a bone marrow transplant. He died at home just after his eighteenth birthday. His parents, Sheila and Ed Thomson, started a memorial fund at UCSF to honor his life. This money was earmarked for "supportive care," i.e., providing services or resources that could ease the burden for families with dying children. After we further defined the concept of a family bereavement retreat, I approached the Thomsons with the idea and they said, "Oh, that's perfect!" They felt very strongly that this was how the funds should be used. I told them that we might bring the account close to zero if we developed the retreat the way we ideally envisioned it, but they said, "Use it all. We'll raise more money." Having that money really broadened the range of possibilities of what we could plan for the weekend.

SLS: *What kind of institutional support have you had from UCSF Children's Hospital?*

RK: The institution believes that the program is very worthwhile and supports our efforts in a number of ways. Nursing administration's financial contributions have varied with each retreat, based on our requests. For example, they have provided gifts for families and staff, as well as honoraria for the keynote speakers. The institution also absorbs the costs associated with photocopying, mailings, and some administrative support. As the retreat date gets closer, a significant amount of time is spent at planning meetings on and off campus. Staff is afforded a great deal of autonomy and flexibility in determining how they allocate their time. Our institution is very proud of our continued efforts, which are responsible for an ongoing, successful program. In fact, the Bereavement Retreat Weekend received campus-wide recognition this past spring.

KEY CONCEPTS AND GUIDING PRINCIPLES: THE BACKBONE OF THE RETREAT

SLS: *What are the guiding principles used in conceptualizing the weekend? What key elements must be included in the retreat?*

RK: *Privacy*. We feel it is important for each family to have some privacy, so when we looked at places to hold the retreat, we didn't consider facilities that had dormitory-type housing. At the retreat, each family has their own room, with a shared bath at the end of a hall. If families have more than two or three children, then we give them two adjacent rooms. We found a place called Walker Creek Ranch, which is a really beautiful outdoor educational facility in northern California. It is set in lovely rolling hills, about 60 minutes north of San Francisco.

Pairing grief and bereavement mental health specialists with UCSF staff to co-lead groups. Although our staff is quite experienced in caring for dying children and their families, we acknowledged our limitations in terms of addressing families' grief and bereavement needs. We thought it would be valuable to develop programs for parents and siblings that were co-led by UCSF staff and outside facilitators who *specialized* in grief and bereavement support. The presence of USCF staff rekindles established relationships, which had supported families throughout the course of their child's illness and death. The outside mental health professionals offer expertise in bereavement counseling. Pairing these two groups as co-facilitators has strengthened our programming. We have found this model to be very effective.

Comprehensive parent program. Several program components are included in the parent's program. The first is a keynote address, "The Layers of Grief," which sets the stage for the weekend. Parents and young adult siblings attend this presentation. When we began, we tried to find out if there were other groups who were already doing this kind of work and if they had identified the range of topic areas that might be helpful for bereaved parents. Compassionate Friends* had an annual conference, and their program included concurrent, mini-workshops on different topics from which participants could choose. We decided to use this same model for our program, but co-lead each session by UCSF staff and mental health specialists experienced in bereavement issues. These sessions include a variety of topics, such as A Father's Grief, The First Year of Grief, Grief and Marriage, Anger and Guilt, and Supporting Siblings. We have added a new session or two at each subsequent retreat based on the feedback we have received from families.[†]

Free babysitting for children under three years old. We realize that parents cannot take full advantage of the program offerings unless we provide babysitting for the very young children, those younger than three years of age. We wanted parents to be able to participate in these workshops without having a six-month-old in their lap or a toddler running around. We found experienced babysitters, all of whom were 18 years of age or older. At the last retreat, six babysitters cared for 12 young children, including 2 children with special needs.

Comprehensive children's program.[‡] We place the children (ages three and

---

*Compassionate Friends is an organization designed to assist families toward the positive resolution of grief following the death of a child of any age and to provide information to help others be supportive. Visit Compassionate Friends on the Web at <www.compassionatefriends.org>.

[†]See Appendix B, p. 365, for the Breakout Session Topics Handout.

[‡]I consulted with two program coordinators/therapists at the Hospice of Marin to create our children's program.

up) in age-based groups depending on the number and ages of children who sign up for each retreat. We create very specific, age-appropriate therapeutic activities, which include an ice-breaker group activity, an introduction to the project, a specific project with a theme around grief or bereavement issues, and a closing activity. At the most recent retreat, we had 10 project facilitators (UCSF staff and therapists experienced in childhood bereavement) who directed the children's activities along with assistance from "camp counselors," who are also UCSF staff nurses and child life specialists assigned to each age group. Examples of projects include making memory boxes and mandalas or shields of strength. These kinds of activities are interspersed with fun, group-building activities, such as a ropes course, field sports, a creek walk, and swimming.

With each retreat, the children's program has grown in size. For the last retreat, surviving siblings were divided into four groups. The preschool group (ages 3 to 5) had 10 children with three camp counselors; the early school age group (ages 6 to 8) had 8 children with two camp counselors; the older school age group (ages 9 to 12) had 15 children with four camp counselors; and the teen group (ages 13 to 17) had 14 adolescents with three camp counselors.[§]

Family time. We want to make sure that family members have time to connect and debrief with one another. It seems natural that mealtimes should be family time, so children eat all meals with their parents. A square dance Saturday night has proved to be a marvelous way for families to just have fun together at the end of the day.

Remembering the children who died. Families send photographs of their deceased children to us beforehand so that we can make photo buttons for them to wear. It is important to acknowledge that all the children who have died continue to be important family members. Their untimely death is what brings us together as a group. Even though they are physically absent, their presence is keenly felt throughout the weekend.

A nondenominational memorial service called "A Time for Remembering" takes place on Sunday morning and lasts approximately 30 minutes. We gather together in an outdoor theatre-style area while music is playing. Our chaplain leads the memorial service, which includes both songs and readings. The names of the children who have died are read by a group of four staff nurses from the pediatric oncology and bone marrow transplant units. We close the service by placing flowers, either live or silk, on a large barren branch, symbolizing the continuation of life and hope. We encourage family members to think a special thought, prayer, or message for the deceased child as they place the flower on the branch. The memorial used to be at the end of the retreat on Sunday morning, right before lunch, after which time people left for home. At the last retreat we held the memorial service mid-morning, followed by a closing address, and lunch. We made this change because we wanted to end the weekend with an uplifting closing speaker. We were hoping it could be somewhat inspirational for the families, maybe reaffirming that there can be enjoyment of life along with very bittersweet memories.

[§]See Appendix B, pp. 366–370, for the Children's Program Bereavement Retreat schedule.

We think that adding a closing address helped families and staff feel stronger when they left the retreat, and not feel so overwhelmed with sadness.

Time for relaxation, fun, and networking among families. It is important to build in time for relaxing and networking. For parents, we schedule a square dance Saturday evening and a nature walk for Sunday morning. We also hope that families connect and network during mealtimes. During the welcoming orientation on Saturday morning, just prior to the keynote address, we acknowledge that the weekend holds a full schedule with content that may be overwhelming. We encourage parents to skip a breakout session if they need time to themselves. They can take a walk and enjoy the beautiful surroundings or even take a nap.[||]

ORGANIZING THE RETREAT: LOGISTICS AND LESSONS LEARNED

SLS: *Who worked with you initially to put the retreat together?*

RK: A small, multidisciplinary group organized the first retreat.[¶] Our planning group has grown to include about 15 individuals, with representation from nursing, social work, spiritual care, and child life. The final product results from the synergy of everyone's creativity, commitment, and compassion.

No *one* person can plan it all. I am largely the detail task master—I keep track of all the details, figure out all that needs to be done, work out the timeline for getting it done, and make sure that we're on track at different time points. One thing we have found that works well is delegating different pieces to smaller groups of people. We have had several mini task forces of two to three people working on different areas and this has helped make things run smoothly.

SLS: *How are physicians involved?*

RK: Physicians were not represented in the planning phase, although many participated by attending the retreat. They most often come to the memorial on Sunday morning and then stay for lunch. Some of them, who can't make the memorial service, come for dinner on Saturday night and stay for the square dance later that evening. For the past two retreats, two physicians have co-led breakout sessions. The physicians have become more involved over time and are very supportive of our efforts.

SLS: *Do you have any insight as to why it's hard to get all the clinical staff to participate?*

[||]See Appendix B, pp. 371–372, for the Family Bereavement Retreat Program Schedule.
[¶]The planning committee for the first bereavement retreat in June 1994 included Linda Abramovitz, MSN, RN, Adrianne Burton, MA, RN, Sarah Gordon, BSN, Robin Kramer, MS, RN, PNP, Judith Laughlin, LCSW, Cathy Portje, MSW, Rev. Rodney Seeger, MDiv, BCC, and Janet Veatch, MS, RN.

RK: There are multiple reasons why all the staff do not participate. Some people are very protective of their private time. Sometimes, unfortunately, people just feel uncomfortable or uneasy with bereaved families. I suppose that they feel that it is too depressing. Also, when staff members have experienced a recent serious illness or death in their own families, some have chosen not to participate. We have been very supportive of that decision. Then, of course, there is a group of staff who must work at the hospital that weekend, so they cannot attend. Over the years, as staff members have learned more about the retreat weekend, their level of participation has increased.

SLS: *How many families do you invite to the retreat? How many attend?*

RK: We invite all families whose child died within the past five years and who speak English (even if it is a small amount) or Spanish. All mailings are translated into Spanish. Some children come to UCSF Children's Hospital from all over the country or world for special treatments. If they were primarily treated elsewhere and only came here for specialized treatment, then we do not invite them. We probably had about 45 adults and 30 surviving siblings at the first retreat in 1994. The number of participants has grown at subsequent retreats. We probably invited close to 110 families for our June 2000 retreat. We were expecting 78 parents (from 45 families), but only 60 actually attended (representing 37 families). That is a 23 percent cancellation rate, in term of parents, or 18 percent in terms of families, which I believe is higher than for the previous retreats. Some families called several days before to cancel and others just didn't come or only the mother came with the children. We were expecting 79 children, including young adult siblings, but only 59 came. A large cancellation or no-show rate makes it difficult to coordinate resources based on accurate numbers of expected participants.

SLS: *Were there any changes made to the basic structure from year to year?*

RK: Starting with the third retreat, we decided to find a way to include Spanish-speaking families. We hired one of our medical interpreters to provide simultaneous interpretation of the opening keynote address from English into Spanish, with headphones for the Spanish-speaking participants. In addition, we found bilingual therapists to lead a Spanish-speaking support group.

We have simplified the process of choosing breakout session topics over time. The first year we asked adults to select their top three choices from a list of 10 topics on the registration form. It proved to be quite a chore to collate these choices, figure out which topics we were going to offer at each of the three breakout sessions, and then to assign people to their first three preferences. In subsequent years, we have simply offered seven to nine choices for each of the three breakout sessions and let people choose what to attend. We have come to learn which topics are the most popular and try to include them twice during the weekend. At the June 2000 retreat we offered a writer's workshop as a strategy to help parents to work through their grief.

At the last three retreats, we have given each family a gift. The gift is a welcoming gesture, as we leave a card with the gift in each room for the family to find on their arrival. The gift also serves as a memento of the weekend to take home. Many people believe the butterfly represents life in the hereafter when one's spirit is set free. We have seen many families who have had a loved one die gravitate toward butterfly objects. One year, I found a little pewter butterfly stand holding a rose quartz egg (rose quartz is a symbol of love), which we gave to the families. In 2000, my colleague, Janet Veatch, found beautiful blue and white porcelain butterfly boxes to give to the families.

SLS: *Is it hard for the families to leave the retreat? What kind of follow-up do you have after the weekend?*

RK: We do try to warn the parents as they leave that there might be a little bit of a letdown. Throughout the weekend they have been in an environment where they felt comfortable and safe in talking freely to people who have had similar experiences. They were able to renew old friendships with staff and make new friends. Then they have to go back to their everyday lives where they do not have the same level of support for their grief. We address this difficult transition with families before they leave. We also send a follow-up note about a week after the retreat, acknowledging that it may have been difficult when they first returned home. We let them know that we are thinking of them and that we are very glad that they came to the retreat weekend. We encourage them to feel free to contact us should they have any questions or if any issues come up that they think we might be able to help them with. We often get personal notes from families after the retreat to thank us for providing this helpful weekend.

STAFFING AND COST OF THE BEREAVEMENT RETREAT

SLS: *Are the people who staff the retreat paid, or do they volunteer their time?*

RK: Outside bereavement specialists receive a $150 honorarium for co-leading a 90-minute support group. This really represents a small token of our appreciation, because the outside facilitators spend the better part of their weekend day involved in the retreat. About 80 percent of the therapists return year after year because it has been such a positive and rewarding experience. They feel very strongly that their participation has been worthwhile for families as well as for themselves.

All the approximately 25 UCSF staff members volunteer their time. I suspect that some people take compensatory days to offset the time that they spend at the retreat over the weekend. But during the planning months, many people put in extra hours at both work and home and are not compensated for this extra time. This is one of the biggest limitations of the retreat. It takes an enormous amount of effort to plan such a complex weekend. It would be difficult to offer it more frequently than every two years because of this reason. The retreat is a labor of love.

SLS: *How much does this kind of retreat cost? What sort of fund raising do you do in order to make sure that it happens?*

RK: The direct costs associated with the most recent retreat were approximately $16,000 to $18,000. Most of this figure represents the room and board for families and staff and the honoraria for the outside bereavement facilitators for the adult and children's programs. It also includes administrative supplies, snack foods, and art supplies.

The Patrick Thomson Memorial Fund has consistently covered the majority of the weekend's costs. We have not really instituted formal fundraising efforts, although several pharmaceutical companies have made donations on a regular basis. For the third retreat we applied to the National Children's Cancer Society, which gave us a generous grant to support the program's overall costs.

For our last retreat we had an unexpected donor, Wish Upon a Star, a local organization that grants wishes to children with life-threatening illnesses. The organization wanted to augment the support that they had already provided for many of these same families. Their generous donation helped cover the costs of honoraria for guest speakers and room and board costs for the families.

STAFF PREPARATION AND TRAINING

SLS: *Do you have any special training for the staff in preparation for the retreat?*

RK: Before the retreat, the children's program subcommittee meets four to five times as a large group and two to three times in smaller work groups to plan and discuss all the details of the various activities, including the necessary supplies. This subcommittee consists of five UCSF staff (two advanced practice nurses, one social worker, and two child life specialists) and five consultants who have an expertise in childhood bereavement (from two Bay Area hospices and a local college BSN nursing program).

Over the years, we have developed a core group of outside facilitators who have participated in multiple retreats. We try to pair them up with members of the UCSF staff with whom they have worked before. We do not require that co-facilitators meet ahead of time, but we encourage them to speak by telephone. We respect the fact that people have limited extra time and that they are professionals. Many do meet prior to the retreat, especially if they have not worked together before.

The training and orientation for staff who are not on the task force are mostly informal. The one group for whom we do target some specific preparation is the UCSF staff members who serve as *camp counselors* in the children's program. The task force member in charge of coordinating these staff provides them with an overview of the weekend, explains their role, and reviews the list of children that will be in their respective groups. The camp counselors receive the detailed children's program agenda to guide them through the weekend's activities. We do not have any specific grief and bereavement discussions before or after the retreat in terms of critical issues and the feelings that may be evoked. Although these camp counselors are experienced pediatric oncology nurses and child life specialists, more formal orientation training and debriefing would be optimal. We hope to address this for our next retreat.

STAFF DEBRIEFING

About 10 days after the retreat, we have a UCSF task force debriefing and evaluation session. We believe that there might be a benefit from having a short debriefing at Walker Creek Ranch immediately after the retreat, particularly with the camp counselors from the children's program. It has been apparent that a processing piece, in which the staff could sit and talk about the kids, what happened during the weekend, or what the families might be experiencing, would be helpful.

Asking staff to stay an extra hour or so Sunday afternoon, when they have just spent their weekend volunteering at the retreat, may be expecting too much. We will have to find ways to streamline, clean up, and efficiently debrief with staff so that they can get back to their own families.

EVALUATION AND FEEDBACK

SLS: *What kind of feedback have you had from the people who have been to the retreats, both staff and families?*

RK: Parents, staff, and the children fill out program evaluations that rate the accommodations and each specific activity in which they participated. We also include several open-ended questions about what they enjoyed the most and least, what they would like to see added at future retreats, and their overall impressions. The responses have been overwhelmingly positive. The feedback has indicated that our model and structure for the weekend seem to be meeting people's needs. I'd like to share a sampling of quotes from the different groups of participants— their own words summarize their impressions better than I can.

Outside bereavement co-facilitators' overall impressions of the retreat:

"I thought it was extraordinary. I was deeply touched by the whole experience. I felt privileged to be a part of it. I saw that the participants looked more relaxed by the end. Their expressions seemed lighter. Thank you for this opportunity."
"powerful and meaningful . . . "
"filled an important need for families"

Parents' comments:

"I left the retreat feeling good about where I am in my grieving with my son's death. I gained that mostly over the weekend."

"The family retreat offered me a place to openly mourn the death of my son. My grief was validated and my struggle was shared by others who truly understood the journey. It was a valuable support system."

Comments from children and teens:

"Sometimes kids (teens especially) don't understand the importance of talking about feelings, and they need a push—like the Rock Ceremony—I'd like to have more things like that."
"I loved the arts and crafts and the rooms and being with others."
"I liked everything. It was fun and we should do it again next year. I want my Dad to come."
"It was fun—the way that we got our own little groups and just had fun."

Several of the teens said that the worst part of the retreat was "having to leave"!

SLS: *Are you measuring any outcomes?*

RK: In terms of outcome measures, we have not done any pre- and post-testing to look at changes in areas such as coping, depression, or family functioning. However, recognizing the importance of outcome measures, I have been meeting with Betty Davies, PhD, RN in the School of Nursing at UCSF. We are trying to plan a bereavement research study that will involve the families at the 2002 retreat. I hope that we will be able to have more specific outcome data in the future by studying the impact of the retreat itself, as a bereavement intervention.

SLS: *How would you say the camp experience has affected your approach to bereavement and your clinical work at Children's Hospital?*

RK: I have come to appreciate how complex the bereavement and healing process is for families. I am committed to ensuring that the bereavement retreat weekend continues to occur every 18 to 24 months.

Shortly after the retreat in June 2000, I had an epiphany. I believe that what happens before the child dies, including the palliative care phase and how the transition from cure to palliation was managed, plays a critical role in families' bereavement experiences. We are zealous in our efforts to cure children—we use sophisticated diagnostic techniques, antibiotics, transfusions, radiation, surgery, and multiple chemotherapy regimens in our efforts to cure children. We need to have that same kind of zealous approach for effective symptom management and psychosocial support during the palliative phase of care. So, once I had time to regroup after that retreat, I decided I wanted to start a palliative care task force to look at how we might improve pediatric end-of-life care at my institution. I think that it should not be just for oncology patients; *all* pediatric patients need to be included. Although I have always had a strong interest in end-of-life care, the 2000 retreat really launched me in the direction of starting a pediatric palliative care program at UCSF Children's Hospital.

LIMITATIONS OF THE RETREAT MODEL

SLS: *What are the barriers to designing and implementing the retreat?*

RK: It takes an enormous amount of work to plan, organize, and implement this kind of event. We all agreed that the bereavement retreat was a great idea, it was needed, and it was the proper way to spend the funds from the Patrick Thomson Memorial account. But the question was how we could take on more work when we can barely get all the work done that we already need to do.

So, one of the key limitations of our program has been the amount of extra work that it entails, much of which is volunteer. Perhaps having access to a cadre of bereavement professionals who are willing to work for a token fee for the weekend is also a limitation to the program's being replicated on a broader scale in other parts of the country. However, the flip side of these possible limitations is that we succeed in spite of the amount of effort that it requires, which suggests that the program meets staff needs as well.

Another limitation of the program is our inability to support families who do not speak English. Unfortunately, we have had to exclude families who speak a language in which we do not have interpreters or fluent, trained therapists. In addition, we have not been able to help families who choose not to attend. Although we would love to expand our bereavement program by using additional ongoing interventions, we just do not have the resources, in terms of manpower and finances, to do so at this time.

ADVICE FOR REPLICATION: THE IMPORTANCE OF STRUCTURE

SLS: *What kind of advice would you give to other people who wish to replicate this kind of program?*

RK: I would suggest that they start with a large task group to share the planning and implementation responsibilities. They need to start by answering important questions, such as these: What kind of weekend do we want it to be? What are the basic principles that we want to incorporate? Do we have institutional support? What resources do we need to identify to help us to build a successful program? Then they just need to get started, working about one year in advance of the event.

The part that becomes very tedious and time-consuming is the administrative coordination of the program. I would advise others to get ongoing administrative support—people who can help with certain responsibilities, such as setting up meetings for the planning group and with outside consultants, organizing mailings, and handling various aspects of all the correspondence. Additional tasks could include collating descriptive statistics of who *does* and *does not* participate in the program. This kind of assistance would be tremendously helpful.

The other piece of advice I'd like to offer is to emphasize a structured approach to the weekend. We try to be as flexible as possible within a structured framework of presentations and mini-support groups that are run by staff experienced in bereavement issues. We always give parents the option of participating in as much or as little as they are comfortable with while they are at the retreat. For example, we have an opening introduction and welcome, and we say to them, "If you need to leave this keynote address, get up and leave. That's perfectly fine. If you go to one workshop and then find you need to take a break, skip the next breakout session. Go take a walk. Go take a nap. Participate at whatever level feels comfortable. We are all here to support one another." We stress this message over and over again throughout the weekend. If parents signed up for one workshop two weeks ago and now they think that they want to go to a different one, they can make the change. I believe it is helpful to create and offer a structured series of events and then be prepared to be flexible, because participants' needs and readiness to engage in the activities will differ.

CONCLUSION

SLS: *Can you summarize what you hope that families take away from this kind of intervention?*

RK: I don't have any grand idea that families come to terms with their grief at the retreat or that one weekend radically changes their lives and where they are within their healing process. What I hope it does is help to move them a little along the way, particularly for families who might have been feeling immobilized or that just couldn't pick themselves up. Sometimes people can feel so overwhelmed and so alone that they don't know which way to turn. My hope is that this weekend acts like a compass, to point them in the right direction. I hope that the retreat helps families to find the path to healing and that it gives them some insight, strength, and support to be able to continue moving forward.

> *Sometimes people can feel so overwhelmed and so alone that they don't know which way to turn. My hope is that this weekend acts like a compass, to point them in the right direction.*

On Creating a Healing Story: One Chaplain's Reflections on Loss, Grief, and Bereavement*

CHRISTIAN JUUL BUSCH

Rigshospitalet
Copenhagen, Denmark

When you tell a story, you mend things that are broken.
—Karen Blixen (Isak Dinesen)

Danish novelist Karen Blixen is describing a key existential and spiritual truth that lies at the heart of the practice of palliative care. Story—language—provides a means of healing something or of creating something new. I will paraphrase Gregory Bateson, whom I credit with formulating the following idea that has informed my work: Until you have said what you are thinking, you cannot think about what you have said![1]

This essay derives in part from my experience as a hospital chaplain at Rigshospitalet in Copenhagen, Denmark, where I have worked for 15 years with patients who are gravely ill and with bereaved family members. I would like to reflect on how we can support people in saying the things that they are thinking and, subsequently, how we can help and challenge them into thinking about what they have said.

First, I will review certain theoretical concepts that inform the ongoing discussion about loss, grief, and bereavement and our attitudes toward patients and relatives in palliative care. In this review, I am very much inspired by the work of the British sociologist Tony Walter. Next, I will proceed to look at some of the ways in which patients and relatives often speak about loss toward the end of life and

> *I would like to reflect on how we can support people in saying the things that they are thinking and, subsequently, how we can help and challenge them into thinking about what they have said.*

*This essay is based on the talk "The Healing Story: Bereavement, Loss, and Grief," given by the author at the VIIth Congress of the European Association for Palliative Care in Palermo, Italy, on 4 April 2001.

grief after the loss of a loved one. My intention here is to demonstrate how an existential attitude toward loss can enable us to help people to express their thoughts—i.e., to say what they are thinking. Finally, I will provide an example from my own practice, working with a group of bereaved family members of deceased children, of how to guide and support patients and relatives in creating a story frame. Given a starting point grounded in an existential understanding of loss, I will illustrate how telling a particular story helped one mother to reflect on the meaning of her child's life and her own grief—that is, to construct a healing story.

ONGOING DISCUSSION OF LOSS, GRIEF, AND BEREAVEMENT

One of the most influential theories in loss, grief, and bereavement over the past decade is that of William Worden, which identifies four tasks that the bereaved must accomplish:[2]

1. Accept the reality of the loss
2. Experience the pain of the grief
3. Adjust to an environment without the deceased
4. Relocate the deceased and move on with your life

Worden's theory emphasizes breaking the emotional bonds with the dead person and letting go of the deceased as the necessary route to adjustment.[3] The translation of this theory into practice has focused largely on helping the bereaved to open up to and articulate their emotions.

Practitioners working in the field of bereavement have taken it for granted that the task of working through and experiencing the pain of loss is necessary if the bereaved person is to let go and move on. But is this right? Do all bereaved people let go and move on?

I find this model too narrow to accommodate the wide range of human experience as I've observed it. Others have also critiqued this theoretical framework for understanding grief and bereavement. Margaret Stroebe notes that there is very little scientific evidence on the grief work hypothesis and that the studies that bear on this issue yield contradictory results.[4]

Tony Walter expands this critique as he describes a shift from a modernist era, in which counselors expertly manage a predictable grief process, to a more postmodern individualizing of loss and grief and a rejection of grand theory.[5] The current discussion among researchers indicates that clinical praxis needs a more nuanced framework than it did earlier.

Research increasingly indicates that a person's path through grief owes more to personality and habitual strategies for coping with stress than with any universal "grief process."[4] My experience working with the bereaved confirms this close connection between a person's outlook and personality and the way that the person expresses grief. For some people, the proper or appropriate expression of their grief is expressing endless grief. For others, repression of feelings is what feels most appropriate. The important message here is that each person's way of expressing grief is possibly the best way for this person.

To my mind, no one fundamental theory pertains to the experience of all bereaved persons. Rather, it is a question of drawing out different grief patterns.[6] This can be accomplished in a number of ways.

> *Research increasingly indicates that a person's path through grief owes more to personality and habitual strategies for coping with stress than with any universal "grief process."*

Wortman and Silver discerned three fundamental patterns based on their review of the literature. All three are equally valid approaches:

1. Moving over time from high to low distress
2. Never showing intense distress
3. Staying in high distress for years[7]

Although we as professional caregivers generally assume that it is better to release emotions (i.e., moving over time from high to low distress or staying in high distress for years) than to repress painful experiences (i.e., never showing intense distress), there is little evidence to confirm this conclusion. Walter notes that it can be fruitful to repress painful experiences.[6] Wortman and Silver point to the fact that the bereaved who do not feel struck by a crisis and consequently do not release their emotions seem to be doing no worse in the long run.

This discussion of patterns of grief leads to the related and pertinent discussion of whether bereaved people should "let go" or "keep hold" of the deceased. The current debate focuses on the possibility of a middle course, an oscillation between "letting go" and "keeping hold." "Oscillation," or "the swing of the pendulum," is a very important concept in describing the current tendency in bereavement research.

Shapiro notes that children generally oscillate between forgetting and remembering: "For children, the unremitting pace of adult grief is too intense, too much an interference with the necessary work of growing up. Children are more likely to put their grief down and pick it up again."[8]

In a recently published book on children's grief, Stine, a 14-year-old Danish girl, who lost her mother and her best friend to cancer, expresses this rapid oscillation in and out of grief. Stine wrote, "I began to think that I was bad luck. Everybody around me was going to die. . . . At [one] time I considered taking my own life because the pain was too great, but I soon changed my mind. The following weekend there was a [horse] rally, and I didn't want to miss that."[9] Her grief is intense, and so is her ability to forget. She swings like a pendulum between remembering and forgetting. It is not a question of one or the other. The bereaved have to move back and forth between emotionally founded grief work and a task-focused learning of new roles and skills. These two important tasks cannot take place at the same time. I have noticed a growing awareness of the need to find a language that accommodates this kind of individualization of the experience of grief. This attention to language and the pattern of oscillating between holding onto and letting go of grief is also important in my work with patients who are gravely ill or dying.

HOW CAN AN EXISTENTIAL PERSPECTIVE ENHANCE PATIENTS' ABILITY TO THINK ABOUT WHAT THEY HAVE SAID?

How do we transfer this principle of oscillation and the swing of the pendulum to the way patients speak of their losses? Listening to patients, I have found many converging points.

How do we express, from an existential point of view, what a person loses when he or she becomes incurably ill? Kjeld Holm, the Danish philosopher and bishop, has described such a loss in the following way: "The understanding of who you are, and consequently, the fundamental principles of your life, are destroyed or cannot be maintained."[10] The purpose of the existential/spiritual conversation is to generate, via this conversation, a renewed understanding of the dying person's changing meanings of life.

Have you ever heard a patient say, "The way I understand myself has been destroyed"? I have not heard that sentence, not even when I have had conversations with ministers or philosophers who were incurably ill. Then how do people speak of their understanding of themselves? Here are some examples from patients and relatives with whom I have worked:

"I have *always* been well, I have *never* been ill before." *Always* and *never* can be used in many different situations, but in conversations with seriously ill people, *always* and *never* frequently signal a key point in a person's fundamental understanding of life and of the self. As such, it is worth listening for these signals, as they may presage an utterance that illustrates how that person understands herself. This moment can also become a moment for a potential question about the understanding.

Let me illustrate with the following example: A 19-year-old professional athlete, one month before his death from leukemia, said, "I have *always* said: 'As long as you go out there and fight, you will win!'" If I ask him, "And how is it right now with that saying of yours?" I invite him to reflect on his actual situation, and he may start talking about his feeling of powerlessness and anxiety. "I have *always* said: As long as you go out there and fight, you will win!" describes his normal feelings of being in control. The question invites him to think about what he has said.

Realizing that life generally moves and exists within two opposing poles can inspire the hope of not being trapped in either false control or in powerlessness. The young athlete did swing like a pendulum between control and powerlessness. A life focused solely on positive aspects is equally as amputated as a life that only sees negative ones. A lived life is in constant motion between joy and sorrow,

hope and hopelessness, control and powerlessness, gratitude and bitterness, humor
and gravity. These swings of the pendulum are manifestations of movement and
life.[11]

In almost every conversation with patients and relatives you will find examples
of the way in which patients swing between onerous, heavy thoughts and light-
ness, between resignation and hope, or between despair and gratitude. The Swedish
oncologist and psychiatrist Loma Feigenberg listed the following opposing cate-
gories or dimensions that patients move
between like a pendulum:[12]

> *A lived life is in constant motion between joy and sorrow, hope and hopelessness, control and powerlessness, gratitude and bitterness, humor and gravity. These swings of the pendulum are manifestations of movement and life.*

In here	Out there
The right to know	The right not to know
Loss	Gain
Hope	Hopelessness (despair)
The will to live	The wish to die
Rebellion	Submission
Control	Powerlessness
Joy	Sorrow
Gratitude	Bitterness

One moment the patient concentrates on the changes happening *inside* him and
is preparing for his death; in the next moment he concentrates on the feeling that
something happens *to* him. Noticing these swings and seeing them as part of the
process can perhaps help patients. We acknowledge and confirm the patients'
conflicting experience. We can note that we did see how the patient made the
movement from resignation to hope or from despair to gratitude.

HOW CAN WE CREATE A STORY FRAME THAT LEADS TO A HEALING STORY?

In a paper entitled "A New Model of Grief," Tony Walter argues that bereavement
is a part of a never-ending and reflexive conversation with self and others through
which the late-modern person makes sense of their existence.[5] In other words,
bereavement is part of the process of (auto) biography. The biographical imperative—the need to make sense of self and others in a continuing narrative—is the
motor that drives bereavement behavior.[5]

The language of spirituality and of the existential aspects of palliative care is
very much based on narratives, on metaphors and stories. When Aristotle talks
about "the gift of the metaphor," he is speaking about how metaphor can open

a passage to a sudden recognition and understanding of a previously hidden truth.

Meaning exists not as something given, but as something that comes into existence when you take the things that happen in your life seriously. Active reflection on one's experience creates meaning. Meanings can be ambiguous and should, in some instances, be approached ambiguously.

> *Meaning exists not as something given, but as something that comes into existence when you take the things that happen in your life seriously. Active reflection on one's experience creates meaning.*

How can we help patients and relatives to tell a story with which they can mend things that are broken? What can we, as professionals, do to help them to say what they think so that they can think about what they have said? I will now describe a process that offers one way of helping patients tell or find healing stories. This process can lead to the creation of an individual story about loss, grief, and bereavement.

I was working with a group of parents, of whom had all lost a child to cancer. These parents all felt this loss, death following a painful disease, was senseless and unjust. During one of our sessions I told the following story, "The Roads of Life," from *Out of Africa*[13] by Karen Blixen (Isak Dinesen), to the group:

The Roads of Life

When I was a child I was shown a picture—a kind of moving picture as it was created before your eyes and while the artist was telling the story of it. This story was told, every time, in the same words.

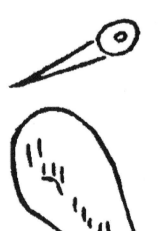

In a little round house with a round window and a little triangular garden in front there lived a man.

Not far from the house there was a pond with a lot of fish in it.

One night the man was woken up by a terrible noise, and set out in the dark to find the cause of it. He took the road to the pond.

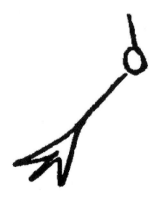

Here the storyteller began to draw, as upon a map of the movements of an army, a plan of the roads taken by the man.

He first ran to the South. Here he stumbled over a big stone in the middle of the road and a little farther he fell into a ditch, got up, fell into a ditch, got up, fell into a third ditch, and got out of that.

Then he saw that he had been mistaken, and ran back to the North. But here again the noise seemed to him to come from the South, and he again ran back there. He first stumbled over a big 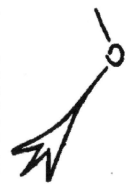 stone in the middle of the road and a little farther he fell into a ditch, got up, fell into another ditch, got up, fell into a third ditch, and got out of that.

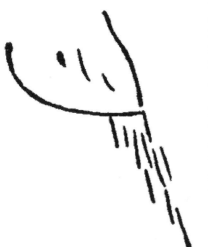

He now distinctly heard that the noise came from the end of the pond. He rushed to the place, and saw a big leakage had been made in the dam, and the water was running out with all the fishes in it. He set to work and stopped the hole, and only when this had been done did he go back to bed.

When now the next morning the man looked out of his little round window—thus the tale was finished, as dramatically as possible—what did he see? A stork!†

Karen Blixen, reflecting on the meaning of this story, then wrote:

I am glad that I have been told this story and I will remember it in the hour of need. The man in the story was cruelly deceived, and had obstacles put in his way. He must have thought: "What ups and downs! What a run of bad luck!" He must have wondered what was the idea of all his trials, he could not know that it was a stork. But through them all he kept his purpose in view; nothing made him turn around and go home, he fin-

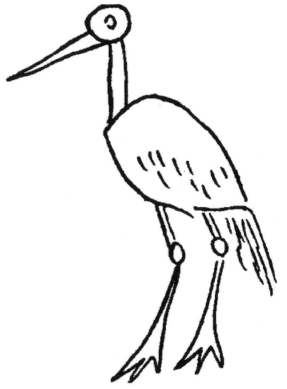

---

†Stork illustrations from *Out of Africa*, by Isak Dinesen. Copyright © 1938 by Random House, Inc. Copyright © renewed 1965 by Rungstedlund Foundation. Reprinted with permission.

ished his course, he kept his faith. That man had his reward. In the morning, he saw the stork. He must have laughed out loud then.

The tight place, the dark pit in which I am now lying, of what bird is it the talon? When the design of my life is completed, shall I, shall other people see a stork?[13]

At first glance, this is an absurd story. It seems completely senseless and ironic that a stork should represent the meaning of life. However, the fact that the story is absurd is actually an advantage, because it means that the reader or listener can construct and tell his or her personal story and meaning within that story.

Not long after I told this story during a group support meeting for these bereaved parents, I received the following letter from one of the parents, a mother, who expressed the significance of her son's life in the light of Karen Blixen's story. She wrote:

> I do not care much if I never see the stork myself; but I hope that my son saw *his* stork before he died. I have seen my boy's stork and it is incredibly beautiful. He fought for his life for five years, and while he fought he gave so many people so much love that we will always carry it with us. His life was more intense than it was short, and his soul was stronger than his body was weak. I cannot possibly find meaning in my son's death, but the meaning of his life turned out to be the abundance of love he gave and the love of life he expressed, and this has influenced everybody he knew. And they will always be influenced by this. I think that is a very beautiful stork. . . .
>
> Yes, I would like to thank him for the time we had. And then I would write a little about the world's greatest kid, whom I miss and mourn and love. But when I die the void and the mourning will vanish—as opposed to the love that will always be here!

The story about the stork obviously provided this mother with a frame to talk about the meaning of her son's life. It created a language in which she could talk about him in a new way. This is one of the important aspects of existential and spiritual care: to create an "open frame" in order to enable the patient or the bereaved to tell his or her individual story. I have used this example to demonstrate one way in which narratives can provide such an open frame.

If one succeeds in defining an open frame, it will be possible to help the bereaved to express how they "let go" and "keep hold" at the same time. Rather than experiencing the memory of the dead as painful and as a burden, bereaved people can experience warmth and pleasure from "keeping hold" of the memory, in the same way that this mother talked about the *love* and *pain*.

Tony Walter confirms that these relationships can continue to be crucial in the lives of the bereaved. He notes that people who have lost a close relative or friend retain a rather distinct image of the importance of the dead person in their lives for an extended period. The deceased can play one of the following four roles in the life story of the bereaved:

1. The deceased is a role model for the bereaved.
2. The deceased is someone who gives advice in particular situations.

3. The deceased is someone who outlines the basic values in life (this role is in particular granted dead children).
4. The deceased is a treasured part of the biography of the bereaved.[5]

One of Karen Blixen's most important mottos was, "Je répondrai," literally meaning, "I will give an answer." In other words, whatever challenges or troubles she met, she would respond to them. I find that this motto fits my own approach to palliative care. Patients and their families have widely different life experiences, hopes and fears. Whenever we meet people, we need to strive to cope with their situations, and never ever give up trying to find a way to help them. It is patients and families who should define what is helpful, rather than rigid theory that prescribes one right way to grieve the loss of a loved one.

REFERENCES

1. Bateson G. *Mind and Nature: A Necessary Unity*. New York: Bantam Books, 1979.
2. Worden JW. *Grief Counseling and Grief Therapy*, 2d ed., London: Routledge/New York: Springer, 1991.
3. Walter T. *On Bereavement: The Culture of Grief*. Buckingham, UK and Philadelphia: Open University Press, 1999.
4. Stroebe M. *Coping with bereavement: A review of the grief work hypothesis*. Omega (1992-3)26(1):19-42.
5. Walter T. A new model of grief: Bereavement and biography. *Mortality*. 1996;1(1): 7-25.
6. Walter T. *The Revival of Death*. London and New York: Routledge, 1994.
7. Wortman C, Silver R. The myths of coping with loss. *Journal of Consulting and Clinical Psychology*. 1989;57(3):349-357.
8. Shapiro E. *Grief as a Family Process. A Developmental Approach to Clinical Practice*. New York: Guilford Press, 1994, 14.
9. Rølmer S, Olesen P (eds.). *Børn om mors og fars død*. Copenhagen: Kroghs Forlag, 2000, 30-31.
10. Holm K. Sorgens sprog. *Trak af den principielle sjælesorg*. Copenhagen: Forlaget Aros, 1986.
11. Svarre HM et al. *Courage to Be: Teaching Material on Dialog with Cancer Patients*. Copenhagen: Danish Cancer Society, 2000.
12. Feigenberg L. *Terminal vård—et metod för psykologisk vård av døende cancerpatienter*. Lund, Denmark: Liber, 1977.
13. Dinesen I. *Out of Africa*. New York: Random House, 1938, 251-253.

Saying Goodbye, Saying Hello: A Grief Sojourn

DAVID BROWNING, LICSW, BCD

Lunenburg, MA

> *You say goodbye and I say hello*
> *Hello hello*
> *I don't know why you say goodbye, I say hello*
> *Hello hello*
> *I don't know why you say goodbye, I say hello.*
> —Paul McCartney

Like many of my generation, I lived my adolescence with a constant stream of Beatles' lyrics flowing through my consciousness. Many years later, this simple goodbye/hello refrain took on real existential bite. But I have gotten ahead of myself. This is the story of my expedition through grief, my own bereavement narrative.

When I was 13, busy learning about girls and how to be my own person, my mother lay in the bedroom of our house, dying of lung cancer. She died the gradual death familiar to families in which cancer has paid a visit. There was something cruelly ironic about having to reconcile the experience of living with a decaying mom while my own body was exploding with teenage desire. I was bursting into view, and she was fading.

> *There was something cruelly ironic about having to reconcile the experience of living with a decaying mom while my own body was exploding with teenage desire. I was bursting into view, and she was fading.*

There was no room for grief in a household of three boys and a father who, in his own encounter with grief, set the best example he knew: you pull yourself together; you get on with life. I remember little in the way of emotion or consolation, but I do remember the numbness. My mind remembers the numbness; my body remembers the numbness. The physical and emotional memory I carry of the months following the death is one of floating in a cloud of gray gauze: alone, desolate, but fully cushioned from pain.

Fast forward twelve years. *I am living on my own, working, socializing, but not really enjoying life. I know something is wrong, but I'm not exactly* *sure what it is. I contact a therapist, an older man who is known to have a gentle and thoughtful nature. The numbness I have come to know so well gives way to a deep mine of emotions. My new escort conveys with his warmth and presence that he will suffer with me whatever pain is unearthed. As the excavation proceeds, I struggle to reestablish what had been a long-interrupted communication with my mom. The conversation commences with fury. I write the following on May 9, 1977, my 25th birthday.*

On Visiting My Mother's Grave

If I could snatch you from your grave
If I could shake you from your slumber
If I could speak with you for five minutes
If I could hold your hand
If I could have your love
If I could only feel it
If it could only guide my days
If I only had it to fall back on
If you could be there when I need you.

Your death was vicious—and senseless.
They had no right
You had no right
To leave me alone.
You took away my bearings
And I have been detached
From people
From living
From myself.

I have been afraid to live or to love.
You took my joy with you
And if I dare to live or love again
To do so with abandon
I again take the risk
Of my joy being snatched away
Recklessly
To be buried in a box.

Safer to exist cautiously.
To not risk my love on living
Or risk my life on love.
Better to construct my own world
Of maximum security.
A maximum security prison
Where the only one
That can be dangerous to me
Is myself.

My therapist provided a loving, paternal space in which to discover the many painful parts of myself that had been sequestered outside my consciousness. I began to learn how central the pain was to my identity, yet how marginally I understood it. I also learned the professional language of the day: "grief work," "working through," "closure," "saying goodbye," and "moving on." I learned that grief was a process that one goes through, with a beginning, an end, and stages in between. I gleaned from all this that my therapeutic assignment was essentially to remember Mom, feel the pain, say goodbye to her, and move on with my life.

But there was a problem. Not with the remembering part, or the pain part, these parts came along well. It was the notion of saying goodbye that I had trouble with. In the process of connecting to my pain, I felt alive in ways I hadn't experienced in many years. The grief affirmed for me the love I had for Mom. However painful it was, it was simultaneously immensely reassuring and liberating.

Fast forward ten years. *I enter counseling for a second time, again with a male therapist, but one that is closer to me in age than the first. By this point I am married, the father of two young daughters, newly graduated from social work school, and engaged in my own practice of psychotherapy. Grief has become a familiar part of my emotional landscape. One looming aspect of the grief is a well of guilt that I do not fully understand. I have a nightmare that I am driving a car, my daughter in the back seat fastened in her carseat. I lose control of the wheel and we are heading for a cliff. I reach frantically for my daughter, but can't save her.*

Another problem is showing up in my personal world. I am keeping distance in relationships that should be intimate—my wife, my children, my friends. I am not allowing myself to be as close as I want to be, nor as close as they need me to be.

In the midst of the guilt and the distance, I struggle to find a stronger connection to Mom. I keep a journal of personal reflections; sometimes I write letters to her. It dawns on me one day that if I want more of a relationship I might need to generate some correspondence in return.

Dear David,

I want you to forgive yourself for any wrongs you think you have done. I want you to love again, with all your heart. I want you to feel safe and strong in keeping your heart open as much as you can. I tried to be the best I could in my life and that meant, first, accepting my pain and, second, finding the inspiration and support to live through it and beyond it.

By staying away from your grief, you have moved so far from your experience, from living life to its fullest. Open your heart, and I will be with you always. Close your heart, and you will lose your connection to me. I have given you the gift of love. In your grief is that love, and in loving is that grief. But your sorrow is a road that takes you to your joy, and it is a road that welcomes you.

To be on this road, you must give some things up. Foremost, you must give up your guilt, because it is guilt that keeps us apart, and that distances you from all that you love. It keeps you out of the world and inside yourself. You must choose to let go of all the guilt in the interest of life. You are strong enough to face your life without guilt, and to look life square in the eyes and say, "I belong here."

Make better friends with the pain that washes over you when you allow our connection to be. The greater the friendship you can make with your pain, the more natural will be your connection to your own loving nature. Then I will become an emblem for you of love and life, rather than of distance and death.

And remember, I am here when you need me.

> Love,
> Mom

My therapist helped me to understand how my grief was holding me emotionally in the past, and preventing me from investing myself fully in the present. He helped me to see how my emotional makeup was keeping me detached from the relationships that meant the most to me. I learned that I had internalized a deep sense of guilt from the events surrounding my mother's death, and that I feared on an unconscious level that I could not prevent disaster from occurring to the people I loved. The grief had become my avenue to feeling more alive and connected, yet it was keeping me detached from the circle of people who loved me. It seemed it should be time to "move beyond" the grief. It seemed it must be time for "closure." It seemed to make sense. Nevertheless, I resisted.

Fast forward seven years. *My oldest daughter is entering adolescence; my wife and I are inching toward midlife. I am busy counseling, teaching, and consulting in the bereavement field. I am beginning to see my grief as an eminent and powerful visitor, but one who has outstayed his welcome. I contact the therapist I had seen 17 years prior and agree to a predetermined number of sessions to work on the specific goal of setting loose this grief that has been such a familiar companion. The therapy is organized around designing, implementing, and processing a ritual involving "letting go."*

I carry out the four stages of the ritual over several weeks. First, I write on a piece of paper a list of the many ways that my grief is holding me back in my life, and make a commitment to let it go. Second, I burn the paper. Third, I spread the ashes in the ocean, at a spot that has special emotional meaning for me. Fourth, I find a picture of my mom and myself, have it enlarged and framed, and set it out in a prominent place in our home. (Prior to this, I did not have any photos of the two of us that were displayed in the open for others to see.) Afterward, I write:

Awaken

> Your death demolished my certain world,
> Your dying left me bereft;
> Your life was like an evening star,
> You came, you sparkled, you left.

You left me with my tarnished world,
Imperfect and out of joint;
But maybe that's the secret,
Maybe that's the point.

It's easy to love a childhood dream,
Made perfect by passage of years;
Much harder to love in the present,
With our doubts, our failures, our fears.

Grief can beat in a merciful rhythm,
Keeping time to a life-healing dance;
Yet at times it is served as a tonic,
Inducing a death-tainted trance.

So these ashes I spread on the water,
Resolving an old spell to break;
Not happy, not sad, not overjoyed,
Just choosing to live life awake.

This third therapy experience helped me to integrate and make meaning of my mother's death at a new level. Inherent in the ritual was an insight that, until that point, had eluded me. By spreading the ashes, I was not "saying goodbye" to Mom; nor was I "reaching closure" in my connection to her. I was making a commitment to no longer be defined by my grief. I was choosing to let go of the pain the best I could, and in so doing, to change the shape and texture of the continuing bond with my mom. In deciding to let go of my grief, I was creating the space for deeper relationships with all the people I love, *including* my mom.

There was a pivotal moment in the last therapy experience, one of those "a-ha!" events that sometimes occur when good psychotherapy is working its magic. At the time this happened I was 45, the same age as Mom when she died; my older daughter was 13, the age I was when Mom died. We were discussing the days surrounding the death when a memory came to me that I had previously kept from consciousness. I recalled the occasion, soon before she died, when Mom stopped talking to my brothers, Dad, and me, and turned her back to face the wall. (I have since learned that this is not an unusual happening. A dying person will often need to detach from loved ones shortly before death, perhaps to summon energy for the next passage.) Four thoughts or feelings occurred almost simultaneously. First, I remembered the anguish I felt when my Mom turned away from us; second, I imagined how my daughter would feel if I were dying and turning away; third, I imagined how it would be for me to be in that situation with my daughter; and fourth, I imagined how my mom must have felt, leaving three teenage sons and a husband.

I was overwhelmed with compassion for Mom. It was the first time in 30 years that I was able to set my own grief aside and empathize with hers. It was the first time that loving her could take precedence over my private experience of grief. It was the point when the frozen bond began to thaw.

It's Time

When you died, I wasn't ready.
I had to freeze you in time and space.
Like a child, grasping a popsicle,
Unwilling to acknowledge
The certitude of its melting.

Now it's time
(*Did we know it could take so long?*)
Thanks for staying frozen for me
(*What mothers will do for their sons!*)
But the meltdown is long overdue.

Today it is clear:
There are more pressing things to do
Than to deny our spirits their destinies.
I must get on with living;
You must get on with death.
Me, I intend
To free my heart
For . . . who knows what?

You, dear mother,
I imagine rising . . . rising . . .
Doing whatever it is
Angels need to do.

What does it mean to love someone after they die? Grief is a reflection of love, but the love I was feeling was a boy's love for his mother. The bond I was hanging on to was a boy's bond with his mother. Mature love is different from a child's love. Mature love requires that you set your own needs aside in caring for another. That day in my therapist's office, I shared for the first time in my mother's pain. The bond that had been so fixed and frail began to feel less clingy, more reciprocal, more flexible, more grownup.

Looking back, I see that learning to grieve was a vital, liberating, and cathartic process for me. I was able to connect to life and to my own feelings in whole new ways. When I was grieving, I was feeling the boy's love, and I was feeling alive. Grieving was my avenue to living again. Over time, however, it became clear that the very process that had been fundamental to my growth had become an obstacle to further growth. To connect to myself, I had learned to hold tightly to my grief. To connect to life and to others, I had to learn how to let it go. Grief had become familiar terrain, reliable territory. To let it go meant to move into life as it is, with all its uncertainty and unpredictability, as well as its joy.

> *To connect to myself, I had learned to hold tightly to my grief. To connect to life and to others, I had to learn how to let it go.*

In retrospect, I believe concepts like "saying goodbye," "finding closure," and "moving on" became stumbling blocks. All the knowledge I garnered from therapy, from the culture, and from my own professional training made me feel that "successful" grieving required me to say goodbye to Mom. I knew I needed to say goodbye in one sense; but, in a more important sense what I needed most was help in saying hello. Rather than severing a bond that was frail to begin with, I needed permission to nurture, strengthen, and deepen the connection to my mother. I needed support in constructing a richer and more flexible image of my mom that could evolve over time, so that the bond could mature accordingly. When I was finally capable of empathizing with my mom's pain, it became clear that the bond could be transformed. When I could say goodbye to my grief without saying goodbye to Mom, I was free to love more fully in the present.

It is in this context that the Beatles' lyrics take on their special meaning. The hello is much more robust and expansive than the goodbye. I say goodbye to the dominion of grief in my life. I say hello to my friends, my loved ones, and the infinite possibilities. And I say hello, in a new and tender way, to Mom.

Promising Practice

Reaching Out to Bereaved Family Members

An Interview with KATHY CARROLL, BSN, RN

St. Vincent's Hospital and Health Services
Indianapolis, Indiana

St. Vincent's Hospital and Health Services, which includes the 650-bed St. Vincent's Hospital and the 200-bed St. Vincent's Carmel Hospital, both located in Indianapolis, Indiana, has been involved in a nationwide effort to improve end-of-life care as part of Supportive Care of the Dying: A Coalition for Compassionate Care.* This coalition began in 1994 by Catholic health systems in Oregon in response to public outcry for legalized physician-assisted suicide. Since then this group has conducted nationwide focus groups of patients, bereaved family members, and professional caregivers to understand what is important in end-of-life care to these different stakeholders.[1]

As a result of its participation in this early focus group, research staff at St. Vincent's Hospital and Health Services began to develop some new comprehensive holistic health care services, including a Bereavement Care Track. This track offers next of kin of all those who died at either of these hospitals some free support services and referrals during the first year after death. In July 1997, Kathy Carroll, BSN, RN, initiated a pilot Bereavement Care Track in three units (the intensive care unit (ICU), the cardiac recovery unit, and the oncology unit), and in 1998 expanded these services to a few more units at St. Vincent's Hospital.[2] Now this service has expanded to cover the entire system, which has on average 88 deaths per month; of these, the majority occur at St. Vincent's Hospital, with only five to eight deaths per month occurring at Carmel Hospital. The Bereavement Care Track services are distinct from most in that a nurse and team of hospital staff volunteers (nurses and other professionals) make three phone calls to next of kin, at three to four weeks, three to four months, and six to seven months after death, respectively. During these calls volunteers inquire about family members' emotional and physical state and offer support services. Similar to most bereavement services, they mail out

---

*Supportive Care of the Dying publishes a quarterly newsletter, as well as researching projects and developing and testing new tools for members before they are offered to the public. For more information see <www.careofdying.org>.

a series of brochures at specific times during the first year after the death. A separate bereavement program, the infant loss program, has been in place at St. Vincent's since 1983. Ms. Carroll serves as bereavement care coordinator in both programs and has used lessons learned in the infant program to roll out this new effort to provide more proactive bereavement support system-wide. In the following interview with Anna L. Romer, EdD, Ms. Carroll describes the design and implementation of this new program, as well as what the particular phone calls entail and what staff at St. Vincent's has learned from bereaved family members about this service.

Anna L. Romer: *What is the main goal of the Bereavement Care Track?*

Kathy Carroll: The main goal of this intervention is to provide a resource and support through the grieving process to family members who have had a loved one die here.

ALR: *Can you describe how you identify all the deaths in your system?*

KC: The deaths in our system are identified through the security department. As a body and the accompanying paperwork are brought to them, they enter the deaths into the computer system, which feeds into my Access database program. So when I enter this death database, the information I find is: The first and last name of the person who has died, the date of the death, the unit that the person was on, the next of kin, and this person's address.

ALR: *Who identified this next of kin?*

KC: We ask patients to name someone local as next of kin when they are admitted. It is not necessarily a spouse or blood relative. There have been many times that I've called the person listed as "next of kin" and that person has said, "You really need to call this person because I just happened to be the caregiver at the time and his daughter is in Texas. So you probably need to call her." And I do then call the daughter in Texas. I have made calls throughout the United States, but I haven't called overseas yet. Figure 2 shows, step by step, the essential elements of the Bereavement Care Track.

ALR: *Could you explain the role of the physician end-of-life committee in the design and implementation of this program?*

KC: Sister Sharon Richardt, director of the St. Vincent Mission Services department, instigated the initial meeting to discuss the possible development of this program. The End-of-Life Committee, a physician-directed committee with members from throughout our institution, and of which Sister Richardt is a member, has overseen its development. The committee members continue to provide input and receive reports on every aspect of bereavement care. The bereavement task force, with members from Hospice, Pastoral Care, and the Infant Loss Program, of which I am a member, designed the actual program.

Essential Elements of the Bereavement Care Track

- *When death occurs:* Pastoral care provider or nurse gives "At the Time of Death" brochure to families.
- *Three to four weeks after death:* The bereavement care coordinator, bereavement care volunteer, or chaplain makes initial phone call to next of kin. We send out a sympathy letter with a personalized greeting, signed by the CEO of St. Vincent's and our Daughters of Charity Administrator, and a brochure listing support groups in the area.
- *Two to three months after death:* Bereavement care coordinator sends brochure on the dimensions of grief, along with a return post card listing seven educational brochures available on request, a checkbox to request information on the community support programs in their specific area, and an option for no further contact.
- *Three to four months after death:* Bereavement care coordinator or volunteer calls next of kin for second time. Pastoral care department hosts quarterly memorial services and invites family members to attend.
- *Four months after death:* Bereavement care coordinator sends out "A Time to Heal" brochure.
- *Six to seven months after death:* Bereavement care coordinator or volunteer makes third phone call to next of kin; this is the last scheduled phone call.
- *Nine months after death:* Bereavement care coordinator sends "As Time Progresses" brochure, a second personalized sympathy letter, and a satisfaction survey.
- *One year anniversary of death:* Bereavement care coordinator sends "Am I normal?" brochure along with a third personalized sympathy letter.

Figure 2.   Essential Elements of the Bereavement Care Track

During the creation and pilot stages of this program the bereavement care coordinator was housed in our Mission Services department. Once this program became system-wide, the program home was transferred to St. Vincent Hospice. The hospice is part of our health system, providing hospice care to patients who qualify.

THE INITIAL PHONE CALL

ALR: *Tell me about the initial phone call that you make to these family members. Is it a surprise or anticipated?*

KC: If the next of kin has read the brochure, the call would not be a surprise; often, however, they haven't read the brochure, so it is. The "At the Time of Death" brochure, which the nurse or chaplain provides to the family when the patient dies, lays out the follow-up care that we provide, including the phone calls.

ALR: *Do you know the details of the death when you make the call?*

KC: No. At St. Vincent's Hospital, it's a cold call. Most of my volunteers are not comfortable enough to make the first phone call when we don't know the cause of death. I've been doing these calls for so long that I no longer feel uncomfortable if a person says the death was a suicide. Some attempted suicides arrive at the hospital still alive, and then die. So we are making calls to next of kin of all the deaths that occur or are dealt with in any way at the hospital.

St. Vincent Carmel is an acute care hospital with approximately five to eight deaths per month. Chaplain Carey Landry, one of the two chaplains at St. Vincent Carmel Hospital, has done an excellent job leading the Bereavement Care Track program there. I send him the lists of all the patients who have died at Carmel and the initial phone call contact information. Chaplain Landry has recruited ten volunteers and he assigns them to do these initial phone calls, as well as doing some himself. He knows who has died and what they've died from, so he can give the volunteers a few more details. He then sends me back a list of who has been assigned to whom.

STRUCTURE AND CONTENT OF INITIAL CALL

ALR: *How long do most of these calls last?*

KC: The first phone call can last up to 10 minutes. Since the pilot in 1997, I have tracked how many minutes, on average, each call takes. For instance, in July 2000, the average initial phone call lasted 5 minutes and 36 seconds. The average three-month phone call for that same month was 4 minutes and 38 seconds. I notice that they drop maybe a minute or two each time that I call. I attempt to call people twice. After the second call, if there is an answering machine, I leave a message with my office phone number. My phone has been rigged, so that my beeper always goes off when I have a voicemail. I'm constantly checking my voicemail.

ALR: *What do you say in the first call?*

KC: In the first phone call I say, "Hello, my name is Kathy Carroll and I am from the St. Vincent's Hospital in Indianapolis, where I coordinate a program called 'Bereavement Care'." Some people don't know what bereavement means, so I wait to hear what kind of reaction I get. If there's no reaction, I ask if the person understands what I mean—sometimes he or she will say "Yes" and sometimes "No." So, then I explain a little bit about what bereavement means.

Then, I explain what the program consists of, that it includes mailings and phone calls. I make sure that they understand that they are under no obligation to participate and they don't have to do anything with the mailings. I give them every option about what they would like to receive or if they would prefer no contact at all. I provide a number to call if they have a question that comes up. For example, if a grandchild has a question about grief and they're not sure how to answer it, they can call us. I emphasize that there is absolutely no cost to the family or partner for our assistance, and we would love to be able to provide them with anything that they need. Currently, our support groups are free. In terms of individual counseling, it depends on what the individual needs. One of our pastoral care associates or I can meet once or twice with an individual for free. However, if the individual or family members are seeking more long-term counseling, we refer them to a grief counselor in the community, who may charge a fee.

ALR: *How do you provide services to people in adjoining states?*

KC: The services remain the same to those family members living in adjoining states. When I make the initial phone call, I always tell these folks that the first brochure refers only to support groups offered in the Indianapolis area, but that the rest of the brochures are educational in nature and can be applied to anyone, anywhere.

FAMILY MEMBER CONCERNS

How the call evolves depends on the response. If the person appears talkative, I'll ask them about the loved one. I might say, "I know your wife died, and I'm very sorry about your loss. Can you tell me a little bit about what happened?" I just open the door. Some people shut the door really quickly. Most people are talkative, and they go into a lot of detail about what happened.

Then there are a number of people who don't know what happened. They can't explain the death. I think that this is one way that the calls can be truly helpful. Sometimes they'll have medical questions, and my nursing background does help. I'm not familiar with some conditions because my own background is in labor and delivery, gynecology, and oncology. If the deceased had open heart surgery, and because they use some terms that I don't know, then I usually refer them back to the physician. I'll tell them that they have a right to call the office and make an appointment. If they really don't understand it and it's *important* for them to understand more detail, they should feel free to call the office and set up an appointment with the physician.

ALR: *Do you ever facilitate that yourself, or do you leave the follow-up to them?*

KC: I encourage them to go back to the physicians. I see my role as primarily one of listening to families and coaching them a bit. On rare occasions, I do intercede and take action on the family's behalf.

ALR: *Do families have questions about getting death certificates or autopsy results during the initial call?*

KC: Many families ask where the death certificate is. Getting a death certificate can take eight weeks. Unfortunately, families need the death certificate in order to access any insurance money or for any other paperwork to progress. This can be a real hardship for older folks. Sometimes there has been an error in completing the death certificate and then it takes longer.

ALR: *Are you able to speed up that process for them?*

KC: I know the process and can explain it to families. In general, funeral homes handle the death certificates. I suggest that families call the funeral home because the funeral home director is the spokesperson and advocate for the family. I encourage families to let funeral directors know that not having the death certificate is a real problem. The director should let the physician's office know that the family needs the death certificate and they may need to keep calling. If the families have not involved a funeral director, the death certificate stays on file at the hospital and they can request it directly.

Autopsy results are never sent to the funeral director. The autopsy results are sent to the physician who ordered the autopsy. Some physicians are good about calling the family and explaining these results or inviting the family to come in to the office to discuss them.

If families are having trouble getting or understanding autopsy results from the physician, another strategy I suggest is that they call their own primary care doctor and make an appointment. The bereaved family member might say to his or her doctor, "Can *you* explain to me what happened to my husband? Can *you* call my husband's doctor and get the autopsy results?" The intercession of the next of kin's own doctor with the physician who has the autopsy results can be especially useful if the family member does not live here in town. It may be that doctors respond well to requests from peers. The primary care doctor can be helpful even though he or she was not involved in the care of the deceased. As a medical person who knows the family member, he or she can explain the terms, and translate the autopsy results into a layperson's language.

ALR: *Are you connecting people with their own primary care teams? Is there an explicit component of this program to attend to the health of the bereaved?*

KC: If the person is open and we're conversing during the initial phone call, I usually ask about contact with his or her primary physician. I go into some of the details of what grief feels like physically, because most people don't understand that. People often don't know that grief may make them feel more tired and/or may affect appetite and sleep. There are a number of physical symptoms of grief. Some people tell me that they had no idea that these physical symptoms were part of grief. It helps to normalize and validate this experience. So I usually encourage them to go see their physician, have their annual checkup, and keep in contact with their primary care physician.

ALR: *What other kinds of issues, in that first phone call, do family members raise?*

KC: Some family members have financial questions about the next steps. Sometimes I direct them back to their own family members. I try to decipher which family member could be an asset to them; it may be a niece, a nephew, or a child. If I am speaking to an older lady who is confused about her finances and she appears overwhelmed, "I've got these doctor bills," sometimes I can determine that they are not bills. I'll have the person open it up, and it might say at the bottom, "This is not a bill," but she hasn't even looked that far. But I usually encourage the person to involve someone else in their financial considerations because it can get very confusing, especially when a person is in the throes of grief. Even when death is anticipated, grief at the loss of a loved one can be overwhelming.

> **Even when death is anticipated, grief at the loss of a loved one can be overwhelming.**

ALR: *Do you intercede on the family's behalf with the hospital's billing department?*

KC: I try, but at the three- to four-week mark, families usually don't even have a bill yet. Sometimes by the three-month phone call, a family will be having trouble with the billing process. I will then call the director of billing here and ask her to work with them.

ALR: *Do you ask them an open-ended question in the first phone call about the quality of care that they got when their relative died, or anything like that?*

KC: No. Nine months after the death, we send a questionnaire about quality care to all of the next of kin that we've been able to reach. We don't see the Bereavement Care Track as a quality improvement effort, per se, although I do handle questions and problems and do follow-up. The focus of these calls and written materials is on supporting the bereavement process of these family members. I don't want people to be afraid to talk to me because they're afraid that I'm going to report everything that I hear. I usually tell family members that I can contact unit directors if they wish, but, otherwise, what they say is confidential.

ALR: *Do you hear any anger about the care of the deceased?*

KC: I think I diffuse a lot of anger. Some people have complaints, and from the stories that they tell me, I would have complaints, too. I listen. I try not to be defensive at all, because that's not going to help. Then I make suggestions about how I might follow up. "Would you like for *me* to contact the nursing director and have her talk to this specific person about the care that your loved one received?" I give them control and let them know that I *will* follow through, and then I call them back and let them know what I've done.

For example, I had one lady complain about how dirty the lounge was on one of the units. So I called the nursing director and told her that I had a real complaint about the cleanliness of the lounge in her unit. I said, "Would you like to go look at your lounge, or do you want me to come over and just kind of glance at it? This lady had some specific complaints." The nursing director called me back two hours later and said, "It's filthy! We have housekeeping up here right now taking care of everything!" Then I called back the family member with the complaint and told her what we had done. If people want to write a letter of complaint, I tell them to whom they should write.

ALR: *What percentage of calls require this level of responsiveness on your part, that you make a follow-up call and then get back to the family?*

KC: I would estimate that about two out of the initial 80 calls that we make at St. Vincent's each month require any type of follow-up. We have not had to make any follow-up phone calls for the families called from Carmel.

DIFFERENCES BETWEEN CALLS AT DIFFERENT TIMES

ALR: *In terms of different times, the three-month, four-month, or the six- and seven-month call, you said they tend to get shorter as time goes on. Are there any other ways in which the calls differ over time?*

KC: At the three-month mark, I talk to them about their "fog." By fog, I mean a kind of shock and numbness. I ask if it is clearing at all and if they notice anything different. I also ask if they are experiencing a "new normal." They've gone through the initial shock. Other people in their lives are starting to back away, probably. It's not that they don't care, but they are getting on with their lives. Most of the bereaved family members I speak to are older; they describe their adult children as busy. I ask them, "How are *you* grieving? Do you think your kids are okay?" Or, "Where are you as the family matriarch, or patriarch? How are you dealing with everything? Are your kids still being as supportive as they were? How are they doing that? Is there anything else that you feel that you need?" But, eventually, by the six-month phone call, we're talking about getting out, just a little bit. I ask how they are handling phone calls to go out to eat and if they are ready for social engagements yet. "What are you doing to activate your life again? Are you ready to do that yet?" It's fine if they are not. But, eventually, I assure them that they will get to that stage.

OTHER RESOURCES OFFERED

ALR: *What other kinds of resources do you offer these bereaved families?*

KC: When we developed this program, we decided that it was not worthwhile to reinvent the wheel, so we refer the adults, teens, and children to existing support groups led by our hospice. I also have a variety of community resources to which I can refer families: spouse support groups that are open-ended in duration, an excellent community-based children and teen center that works with people in grief. We refer families there because they also provide individual counseling. So, for example, if it's a young parent who has some children of grade-school age, and she needs some extra assistance and is not sure how to do all this, she can take her children there. They can participate in a support group, while she can receive individual counseling. We have lists of individual counselors who specialize in grief and loss issues. We have an annual weekend retreat for grief called "Camp Healing Tree" for children, ages 7 to 17. Staff from four hospitals in the community work together to prepare for and conduct this weekend retreat for bereaved children. Each child is paired with a bereavement volunteer for the weekend. We have an educational series for families about dealing with grief around the holidays.

We have another volunteer group here at the hospital, the senior partner program, staffed by volunteers who are seniors themselves. On occasion, I have put a couple of elderly bereaved family members in contact with this group because they are isolated, have no relatives, and want to receive calls *daily*. Members of the senior partner program will call and check on them or pray with them. They will do whatever the person wants. I've used the program about four or five times in the four years I've been running the Bereavement Care Track. So we have a variety of activities and resources for bereaved friends and families.

EVOLUTION OF THE PROGRAM

ALR: *How did this structure evolve from the pilot program?*

KC: Starting with a small pilot program has been essential to our success. In the pilot, the first phone call to bereaved family members was originally scheduled at three to four months after the death and we only made two calls. But we received feedback from families on the questionnaire that we sent out saying that the first call came too late. So I shared these comments with members of the End-of-Life Committee, and we decided to try calling bereaved family members three to four weeks after the death.

Originally, we mailed the satisfaction/quality improvement questionnaire three months after the death. Our response rate was terrible—only 8 percent of the approximately 88 next of kin to whom we sent questionnaires responded—in other words, we received about seven questionnaires. Then I talked to the hospice staff to find out how long after death they send out their satisfaction survey. We learned from their experience and began sending it out at the nine-month mark, and we now get a 16 to 24 percent response rate—about 14 to 21 questionnaires.

VOLUNTEER CORPS OF HOSPITAL STAFF

Until we expanded the Bereavement Care Track to the entire system, I made all the calls. Then, in July 2000, I teamed with pastoral care to recruit and build a volunteer corps of hospital staff. Our goal has been to recruit staff from every unit, and we have been successful in 80 percent of our units. The involvement of the pastoral care department evolved simultaneously with the expansion of the program. We only had seven volunteers in place at St. Vincent's when we began to implement the program across the system. We now have 43 volunteers across both hospital settings. The recruitment and training is ongoing and continues to grow.

ALR: *How did you recruit paid staff to volunteer additional time? Explain the role of pastoral care staff in this process.*

KC: Sister Sharon Richardt suggested that the pastoral care associates at both St. Vincent's Hospital and St. Vincent Carmel should do most of the follow-up phone calls to families who had had a loved one die at the hospital. She presented this idea to the pastoral care director in July 2000. I didn't think this idea was feasible, given how many other tasks they handle. So, I went to the pastoral care department and we brainstormed together how to avoid their taking on an extra burden, which they do not have staff to cover.

Together we came up with the idea of recruiting staff from all the units in the hospital to volunteer to do some calls. Each pastoral care provider was to get in contact with me and *either* set up an in-service on the units with which he or she was identified or give a 10-minute talk at unit meetings about what bereavement care means and how staff can volunteer for the program. We have been recruiting volunteers for a year now, and 80 percent of the units have some volunteers who work with me to make these follow-up phone calls.

ALR: *Are you conducting the calls for the deaths on the remaining 20 percent of the units?*

KC: Yes. Some units, our ICU, for example, have an average of 16 to 20 deaths per month. So, even the five volunteers in ICU can't keep up. The units that do not have any volunteers are those that have not yet been made aware of this opportunity; on these units, the chaplain has not yet made arrangements for me to come and provide their unit associates with an in-service or information at their unit meeting.

ALR: *What motivates paid staff to give extra time to volunteer in the bereavement program?*

KC: Service is one of our core values here at St. Vincent Hospital and I feel that many associates find this type of volunteer work personally rewarding. We have a program at St. Vincent's called ACTS, or Associates Called To Serve, which is a group made up of anyone associated with St. Vincent's who volunteers, in any capacity. The program tracks how many hours associates contribute, as well as exactly what they are doing. Associates active in the ACTS program can certainly include this information on their annual evaluation.

ALR: *Is there an unwritten expectation that everyone will volunteer?*

KC: No, not really.

ALR: *What makes them volunteer?*

KC: Part of the reason that they volunteer is the way we have presented the progam. I try to frame this activity as a way to stay connected with families with whom staff members have become involved. I feel it creates some closure for the professional caregivers, which is usually missing for them when a patient dies. This program allows the professional caregiver to call this family two or three times and make sure that everybody's doing okay. I don't give any volunteer more than five phone calls a month, total.

The staff who choose to volunteer, especially those working in the cardiac or intensive care units, find it brings some real closure for themselves. They really have *liked* being able to stay in touch with these families. I had a nurse who had to stop volunteering because of her involvement in a master's degree program; the other day she came up to me and said, "I just can't believe how much I've missed making those phone calls." Now that she's completed her program, she's asked to volunteer again.

TRACKING CALLS

ALR: *Do you have a system for tracking all the calls?*

KC: Yes. Each month, I monitor whether a scheduled phone call was made and its outcome. After each contact, I also note whether the family has requested no further phone calls or contact.

I have a spreadsheet program that helps me to track each volunteer and all the contacts that have been made. First, I track all the six-month calls, then all the three-month calls, and then I know who is free to do any initial calls other than myself. I send out a form to each volunteer. Information about the deceased, the relationship of the next of kin, how old the person was that died, the gender, the name of the next of kin, and the phone number is all at the top of the form. The form also includes details of earlier phone contacts. For instance, if I'm asking a volunteer to make a six-month phone call, she can look back on this form to see what happened at the initial phone call and during the three-month phone call.

I send out assignments each month. Some volunteers have told me that they will inform me when they have a family with whom they have worked, whom they want to follow for bereavement care. So, some volunteers only work with families of patients who died on the particular unit on which they work. At St. Vincent's Hospital, seven volunteers have requested to do one-month, three-month and six-month phone calls. These volunteers want to follow a family from the very beginning.

ALR: *How do you track what happened on the call?*

KC: I ask volunteers to write a synopsis of the conversation and send it back to me, on a feedback form. It includes information about how the family feels that they're doing. For example, the volunteer will note if everyone is sleeping and eating, if the family is, in fact, receiving the brochures, and if the family member wants to keep receiving written materials. Volunteers also note any particular actions that they have taken or if any family member is sick. When the volunteer or I call back the next time, we ask how that family member is doing.

Most volunteers don't have access to the database because of confidentiality. I have two volunteers dedicated to data entry who work with me three hours per week. Together we enter this information into the database.

Keeping the database up to date and tracking who has done what are both administrative pieces that are essential to the project. If I've sent one volunteer two sets of bereavement calls and I haven't heard back from her for two months, I need to call her and ask what's going on. Sometimes volunteers are afraid to admit that they are behind on their calls. If it isn't working, I ask them to send the forms back to me.

ALR: *For what percentage of total deaths per month does either you or a member of the volunteer corps actually complete the initial call?*

KC: I would estimate that we reach approximately 33 to 40 percent of the total pool with that first call; this means that we speak to 26 to 32 family members. Even when we don't reach families initially, we try again at the three- and six-month intervals.

Of those family members that the volunteers or I actually speak with for the initial phone call, I would estimate that we reach approximately a quarter of them (six to eight) for the three- and/or six-month phone call. Some of these elderly bereaved people leave home and stay with a child or loved one for a time following the death, so they are hard to reach at home. In addition, many of the older folks go south for the winter, so it depends on the time of year as to whether we reach people at home. Some family members are never home and do not have an answering machine, so we cannot reach them for any of the three phone calls.

TRAINING

ALR: *How do you train these volunteers?*

KC: We have a three-hour training session. I review what the volunteers can anticipate hearing people talk about and explain the importance of these phone calls. The protocols for the initial, three-month, and six-month phone calls are in the manual that they receive, as well as the policies and procedures that we have developed for bereavement care here. I review common needs and helping strategies, some common myths about grief and loss, and some of the physical and emotional symptoms of grief. We also offer tips for the evaluation and assessment of risk of suicide or possible indicators that the family member is experiencing a more severe problem in addition to grief. If something in the conversation seems problematic, I encourage volunteers to refer a family member back to me in these cases. I then complete these referrals.

We offer some strategies for phone calls, including reviewing the use of open-ended and yes/no questions and a handout on the principles of reflective listening. We have a tool for assessing one's own performance as an interviewer. It is a set of self-evaluation questions for the volunteer to consider after making a call. We think these materials are important, because even though most of these volunteers are nurses, sometimes their training has not included a thorough introduction to grief.

ALR: *Do you have anything in place to elicit feedback from the volunteers, such as supervision or focus groups?*

KC: Last summer we had a meeting where the volunteers got together and talked about how things were going for them. I invited pastoral care chaplains from throughout the institution to that meeting. Volunteers talked about phone calls and problems that they run into. They have commented on how to handle certain responses from family members or may ask how to handle a certain complaint. I can deal with most of the questions, but I think it is important for volunteers to know that the chaplains are involved in this work, too. In addition, I have a monthly letter that I send out with their assignment for the month. The main purpose of this memo or letter is to keep them updated on any educational opportunities that they may share with the bereaved family members that they are calling. I also use this letter to praise them for their work and to keep up morale.

ALR: *How do the pastoral care associates help?*

KC: Their presence at the meeting reinforces their role as the resource for the volunteers on the unit. Say, for instance, a volunteer has made a phone call to a family member and has a question or concern that he or she hasn't reached me about yet. This volunteer can go to the chaplain and say, "You know I called this person the other night—can you help me with this?"

IMPACT AND EVALUATION OF THE PROGRAM

Perhaps it is not surprising, given these efforts to listen and follow through with families' concerns or complaints, but our Risk Management department did notice differences between the units where the pilot program was in place and other units in the hospital. During the pilot stage of the Bereavement Care Track, Risk Management reported no complaints from the pilot units regarding care received at the end of life. The number of complaints from the other units averaged four to five per year. Although this was not a goal of the program, the pilot program suggests that this in-person contact with families shortly after a death can address anger and disappointment with care in a constructive way. We don't yet know if its implementation system-wide will have an effect on complaints to Risk Management across the system.

ALR: *What do you think is the main impact of this intervention, in terms of the bereaved families?*

KC: The main thing that I hear from people is that the education that they're receiving from the brochures is extremely helpful to them. Based on analysis of the results of the quality improvement questionnaire that we send out at nine months, we have learned that the brochures are helpful. I believe that the brochures help families to feel that their own experience is valid—that they're okay where they are in the grief process. I think people need this reassurance. I would say that this is the biggest thing that the program provides; even more so than the phone calls, per se, it provides people with a resource.

I've found, through my long experience in the perinatal loss program, that if people know that a resource is available, even when a large percent of them don't use it, they feel comforted just knowing that somebody is there. I would say *that's* the biggest thing we offer.

> *. . . if people know that a resource is available, even when a large percent of them don't use it, they feel comforted just knowing that somebody is there. I would say* that's *the biggest thing we offer.*

ALR: *Have you analyzed the open-ended responses in the satisfaction survey? What kinds of things are bereaved family members saying?*

KC: Most of the open-ended responses express thanks for our efforts and the care that their relative received. I have had letters attached describing an incident that still is upsetting to the family. I copy and forward these letters to the relevant unit director. Some families describe complaints about a physician. If it's an incident in the ICU with a St. Vincent's physician, I will actually photocopy the letter and send it to the director of nursing and to the medical director of the ICU so that they can follow up with it. The directors usually get back to me. If I don't hear from them within a timely fashion, I'll ask them what they've done about it so that I can get back to the family and offer some follow-up information. It's so important for families to know that I've read the letter and that the letter meant something.

ALR: *Do you evaluate your volunteers at all?*

KC: I do not have a procedure for evaluating the volunteers for this program at this time. We just encourage them to use the self-evaluation questions in the manual. I have had a couple of volunteers discontinue making phone calls after evaluating their own comfort level and technique.

LIMITATIONS OF THE BEREAVEMENT CARE TRACK

Risk of Burnout

Prior to the development of the volunteer program, I was overwhelmed by the volume of calls. Probably the biggest thing that anybody who is building a program like this needs to be aware of is burnout. I do a lot of teaching about burnout to my volunteers. My volunteers have the option of making only one phone call a year. They are in total control of their time and how much they choose to volunteer. If they want to take the summer off, they let me know. I try to *never, ever* make them feel guilty about whatever they're doing. You can't require volunteers to do what they don't want or can't do.

Chaplain Carey Landry, from St. Vincent's Carmel Hospital, presented how he runs the Bereavement Care Track at Carmel, where they deal with five to eight deaths per month, to the pastoral care department here at St. Vincent's. The chaplains here, at this much larger setting, said, "We can't possibly do all that." Some units have very few deaths, but others are *so* overloaded. For example, the ICU alone has three to four times the number of deaths per month as all of Carmel Hospital. The two part-time chaplains connected with that unit are both wonderful people, but the volume is too great for them to supervise the logistics of distributing the initial phone calls and background information, not to mention making initial calls.

ALR: *What is in place to keep this system viable for you? Are there any other paid staff who are committed to making sure that the calls are made?*

KC: Since the start of the program in 1997, I have to be honest and say I have been close to burnout one time. Luckily, I then went on vacation and subsequently felt refreshed. Unfortunately, there are no other paid associates who are committed to making sure that the calls are made if I need to take time off. However, I do have many allies here at the hospital who are very supportive. As the volunteer program continues to grow, I gain more confidence in the continued success of this program.

ALR: *What might you like to do differently?*

KC: A few bereaved family members probably would benefit from more frequent phone calls or more extended phone calls. For instance, some family members would like to get calls at 9 months and 12 months. I've encouraged my volunteers to let them know that the six-month call is the final phone call, and at that point to ask family members if they *need* a further phone call. And if they *do*, I've got a certain calendar in which I mark down the extra phone calls. When that date comes up, I will send it back to their volunteer or I will call the family.

We also would like to develop our policies and procedures into standards of care for bereavement care across our system. We had an earlier goal of doing so, but have not yet been able to get there.

In thinking about how to improve the program, I think we can strengthen the evaluation and feedback components. Specifically, we need to:

- Offer more ongoing supervision and support to the volunteers
- Offer family members the opportunity to participate in a focus group after the one-year anniversary of the death

STAFF DEVELOPMENT

The Bereavement Care Track is currently expanding into helping our patients and their family members with the anticipatory grief stage of the dying process. Strengthening the hospital staff's knowledge base in this area also will support and improve the care of families before and after the death of a loved one. We need to continue system-wide efforts to:

- Continue education for all staff on compassionate care of the dying
- Educate staff on ethics and futile care and the transition from aggressive curative care to comfort care for the dying

Four times a year, we provide a one-day workshop called Compassionate Care of the Dying for any associate from St. Vincent's Hospital and the affiliate hospitals. The workshop consists of a multidisciplinary panel discussing holistic care at the end of life; a panel of patients and family members telling their stories; a plenary session on ethics; breakout sessions on pain management, ethics, spirituality of dying, and multicultural aspects of dying; group discussions; and care of the caregiver. The burnout issue was discussed at the beginning of the day and at the end.

In addition, we are beginning to work with each "service line" in the hospital on anticipatory grief. Are we serving as patient advocates? Are we providing patients with a safe and peaceful atmosphere in which to die? This is a main topic during the conversations held with the family members following their loss. Did they feel safe? Was their loved one able to die a good death?

ALR: *If you were to advise others seeking to replicate the Bereavement Care Track, what key piece of advice would you offer?*

KC: Start off small. To expand to a full bereavement care program, it might work better to have at least two people sharing the bereavement care coordinator position so that the program does not depend on just one person. I would say, "Take it slow. Be flexible and start with a pilot program first."

REFERENCES

1. McSkimming S, Hodges M, Super A, et al. The experience of life-threatening illness: Patients' and their loved ones' perspectives. *Journal of Palliative Medicine*. 1999; 2(2):173–184.
2. Carroll K. Four point strategic plan for supportive care. *Supportive Voice*. Fall 1998–Winter 1999 at <www.careofdying.org>.

Never Too Young to Know: Death in Children's Lives by Phyllis R. Silverman*

CAROL WOGRIN, RN, PsyD

National Center for Death Education, Mount Ida College
Newton, Massachusetts

Death touches the lives of children regularly, the death of a pet, friend, teacher, parent, sibling. Yet, as a society, we avoid acknowledging this reality. But the fact is that death is always a part of life and frequently affects the lives of children. We also seem to have developed the belief that children will somehow be shielded from the pain associated with loss if we avoid talking with them about death when it does occur. Unfortunately, in response to our discomfort when children do have to endure significant emotional loss and pain, we often leave them alone to manage life's most difficult challenges. For too long, children's grief has been examined and discussed without regard to the way their experience is embedded in their families and the larger social system. Additionally, there is a frequent assumption that the death of someone as important as a parent is likely to derail a child and result in the development of psychopathology.

> *For too long, children's grief has been examined and discussed without regard to the way their experience is embedded in their families and the larger social system.*

In *Never Too Young to Know*, Phyllis Silverman challenges these widely embraced beliefs. She provides a model for understanding grief in children that is embedded in the developmental and social context in which all life's experiences exist. She deals with the complexities of grief in a very clear, logical way and lays out the difficult feelings and challenges associated with adjustment to loss as they are experienced developmentally and within a family context. The overall emphasis of the book is on coping and adaptation. She stresses how important it is for children to be given accurate information geared toward their developmental level and the capacity children have to adapt to crisis and loss when they are given the appropriate support, particularly from a parenting figure, but from the larger

*Silverman PR. *Never Too Young to Know: Death in Children's Lives*. New York: Oxford University Press, 2000.

social system as well. So, while the death of a loved one does become a part of the fabric of a child's life and who that young person is, it does not typically result in abnormal development.

Never Too Young to Know is well organized and easy to read. The book is divided into three main sections. Part I provides a theoretical basis for understanding grief in children. In this section, Silverman examines historical factors that have molded the ways in which we view death, as medical technology has resulted in keeping people alive much longer, successfully treating formerly life-threatening illnesses, and moving death out of the home and everyday life. She also describes the ways in which, in keeping with other social changes, our theoretical and social understanding of grief has evolved. For much of the last century, models for understanding grief were heavily influenced by Freud, who stated that the work of grief is geared toward emotionally detaching from the deceased so that the bereaved can reinvest their energy in new relationships. The influence of these beliefs is still quite prevalent today. It is common to hear people talk about "letting go," "moving on," or "obtaining closure." Drawing from her research with the bereaved, the author offers a new paradigm for understanding the grief process. This paradigm focuses on how we make meaning of our world, the ways in which we hold on to our connections to deceased loved ones, and the dynamic nature of these internally held relationships.

Silverman also stresses the importance of looking at children's experience and expression through a developmental lens. She provides a solid overview of child development, laying the groundwork for understanding the grief process, as well as presenting theory on family systems and family dynamics, since children's worlds are defined and molded by the families and larger social context in which they live.

Part II brings the new paradigm to life through the voices of bereaved children and parents. Vignettes and quotes from many bereaved children and adults who care for them are heavily interspersed throughout the chapters and succeed in painting a clear picture of the grief process and its role in the lives of children and families. In different chapters, Silverman addresses the effect of different types of losses and the various ways in which children cope. Although there are many shared elements among grief reactions anytime that we lose a person we love, there are also differences in responses to grief—from person to person, family to family—as well as elements that are specific to the nature of the loss. When a child loses a parent, the realities of the world that the child lives in are altered drastically, as the entire family will shift to accommodate to this loss. Usually, the remaining parent will seem different, as this parent struggles with his or her own grief. Questions and fears about who will fill the roles of the person who is gone are paramount. When a sibling dies, the loss is yet again distinct. The child loses a particular relationship, possibly a playmate or competitor, someone for whom the child may have cared, a role model, a friend. Often overlooked, but given full attention here, is the experience for children of having a friend die. With each of these types of losses, Silverman describes the ways in which children attempt to cope and adapt to the loss and their changed world. She describes the behavioral expressions of many of the difficult feelings with which children struggle, again drawing extensively from the voices of children themselves and from the parents who observe and interact with them. Through their stories, the reader gains insight into the meaning of various behaviors, such as a child who is lashing out in anger, and an understanding of helpful ways to respond. In keeping with the important role that the connections with the deceased play in this paradigm of the grief process, with each type of loss Silverman offers descriptions from children and adolescents of the positive roles that their ongoing internal relationships play in their development over time.

Although there is information throughout the book on responding to children's grief and helping them to develop important tools for coping with the difficulties that life hands them, Part III has helping as its focus. Silverman describes informal helping, including practical and emotional support, which comes from family and friends, teachers, religious communities, and other elements of the social world of the child and his or her family. She also describes formal helping, such as counseling, support groups, and mutual help groups, emphasizing the importance of the bereaved paying attention to whether support that is being offered truly feels helpful or not, and to trust their sense of what they need.

Several messages in this book are very clear. Grief is a normal, albeit difficult and challenging, part of life. And, as a normal part of life, grief does not usually result in the development of pathology, especially when a child is supported in dealing with the difficult feelings associated with loss. The children in this book tell us so clearly how much they need information and need to be listened to in order to cope with all the challenges of the grief process as they continuously rework their experience as they grow. Finally, we should not wait until a child has experienced a devastating loss to begin to teach them about death. We need to begin addressing death as a normal and guaranteed part of the human condition, so that children and adults alike have experience and skills in coping with life when they are posed with the enormous challenge of adapting to the death of a loved one.

> *. . .we should not wait until a child has experienced a devastating loss to begin to teach them about death.*

Online Bereavement Support

YVETTE COLÓN, MSW, ACSW, BCD

American Pain Foundation
Baltimore, Maryland

There is no doubt that the loss of a loved one can be profoundly traumatic in physical, emotional, and spiritual ways. Bereaved individuals seek help and support in a variety of traditional ways: individual grief counseling, bereavement groups, and peer support groups. But with the expansion of the Internet, many bereaved individuals are taking responsibility for their own emotional needs by using their computers to access online support groups and discussion forums.

Since the early 1990s, when the World Wide Web was made available for public use, grieving persons have easily found diverse online bereavement communities, where there are now many support and discussion forums. Clinical social workers and other mental health professionals have been involved in online discussion and support groups focusing on the many phases of the bereavement process. People with a shared history, shared values, and a variety of interests regarding their grief experiences can connect and carry on a conversation with anyone around the world, all without leaving their own communities. The demand for online services is high, and online group participation continues to increase.

Most of the literature available about online support falls into the category of anecdotal, narrative experiences of participation in virtual communities or sociological studies of computer-mediated communication. Several studies have used qualitative methods. Few studies have looked at clinical interventions or any results of participating in online bereavement therapy or support, as participant or practitioner. A systematic evaluation of group outcomes in online support groups has not been done yet.

Galinsky, Shopler, and Abell acknowledge that technology is beginning to play a small, but important role in group practice and consider the benefits and problems of technology-based groups.[1] Their study is a survey of the nature of their subjects' knowledge, experience, and comfort with technology-based groups. The sample consisted of group practitioners who were members of the Association for the Advancement of Social Work with Groups.

Finn described a pilot project for an online support group and the advantages, disadvantages, and potential for use, as well as the benefit to group leaders and participants.[2] He noted again that there has been little systematic evaluation of computer-based self-help groups and no research about their use as an adjunct to face-to-face support groups.

In a study about computer-mediated support groups, Weinberg, Schmale, Uken, and Wessel asserted that, although support groups can help people to increase their coping skills, only a small percentage of people in a crisis will choose to participate in one.[3] They noted that computer-mediated groups have the potential to serve those who are unwilling or unable to participate in a face-to-face group. Their qualitative study highlighted an online support group pilot project with six breast cancer patients and discussed the advantages as well as limitations of this modality.

Online groups can be conducted in three different ways: as a chat group (or chat room), a bulletin board, or a listserv (mailing list). A chat group is a real-time exchange in which everyone is at his or her computer at the same time using a special program so that the entire group can communicate with each other. A bulletin board (sometimes referred to as a message board) is a program or location (on the Web) where participants can read and write messages at any time, which can then be read by any other participant, remain indefinitely, are posted sequentially, and are often organized by topic. A listserv is a private e-mail group in which each subscriber receives a separate copy by e-mail of each message that is posted and can maintain ongoing communication with other list members who share a common concern. All these groups are available through the Internet at no charge to the participant.

Anyone contemplating starting an online bereavement group or discussion forum must be comfortable communicating in an electronic format. Previous participation in an open online bereavement, mental health, or professional forum helps a facilitator to understand the process from the participant's point of view.

There are practical matters to consider in forming an online bereavement group. Not only must facilitators be comfortable with the technology that they are using, but they must also be knowledgeable about the technology that powers their online group. They must understand how people interact in text-based environments and be aware of issues involved in computer-mediated communication. They must be able to build a community, foster a sense of trust, and guide effective and therapeutic interactions among group members. The definition, role, and scope of responsibilities of the facilitator must first be well thought out. A statement of format, guidelines, duration of the group, and what is expected from participants can be sent out as an announcement. All e-mail exchanges and postings to the group should remain as secure and as confidential as possible. The facilitator should have a stated policy for crises and emergencies experienced by the participants.

Participants must be able to write and express themselves adequately in order to participate in an online group. If the bereavement group is a closed group with limited membership and time span, this can be assessed by e-mail responses to screening questions. Facilitators can recruit from hospitals, clinics, community organizations, or their own agency. Once participants are screened and accepted into a bulletin board or mailing list, they have access to the group 24 hours a day, 7 days a week for the duration of the group. They should be encouraged to send as many messages as they like, as long as the messages are on topic. Because anything can happen in an online group in any 24-hour period, it is very important for the facilitator to log in at least once each workday in order to read postings or e-mail, respond to questions and concerns, and guide the group.

Facilitators must be aware that the physical and verbal cues that are often found in an in-person group are likely to be missing or different in an online group. In addition, the facilitator must pay close attention to language, engagement, and the ways that group members write and express themselves. The facilitator must be more active and sometimes more directive in the group to make up for the lack of eye contact and body language.

Online bereavement support groups have the potential to provide many benefits to the participants. First, participants sometimes develop personal relationships with each other and have individual contact outside the group, sharing information and extending the network of support. Second, the level of intimacy and trust can be greater because participants may feel more comfortable disclosing and discussing their concerns in writing than in person. Finally, because there are no time restrictions, as there often are in face-to-face groups, members of bulletin board bereavement groups can participate as much as they wish at times that are most helpful to them.

However, the text-based nature of the group environment presents a challenge. The written word can be stark and direct; humor and sarcasm can be misinterpreted easily and feelings can be hurt. Participants must be able to write effectively in order to get the maximum benefit from an online discussion. Group leaders must be skilled to facilitate the discussion, mediate conflict, and support all members through writing alone. Clinical supervision and knowledge of resources for conducting online support groups are critical.

Social workers and mental health professionals have written extensively about these benefits.[4-6] More than ever before, online bereavement communities are able to sustain people who step forward to request support and information. Internet users are becoming more and more technologically sophisticated, and online usage and accessibility are increasing daily. This, in turn, fosters the creation and expansion of Internet communities into places where people are not afraid to ask questions, tell their stories, share their grief, or seek help.

ONLINE BEREAVEMENT RESOURCES

Bereaved Families Online offers support for people who have lost an immediate family member.

Cancer Care, Inc. provides online bereavement groups facilitated by certified social workers. <www.cancercare.org/services/online_support.asp>

Grief and Loss in the Workplace provides guidelines and resources for co-workers, managers, and supervisors. <www.umich.edu/~fasap/health/grief/intro.htm>

GriefNet offers numerous discussion and support groups for bereaved persons (in e-mail listserv format) and a variety of resources related to death and major losses.

Grief Recovery Online features message boards, chat groups, and resource listings. Spanish-language groups are available.

Growth House offers an extensive grief and bereavement section, including a chat room and information about general and family bereavement, pregnancy loss and infant death, and helping children cope with grief and illness. <www.growthhouse.org/death.html>

HospiceNet offers extensive information about grief and bereavement, including issues regarding children and adolescents. <www.hospicenet.org/html/bereavement.html>

KidsAid is an online support group for children dealing with any kind of loss. It includes artwork, stories, and poems.

WidowNet is an information and support group resource for and by men and women of all ages, religious backgrounds, and sexual orientations who have suffered the death of a spouse or life partner. <www.fortnet.org/WidowNet/>

STANDARDS OF PRACTICE, ETHICAL GUIDELINES, AND ONLINE RESOURCES

American Counseling Association
Ethical Standards for the Practice of Online Counseling
<www.counseling.org/resources/internet.htm>

Community-Building on the Web
<www.naima.com/community>

International Society for Mental Health Online
Suggested Principles for the Online Provision of Mental Health Services
<www.ismho.org/suggestions.html>

National Board for Certified Counselors
Standards for the Ethical Practice of Web Counseling
<www.nbcc.org/ethics/webethics.htm>

Psychology of Cyberspace
<www.rider.edu/users/suler/psycyber/psycyber.html>

Psychology of Virtual Communities
<webpages.charter.net/stormking/>

SUGGESTED READING

Fink J (ed.). *How to Use Computers and Cyberspace in the Clinical Practice of Psychotherapy*. Northvale, NJ: Jason Aronson, 1999.

Gackenbach J. *Psychology and the Internet: Intrapersonal, Interpersonal, and Transpersonal Implications*. New York: Academic Press, 1999.

Grohol JM, Zukerman EL. *Insider's Guide to Mental Health Resources Online: The Clinican's Toolbox*, 2d ed. New York: Guilford Press, 1999.

LaBruzza A. *The Essential Internet: A Guide for Psychotherapists and Other Mental Health Professionals*. Northvale, NJ: Jason Aronson, 1997.

Rosen LD, Weil MM. *The Mental Health Technology Bible*. New York: John Wiley & Sons, 1997.

REFERENCES

1. Galinsky MJ, Schopler JH, Abell MD. Connecting group members through telephone and computer groups. *Health and Social Work*. 1997;22(3):181–188.
2. Finn J. Computer-based self-help groups: A new resource to supplement support groups. *Social Work with Groups*. 1995;18(1):109–117.
3. Weinberg N, Schmale JD, Uken J, Wessel K. Computer-mediated support groups. *Social Work with Groups*. 1995;17(4):43–54.
4. Colón Y. Digital digging: Group therapy online. In *How to Use Computers and Cyberspace in the Clinical Practice of Psychotherapy*, J Fink (ed.). Northvale, NJ: Jason Aronson, 1999.
5. Schopler JH, Galinsky MJ, Abell M. Creating community through telephone and computer groups: Theoretical and practical perspectives. *Social Work with Groups*. 1997;20(4):19–34.
6. Schopler JH, Abell M, Galinsky MJ. Technology-based groups: A review and conceptual framework for practice. *Social Work*. 1998;43(3):254–267.

Selected Bibliography

Part Four

Selected references by contributors to this part:

American Academy of Pediatrics Committee on Psychosocial Aspects of Child and Family Health. The pediatrician and childhood bereavement. *Pediatrics*. 2000;105(2):445–447.

Campbell S, Silverman PR. *Widower: When Men Are Left Alone*. Amityville, NY: Baywood, 1996.

Klass D, Silverman P, Nickman S. *Continuing Bonds: New Understandings of Grief*. Washington, DC: Taylor & Francis, 1996.

Nickman SL, Silverman PR, Normand C. Children's construction of a deceased parent: The surviving parent's contribution. *American Journal of Orthopsychiatry*. 1998;68(1):126–134.

Silverman PR. It makes a difference. *Illness, Crisis & Loss*. 2001;9(1):111–128.

Silverman PR. *Never Too Young to Know: Death in Children's Lives*. New York: Oxford University Press, 2000.

Silverman PR. Research, clinical practice and the human experience: Putting the pieces together. *Death Studies*. 2000;24(6):469–478.

Silverman PR, Nickman S, Worden JW. Detachment revisited: The child's reconstruction of a dead parent. *American Journal of Orthopsychiatry*. 1992; 62(4):494–503.

Walters T. *On Bereavement: The Culture of Grief*. Philadelphia: Open University Press, 1999.

Worden JW. *Children and Grief*. New York: Guilford Press, 1996.

Other selected references:

Attig T. *The Heart of Grief: Death and the Search for Lasting Love*. New York: Oxford University Press, 2000.

Attig T. *How We Grieve: Relearning the World*. New York: Oxford University Press, 1996.

Bedell SE, Cadenhead K, Graboys TB. The doctor's letter of condolence. *New England Journal of Medicine*. 2001;344(15). 24 October 2001. ⟨www.nejm.org/cgi/content/short/344/15/1162⟩

Bertman S (ed.). *Grief and the Healing Arts: Creativity as Therapy*. Amityville, NY: Baywood, 2000.

Burnell GM, Burnell AL. *Clinical Management of Bereavement: A Handbook for Healthcare Professionals*. New York: Human Science Press, Inc., 1989.

Caserta MS, Lund DA, Rice SJ. Pathfinders: A self-care and health education program for older widows and widowers. *Gerontologist*. 1999;39:615–620.

Connor SR, McMaster JK. Hospice, bereavement intervention and use of health care services by surviving spouses. *HMO Practice*. 1996;10(1):20–25.

Corless IB. Bereavement. In *Textbook of Palliative Nursing*, BR Ferrell, N Coyle (eds.). New York: Oxford University Press, 2001, 352–362.

Davis GF. Loss and the duration of grief. *Journal of the American Medical Association*. 2001;285(9):1152–1153.

Dowdney L, Wilson R, Maughan B, Allerton M, Schofield P, Skuse D. Psychological disturbance and service provision in parentally bereaved children: Prospective case-control study. *British Medical Journal*. 1999;319(7206):354–357.

Eisenbruch M. Cross-cultural aspects of bereavement. II: Ethnic and cultural variations in the development of bereavement practices. *Cultural Medicine and Psychiatry*. 1984;8(4):315–347.

Freedman J, Combs G. *Narrative Therapy: The Social Construction of Reality*. New York: W.W. Norton, 1996.

Gray SW, Zide MR, Wilker H. Using the solution focused brief therapy model with bereavement groups in rural communities: Resiliency at its best. *Hospice Journal*. 2000;15(3):13–30.

Hedtke L. Remembering practices in the face of death. *Forum: Association for Death Education and Counseling*. 2001; 27(2):5–6.

Kagan Klein H. *Gili's Book: A Journey into Bereavement for Parents and Counselors*. New York: Teachers College Press, 1998.

Katz J, Sidell M, Komaromy C. Death in homes: Bereavement needs of residents, relatives and staff. *International Journal of Palliative Nursing*. 2000;6(6): 274–279.

Klass D. *The Spiritual Lives of Bereaved Parents*. Philadelphia: Brunner/Routledge, 1999.

Larson DG. *The Helper's Journey: Working with People Facing Grief, Loss, and Life-Threatening Illness*. Champaign, IL: Research Press, 1993.

Lemkau JP, Mann B, Little D, Whitecar P, Hershberger P, Schumm JA. A questionnaire survey of family practice: Physicians' perceptions of bereavement care. *Archives of Family Medicine*. 2000;9(9):822–829.

Lewis AE. Reducing burnout: Development of an oncology staff bereavement program. *Oncology Nursing Forum*. 1999;26(6):1065–1069.

Lund, DA, Caserta MS, Dimond MF. The course of spousal bereavement in later life. In *Handbook of Bereavement: Theory, Research and Intervention*, MS Stroebe, W Stroebe, RO Hansson (eds.). New York: Cambridge University Press, 1993, 240–254.

Monk G, Winslade J, Crocket K, Epston D. *Narrative Therapy in Practice: The Archeology of Hope*. San Francisco: Jossey-Bass, 1997.

Morgan J (ed.). *Meeting the Needs of Our Clients Creatively: The Impact of Art and Culture on Caregiving*. Amityville, NY: Baywood, 2000.

Oliver RC, Sturtevant JP, Scheetz JP, Fallat ME. Beneficial effects of a hospital bereavement intervention program after traumatic childhood death. *Journal of Trauma*. 2001;50(3):440–446; discussion 447–448.

Oliviere D, Hargreaves R, Monroe B (eds.). Bereavement care. In *Good Practices in Palliative Care: A Psychosocial Perspective*. Aldershot, UK: Ashgate/Arena, 1998, 121–143.

Parkes CM. Coping with loss: Bereavement in adult life. *British Medical Journal.* 1998;316(7134):856–859.

Parkes CM, Relf M, Couldrick A. *Counseling in Terminal Care and Bereavement.* Baltimore, MD: BPS Books, 1996.

Rando TA (ed.). *Clinical Dimensions of Anticipatory Mourning: Theory and Practice in Working with the Dying, Their Loved Ones and Their Caregivers.* Champaign, IL: Research Press, 2000.

Ringdal GI, Jordhøy MS, Ringdal K, Kaasa S. The first year of grief and bereavement in close family members to individuals who have died of cancer. *Palliative Medicine.* 2001;15(2):91–105.

Sandler IN, West SG, Baca L, Pillow DR, Gersten JC, Rogosch F, Virdin L, Beals J, Reynolds KD, Kallgren C, Tein J-Y, Kriege G, Cole E, Ramirez R. Linking empirically-based theory and evaluation: The Family Bereavement Program. *American Journal of Community Psychology.* 1992;20:491–521.

Saunderson EM, Ridsdale L, Jewell D. General practitioners' beliefs and attitudes about how to respond to death and bereavement: Qualitative study. *British Medical Journal.* 1999;319(7205):293–296.

Shapiro E. *Grief as a Family Process: A Developmental Approach to Clinical Practice.* New York: Guilford Press, 1994.

Sheldon F. ABC of palliative care: Bereavement. *British Medical Journal.* 1998;316(7129):456–458.

Sirkiä K, Ahlgren B, Hovi L, Saarinen-Pihkala UM. Weekend courses for families who have lost a child with cancer. *Medical and Pediatric Oncology.* 2000;34(5): 352–355.

Slavitt DR. The treasures of grief. *Journal of Pain and Symptom Management.* 2000;20(5):353–357.

Stevenson NC, Straffon CH. *When Your Child Dies: Finding the Meaning in Mourning,* revised edition. Lakewood, Ohio: Philomel Press, Theo Publishing Co., 1990. Available from Philomel Press, c/o St. Paul's Episcopal Church, 2747 Fairmount Blvd., Cleveland Heights, OH 44106.

Stewart M, Craig D, MacPherson K, Alexander S. Promoting positive affect and diminishing loneliness of widowed seniors through a support intervention. *Public Health Nursing.* 2001;18(1):54–63.

Stroebe MS, Hansson RO, Stroebe W, Schut H (eds.). *The Handbook of Bereavement Research: Consequences, Coping, and Care.* Washington, DC: American Psychological Association, 2001.

Sutton RB. Supporting the bereaved relative: Reflections on the actor's experience. *Medical Education.* 1998;32(6):622–629.

Van-Si L, Powers L. *Helping Children Heal from Loss: A Keepsake Book of Special Memories.* Portland, OR: Continuing Education Press, 1994. Available from Continuing Education Press, School of Extended Studies, Portland State University, P.O. Box 1394, Portland, OR 97207.

Waldegrave J. Settled stories as goals for therapy. *Forum: Association for Death Education and Counseling.* 2001;27(2):7–8.

Weeks OD, Johnson C (eds.). *When All the Friends Have Gone: A Guide for Aftercare Providers.* Amityville, New York: Baywood, 2001.

White M. Saying Hullo Again: The Incorporation of the Lost Relationship in the Resolution of Grief. In *Selected Papers*, M White (ed.). Adelaide, Australia: Dulwich Centre Publications, 1989, 29–36.

Winslade J. Putting stories to work. *Forum: Association for Death Education and Counseling*. 2001;27(2):1–4.

Wolfe B. Grief and the family. *Minnesota Medicine*. 2000;83(5):55–56.

Woof WR, Carter YH. The grieving adult and the general practitioner: A literature review in two parts (Part 1). *British Journal of General Practice*. 1997;47(420): 443–448.

Woof WR, Carter YH. The grieving adult and the general practitioner: A literature review in two parts (Part 2). *British Journal of General Practice*. 1997;47(420): 509–514.

References on coping and first-person narrative accounts of loss:

Doka KJ. *Living with Grief: Who We Are and How We Grieve*. Washington, DC: Hospice Foundation of America, 1998.

Doka KJ. *Living with Grief When Illness Is Prolonged*. Washington, DC: Hospice Foundation of America, 1997.

Doka KJ. *Living with Grief after Sudden Loss*. Washington, DC: Hospice Foundation of American, 1996.

Finkbeiner AK. *After the Death of a Child: Living with Loss through the Years*. New York: Free Press, 1996.

Henderson C. *Losing Malcolm: A Mother's Journey through Grief*. Jackson: University Press of Mississippi, 2001.

McCraken A, Semel M (eds.). *A Broken Heart Still Beats After Your Child Dies*. Center City, MI: Hazeldon, 1998.

Neimeyer RA. *Lessons of Loss: A Guide to Coping*. New York: McGraw-Hill, 1998.

Rosenblatt PC. *Parent Grief: Narratives of Loss and Relationship*. Philadelphia: Brunner/Mazell, 2000.

Part Five

Promoting Better Pain Management in Long-Term Care Facilities

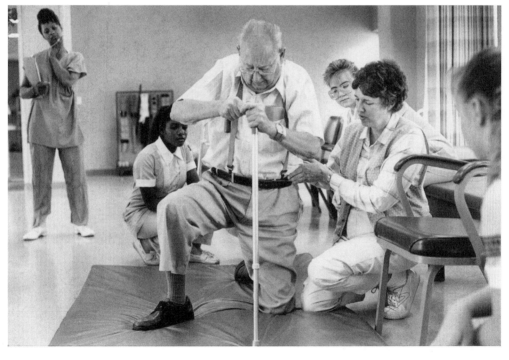

"Learning New Skills"
©1992 Susie Fitzhugh. All Rights Reserved.

Harnessing Power and Passion: Lessons from Pain Management Leaders and Literature

JUDITH A. SPROSS, PhD, RN, AOCN, FAAN

*Education Development Center, Inc.
Newton, Massachusetts*

Anyone who has labored in the field of pain management for any length of time knows that the Wisconsin Pain Initiative (WPI, formerly the Wisconsin Cancer Pain Initiative) has been at the leading edge of improving pain management in the United States. Like E.F. Hutton, when the Wisconsin Pain community speaks, we in the field of pain management listen. The two Featured Innovations in this part of the book illuminate both sides of the intervention experience. Weissman and his coauthors detail the process of designing and implementing an intervention to institutionalize pain management, specifically geared to the needs of long-term care facilities. Mary Arata, a member of one of the teams in this study, speaks candidly about how staff working in long-term care translates the intervention into practice. As a clinical nurse specialist, I was responsible for improving pain management in acute, rehabilitation, and outpatient oncology settings. As project director of Mayday PainLink,* my colleagues and I have been providing technical assistance to teams seeking to improve their institution's methods for assessing and treating pain. Thus, I have had the opportunity to participate in or observe many examples of institutionalizing pain management. Over the years, it has become clear to me that improving pain management is not simply a matter of teaching clinicians knowledge and skills, adopting policies and procedures, implementing quality improvement, and empowering nurses. Rather, it is a complex, clinical, social, and political process, which may explain why we have not seen greater progress in relieving pain in the last two decades than we have.

To ensure that all patients have equal access to pain management and relief, it is important to understand the nature of institutional change. By examining the work of our featured innovators, as well as my own experience as a change agent, I explore the process of institutional change, not just what accounts for success, but, equally important, what holds clinicians and institutions back. To make the processes and challenges of institutional change more explicit, I first review four

*See <www.edc.org/PainLink/> for details.

dimensions of institutions—strategic, structural, technical, and cultural—that change agents need to address to achieve clinical quality improvement across an organization.[1] The featured efforts illustrate what attention to these dimensions entails, and I will discuss factors within each dimension that may influence the success of an initiative. I will then examine the application of these dimensions to institutional self-assessment and action planning. This framework provides one explanation of the "mechanism of action" of institutional change. Just as pharmacologic mechanisms of action help us to evaluate therapeutic, adverse, and idiosyncratic responses of patients to analgesics, I hope this exploration will help readers to evaluate and address staff responses to institutional improvement efforts.

DIMENSIONS OF INSTITUTIONS: AN OVERVIEW

The **strategic** dimension refers to the conditions and processes that are most essential to the organization and provide the greatest opportunity for improvement.[1] The Joint Commission for Accreditation of Healthcare Organization's (JCAHO) pain management standards are, perhaps, the most important incentive that clinical settings now have for ensuring that institutions address the strategic dimension.[†] The **structural** dimension refers to the presence or absence of appropriate mechanisms, such as committee structures, policies, and procedures, to facilitate adoption of evidence-based practices throughout the organization. The **technical** dimension refers to the training and information system issues relevant to the institutional change being undertaken.[1] The **cultural** dimension refers to the beliefs, values, norms and behaviors of individuals within the organization, and the organization as a whole, which can inhibit or facilitate quality improvement work.[1] Adoption of evidence-based practices is influenced by local factors, and so it is critical to study this dimension. Having participated in and observed the process of institutional change, I would add that the cultural dimension also includes the interpersonal factors and emotions that accompany change. Unless all four dimensions are addressed, there will be no long-term organizational impact.

Shortell et al. analyze how the presence and absence of each of these dimensions (strategic, structural, technical, and cultural) affect the result of an organization-wide quality improvement effort. They note that absence of attention to the strategic dimension will lead to "no significant results on anything important"; no attention to the cultural dimension will lead to "small, temporary effects" but "no lasting impact"; the absence of attention to the technical dimension will lead to "frustration and false starts"; and the absence of attention to the structural dimension will lead to an "inability to capture learning and spread it throughout the organization."[2]

To make institutional self-assessment along these dimensions more straightforward, in Table 1 I have categorized elements of the Medical College of Wiscon-

---

[†]See <www.jcaho.org/accredited&organizations/hospitals/standards/revisions/2001/pain&management.htm> for these pain standards and revisions for 2001 and 2002.

Table 1
Dimensions of Change and Strategies for Institutionalizing Pain Management Practices[§]

Strategic	*Structural*
• Facility administrators' buy-in • Regulators' buy-in • Resident and family buy-in • Pain management quality improvement process in place (8) • Explicit facility plan for assessing resident and family satisfaction (7) • Pain management included in facility's mission, patient bill of rights, and other documents • Recruiting influential allies	• Facility needs assessment • Interdisciplinary pain management team (6) • Context-sensitive action plan • Standardized tool for cognitively intact residents (1) • Standardized tool for cognitively impaired residents (2) • Standardized facility pain scale (3) • Standardized pain documentation flow sheet (4) • Explicit pain assessment/management policies (5) • Pain management quality improvement process in place (8)
Technical	*Cultural*
• Assessing discrepancy between current and recommended practice (e.g., knowledge surveys, needs assessments) • Education plan for facility RNs (10) • Education plan for facility LPNs (11) • Education plan for facility nurse assistants (12) • Education plan for facility rehab staff (13) • Education plan for all new facility staff (14) • Explicit education program for residents and families (9)	• Coaching/mentoring of participants • Staff empowerment • Decreased staff frustration • Improved nurse–physician communication and conflict negotiation regarding pain management • Improved teamwork • Creating a culture of advocacy • Identifying one or more institutional pain management champions • Celebrating accomplishments shared with program participants (e.g., testimonials, internal and external publications and presentations, posters)

[§]Numbers in parentheses refer to the indicators targeted by the MCW Program. See Figure 3 on p. 268. My choices here are informed by references 3 through 11.

sin (MCW) pain management in long-term care program according to these dimensions using the program description. Note that the table incorporates both the objective indicators of institutionalized pain management practices targeted by the MCW program[‡] and the general processes embedded in programs of institutional change.[3-11] My own experiences and those of the featured innovators suggest that a critical analysis of these indicators and processes can help administrators and clinicians to understand the "mechanism of action" of institutional change and enable them to identify the areas in which they might have the most success, to anticipate barriers, and limit frustration.

THE STRATEGIC DIMENSION

Institutional commitment has been recognized as a key element in a number of guidelines[10-12] and publications,[3,4,7,11,13-15] but the extent to which institutions have been willing to make this commitment has varied. Institutional commitment can be manifested in a number of ways: administrative buy-in, mission statements, Continuous Quality Improvement (CQI), and resource allocation. It is important to understand who has the power to make decisions. This power may be distinct from administrative buy-in. For example, administrators may approve pain as a CQI indicator, but if you cannot get a key physician's or committee's involvement or endorsement, the progress of the initiative will be impeded. Now I will elaborate on what attention to the strategic dimension means.

The MCW long-term care program and its implementation at Franciscan Woods demonstrate that administrative buy-in is a central element of institutional change. Administrators demonstrated commitment by permitting a facility needs assessment to be done by the MCW staff and by sending facility staff to the MCW program. Facilities that followed through on commitments to assess resident and family satisfaction and incorporated pain management as a quality improvement focus, and initiated a program of resident and family education as part of their action plans were publicly stating that their staff would be accountable for managing pain. This is *strong* evidence of incorporating pain management into the strategic dimension of their organizations. Such accountability is central to pain management initiatives.

Accountability must be established early on in an initiative. There are two levels of accountability: individual accountability for integrating good pain management into one's practice and institutional accountability for making institutional changes that spread the learning throughout the organization. If only some individuals adopt better pain management practices, then only some patients will have pain relief. Practically speaking, leaving pain management up to individuals without any institutional policy for accountability permits two standards of care to exist: that of the champions who implement evidence-based practices and that of those who continue to manage pain using knowledge that is 20 or 30 years old.

[‡]See the Improving Pain Management in Long-Term Care Facilities, Weissman et al., pp. 265-274.

If a champion operates only from his or her own commitment without institutional authority, the initiative and its accomplishments are less likely to survive a change in staffing or workload, or the champion will burn out. The JCAHO pain standards should give facilities a strong incentive to demonstrate their institutional commitment to relieving pain.

> *If a champion operates only from his or her own commitment without institutional authority, the initiative and its accomplishments are less likely to survive a change in staffing or workload, or the champion will burn out.*

The Featured Innovation demonstrates that embarking on a process of institutional change represents a significant commitment of human and other resources. However, it is not clear from the articles what actual financial and resource commitments are required to improve pain management. In reading, one wants to know what it costs—in staff time, resources such as additional analgesic medications needed in the pharmacy's inventory, or materials for initiating nondrug treatments. Nurses would want to know how Ms. Arata's time as a staff nurse was reallocated so that she could lead the successful initiative at Franciscan Woods. Not only must administrators think that improving pain management is a good idea and demonstrate verbal support, but they must also weave it into the process of organizational planning and resource allocation. As long-term care facilities (LTCFs) work to improve pain management, understanding the budget implications will be useful to other change agents.

THE STRUCTURAL DIMENSION

When one considers the institutional structures needed to improve pain management, committee structures, staffing, and policies and procedures come immediately to mind. One of the first tasks undertaken by the Franciscan Woods staff was developing an interdisciplinary work group. I am sure those invited were selected with care. Note that the team included a pharmacist—a key person, since many of the new behaviors require more attention not only to prescribing and administering medications, but also to observing the responses of patients. Also, rehabilitation staff members were included in the process of change. Because physical and occupational therapies can induce pain and therapy staff members make observations of activity-related pain as well as responses to analgesics, these staff members provide important insights into the overall treatment plan. However, it is not enough to establish a team and schedule meetings. Effective committee work depends on qualities associated with the cultural dimension of institutions: good communication, outreach to facility staff and administrators, the recruitment of influential allies, setting priorities, and following through on tasks. One lament I have heard from the innovators I have coached is that some key person who could exert influence on potential allies never comes to meetings or does not follow through on commitments made to the team. Since one purpose of an interdisciplinary team is to broaden the base of support for making changes (a cultural intervention), factors such as interest, reliability, and ability to follow through should be considered when assembling a team.

Other LTCFs might start somewhere else. Some teams have found that making pain management a CQI project or developing and disseminating policies is a better first intervention. These structural interventions can build interest in the topic of pain management. Thus, when an institution is ready to address the problems uncovered by a CQI evaluation or the challenges of consistently implementing a pain assessment standard, a core group of committed staff is ready to work together to make change.

THE TECHNICAL DIMENSION

For nearly two decades, numerous studies have demonstrated that nurses, physicians, and pharmacists lack important pain management knowledge. However, we learned early on that education was insufficient.[16] Pain management is not just a clinical issue, but a political and social process that takes place within a societal and institutional context.[5,14,17] Any effort to change practice must take this into account. Having said that, the technical dimension—giving staff the knowledge and skills that they need—is vital. There is accumulating evidence that the problem of pain undertreatment is a serious concern for the elderly, particularly for residents of long-term care.[18-23] The evidence-based clinical knowledge and skills needed to relieve pain are well defined and are important, but they are not enough. Concomitant institutional changes must be initiated and maintained; otherwise, pain undertreatment will remain an intractable problem. As the MCW program illustrates, clinicians need to be able to communicate effectively, resolve conflicts over pain management productively, and understand the systems in which they work in order to bring about institutional change. The action plan with regard to education should focus on a realistic goal and a timetable for achieving it. It is important to consider what the "market will bear"—i.e., what staff can handle in terms of content and time commitment. Fortunately, a variety of initiatives have led to the development of tools and strategies—essentially, a curriculum for change agents—for institutional assessment and intervention.[7,9,11,24-26] These resources are indispensable to readers who wish to make change in their own facilities.

Educating staff about pain management and change strategies also begins to address the cultural dimension by challenging the values and myths that are at the heart of pain undertreatment (e.g., opioids are bad, the elderly experience less pain, the elderly can't tolerate opioids, the risk of addiction is high). Innovators need to understand that pain management education is not like teaching staff about a new medication or a new piece of equipment. Pain and pain management have multiple meanings and these meanings differ and often even conflict, de-

> *Pain management is not just a clinical issue, but a political and social process that takes place within a societal and institutional context.*

pending on the individual.[27] Pain management education challenges deeply held convictions about the nature of pain and what constitutes appropriate treatment and, in this sense, efforts to improve pain management are *radical*. Indeed, educating staff to re-examine their approaches to patients in pain is really a form of proselytizing. One seeks to *convert* a group to a new way of thinking, not just a new way of doing. The nature of the change will be celebrated and readily adopted by some; others will invest considerable energy in resisting the change; a third group will wait to see which of the first two groups is going to prevail. This understanding of what pain management education means for staff and institutions underscores the importance of addressing the cultural dimension in any institutional change effort.

THE CULTURAL DIMENSION

When one looks at the pain management improvement literature, most of the work has been done on addressing the structural and technical dimensions, with some attention to the strategic dimension. Although there is considerable evidence that the cultural aspects of organizations have an impact on pain management, with the exception of trying to change clinicians' attitudes toward opioids and the risk of addiction, there has been little attention to this dimension of institutions as it relates to improving pain management. Indeed, participants in interventions to improve pain management identify these barriers associated with the cultural dimension: unwillingness to prescribe opioids, regulatory barriers, team communication issues, lack of collaboration between nurses and physicians, and ethical dilemmas.[5,7,8,14,25,28-30] In addition, I believe that the emotions that accompany pain management improvement efforts and the locus of power and decision making are parts of the cultural dimension. Emotions experienced by staff participating in change efforts run the gamut from angry, frustrated, overwhelmed, and helpless to satisfied, successful, supported, and confident. Because there is less information on the cultural dimension of institutions in the literature on pain management, I will discuss it here in some detail.

The cultural dimension is not explicitly identified in the 14 indicators targeted by the MCW program. If one reads between the lines of the two stories about this program in this part of the book, one can see the ways in which the MCW program actually addressed the cultural dimension. The most important evidence of attention to this dimension, perhaps, is recognizing that institutional change is a process that requires support and reinforcement. An implicit goal of scheduling training sessions over the course of a year instead of a one-time meeting was the creation of a mutually supportive, interinstitutional community. I imagine that participants not only consulted with the MCW staff between sessions, but that the participants contacted each other for ideas, support, and commiseration. Such support has been an integral part of other change efforts.[7,9,28]

Ms. Arata notes that at first they were "a little overwhelmed" by the demands of action planning. However, she and her colleagues didn't try to do everything at once. The "technical content" provided in the MCW Program helped her and

> *. . . one of the key strategies for making staff want to change is to provide evidence of the gap between current practice and recommended practice.*

her colleagues see the discrepancy between current practice and recommended practice. Uncovering this discrepancy is one of the most important motivators for changing practice. Staff members want to do a good job, but if they do not know that their practices are outdated, they do not have the motivation to change. In some programs and settings, assessing this discrepancy is done by a survey and then by sharing the results of the survey with the staff.[7,9,28] Thus, one of the key strategies for making staff want to change is to provide evidence of the gap between current practice and recommended practice. Demonstrating such a gap can be used to persuade administrators that they should make pain management a priority, a strategy for addressing the strategic dimension as well.

Recruiting allies is a key element of enhancing the "cultural" support for changing pain management, enabling one to build a culture of advocacy. Members of *all* clinical disciplines and role groups, especially nurses, pharmacists, and physicians, have a part to play in improving pain management. However, it is often difficult to recruit physicians to the change initiative.[31] The absence of physician support is thought to be a factor in less successful CQI efforts.[1] So, developing strategies to recruit physicians may be a key cultural intervention. Once recruited, pain champions are usually involved for the long haul, and all advocates need nurturing. This need can be met by acknowledging and celebrating a team's accomplishments, for example, the storyboard mentioned in the MCW Program. Featuring the team's work or a clinical exemplar in an internal publication or a community newspaper is another strategy. Collecting and publishing testimonials feeds enthusiasm for this labor-intensive effort.

The MCW Program and its participants wisely focused attention on certified nursing assistants (CNAs), the staff members in long-term care with the most direct patient contact. Support staff have not generally been an explicit focus of institutional change initiatives (a notable exception is Chichin et al.[32]), but the innovators recognized that without targeting the involvement of CNAs, any long-term care initiative is doomed to fail. CNAs need to know what to observe, what to report, and what they can do to comfort patients in pain. Indeed, in one report the pain champion told of instructing housekeeping and dietary staff what to observe and report to the nursing staff so that the nurses could respond promptly, even to nonverbal evidence of pain.[33]

Ms. Arata's comments highlight some less obvious elements of culture, which change agents would do well to address. If we unpack the idea of nurse empowerment described by Weissman and colleagues, we develop a deep understanding of the cultural change engendered by the pain management initiative. Ms. Arata's comments reveal the challenges and successes inherent in the process of empowering nurses. She notes that "Initially, we were all nurses." Although an interdisciplinary team is ideal, it may not be realistic or feasible at the beginning. Nurses and nursing staff often provide the critical mass of knowledge, commitment, and talent that have contributed to successful initiatives. The MCW program provided the tools of behavioral change. The information and tools that Ms. Arata and her colleagues brought back to the facility enabled nurses to start behaving similarly around pain management practices. Specifically, they began to use a common language (the pain scale) when speaking to nursing assistants and physicians. They communicated to residents and their families the critical message that pain can be relieved.

Ms. Arata makes an important point about sustaining practice changes: these new behaviors require reinforcement through ongoing monitoring and coaching. Many reports on improving pain management imply the importance of having an internal coach attending to staff and patient responses to the change effort. Ms. Arata noted that difficult patients could activate old values, such as believing that the patient is drug seeking or craving attention. Activating old values can "extinguish" the new pain management behaviors if there is not a coach to help staff to apply the new knowledge to more complex patients. The champion or coach must use these teachable moments to link the "difficult" behavior to a likely problem of undertreated pain. Consider these other situations in which staff may need coaching: When scheduled opioids are used instead of prn[||] analgesics, nurses often need reassurance that they can care for their patients safely when they make this change in clinical practice. Or when staff observe that a particular patient experiences opioid-induced respiratory depression, even though they have been told that this is uncommon, someone has to help them not only to adjust the particular treatment plan, but also to interpret the situation so that staff's fear of causing respiratory depression is not reinforced. In the long-term care setting, concerns about polypharmacy (multiple medications for multiple health problems) in the elderly can conflict or compete with advocating appropriate analgesics. The coach will need to work with staff to mediate these concerns safely, while ensuring patients' pain relief. Thus, an effective coach recognizes both the institutional and clinical dimensions of improving pain management.

These innovators' work suggests that other factors may need to be addressed, such as the quality of communication and conflict negotiation strategies. I have addressed only selected cultural aspects of organizational life. Readers may identify factors that are more salient in their particular situations than the ones I have addressed here. To learn more about organizing groups to effect change, advocacy, and recruiting influential others, readers can visit the Center for Community Change website.[¶]

INSTITUTIONAL SELF-ASSESSMENT, DIAGNOSTIC ANALYSIS, AND ACTION PLANNING

Both the Weissman et al. paper and the interview with Mary Arata make clear that institutional change is essential to ensuring that residents in long-term care set-

---

[||]The acronym prn stands for pro re nata, or "as needed."
[¶]The Center for Community Change website is <www.communitychange.org>.

tings have access to appropriate and effective pain management. The adoption of evidence-based practices is context dependent.[34-37] That is, one needs to think about specific aspects of the institution as well as clinician practices. So, just as assessment is the first step in managing pain, institutional assessment—an evaluation of a setting's strengths and weaknesses with regard to changing clinical practices—is essential to developing an action plan and optimizing the success of an improvement initiative. Although there are several examples of paper and pencil institutional checklists,[9,24,26] which outline the possibilities for institutional interventions, none are organized with the aforementioned understanding of institutional dimensions in mind. Table 2 lists questions by dimension that staff can ask about their institutions. An affirmative answer indicates an institutional strength; a negative answer identifies a potential focus for intervention.

Engaging in a diagnostic analysis can determine what particular strengths exist and in which dimensions. This understanding guides a team's action planning and helps members to establish priorities. Strengths can be leveraged to reap short- and long-term benefits. For example, one might determine that staff does not have the knowledge to assess and relieve pain (the technical dimension) and that there are only a few pain management champions. Whereas, eventually, all four dimensions must be addressed for a change effort to "take," the champions may decide that the action plan priority is to widen the base of support for change. One team with which I worked spent a year getting the backing of the Ethics Committee, one of the most influential committees in the organization.[38] Educational efforts were initiated only after the committee's endorsement and activism ensured that pain relief was an institutional priority. Or, the champions could decide that education is the best strategy to widen the base of support. Another team decided to educate nurses about pain management first. Once nurses began "singing from the same sheet of music" with regard to pain management, it became easier to enlist physicians and administrators in the effort. The MCW program faculty emphasized that they did not require participants to use specific tools or policies; they recognized that a successful initiative must take into account the local conditions. There is no "one size fits all" action plan; even with a mandate to meet pain management standards for accreditation, failure to consider the local conditions will undermine any change effort. Ideally, action plans will target activities that are likely to exert influence in multiple dimensions of institutions.

Ms. Arata noted that they had made progress during the first year of participation, but still had "more to do." This comment underscores the nature of change as a long-term process. It takes time to see results and it may take two to three years for the cumulative effects of a team's efforts to become visible.[28] Such a sustained effort, particularly considering the vicissitudes of modern health care, requires the interpersonal support that comes from being part of a larger community. To do this requires acknowledging incremental progress and celebrating small victories. Champions have a demanding task: to keep the vision of improved pain management on the front burner while coping with competing clinical and administrative demands, such as complex patient needs and staff turnover.

Table 2
Diagnostic Analysis: Questions for Institutional Self-Assessment

Strategic	*Structural*
• Is there an explicit institutional commitment to improving pain management? Is there evidence of this commitment and is the evidence strong (e.g., dedicated staff member, budgeted resources)? • Is there sustained, visible support from key clinical and administrative leaders (e.g., CEOs, department directors, senior physicians, nurse administrators, and managers? • Is your setting accredited by organizations that have pain management standards (such as JCAHO)? • Is pain management recognized as a potential risk management issue? Is pain management recognized as a potential financial risk?	• Is there an interdisciplinary work group to address pain management? • Are there policies and procedures for pain assessment and treatment? • Are there existing committees with clout that can lend support to your pain management improvement effort (e.g., Pharmacy and Therapeutics, Risk Management)? • Do annual mandatory classes (similar to those for CPR or infection control) include the topic of pain management? • Does the formulary include an adequate range (types and routes of administration) of medications for treating pain (e.g., non-opioids/NSAIDs, opioids, co-analgesics)? • Are there resources for implementing non-pharmacologic interventions (tape players, relaxation and music tapes, hot and cold packs, etc.)?
Technical	*Cultural*
• Has the question of which staff can perform what pain management activities been clearly defined? For example, is there a list of observations that CNAs are taught to report? Are there nondrug interventions that CNAs can perform under the supervision of nurses? • Is pain management an emphasis in orientation, in-service education, and continuing education?	• Does the interdisciplinary pain management committee function well? Are communications within the committee, between committee and administrators, and between committee and clinicians effective and respectful? Is there evidence of commitment (i.e., do committee members show up, follow through on activities)? • Has a "power analysis" been done; i.e., has the team identified the

(continued)

Table 2 (*Continued*)

• Do staff need to demonstrate their competence in pain management periodically? • Are physicians (who round less frequently in nursing homes) up-to-date on the LTC setting's pain management efforts?	influential others who will support or resist the institutional change? • Have all staff with patient contact (not just clinical staff, but house-keepers, volunteers, etc.) been recruited into the pain improve-ment effort? Does this group include informal leaders as well as those in positions of authority? • Is there an internal marketing plan for promoting the message that "pain can be relieved"? • Is there a plan to acknowledge and celebrate progress?

CONCLUSIONS

I have tried to illuminate the complexities of institutional change to improve pain management as a clinical, social, *and* political process. The MCW program demon-strates that improving pain management re-quires champions to focus on *developing capacity* and *building community*. Devel-oping capacity means giving staff the knowl-edge, skills, tools, and processes to do the job. This education is not a one-shot inter-vention nor is it sufficient. Providing pain management knowledge and skills and steady attention to integrating them into practice through coaching helps institutions to develop capacity. Building com-munity is accomplished by teaching program participants about the change process and socializing staff to become change agents and coaches themselves, enabling them to reproduce these methods in their own settings. Building a com-munity of advocates does not happen overnight; indeed, one needs to be delib-erate and strategic in the recruitment effort.

> *The MCW program demonstrates that improving pain management requires champions to focus on* developing capacity *and* building community.

Christine Miaskowski, PhD, RN, a nurse researcher and president-elect of the American Pain Society, called for a revolution.[39] I agree. However, revolution alone, like education alone, will be insufficient. To assume the mantle of pain man-agement advocate is to make a commitment to revolution and transformation. What is needed is a revolution in our collective thinking: we must abandon outdated beliefs and must convince ourselves, our colleagues, nursing home residents, and their families that *pain can be relieved*. This is a simple message that must be repeated over and over again. As hard as it is to abandon old ways of thinking, it can be done more easily now than ever before because there is, among many clinical staff members, a sense that we could be doing a better job with pain. However, it is harder (and impractical) to think that we can abandon the systems in which we work. As the work of our authors suggests, we *can* reinvent and transform our practice environments so that they support evidence-based pain management. To reinvent and transform our practice settings, we must understand the institutional factors that sustain the status quo. With this knowledge we can promote changes that engage the commitment of influential others, redistribute power, and spread evidence-based pain management throughout the organization.

REFERENCES

1. Shortell S, Bennett C, Byck G. Assessing the impact of continuous quality improvement on clinical practice: What will it take to accelerate progress? *Milbank Quarterly*. 1998;76:593–624.
2. Shortell S, Bennett C, Byck G. Assessing the impact of continuous quality improvement on clinical practice: What will it take to accelerate progress? *Milbank Quarterly*. 1998;76:607.
3. Spross JA, McGuire DB, Schmitt R. Oncology nursing position paper on cancer pain. *Oncology Nursing Forum*. 1990;17:595–614(Part I); 751–760(Part II); 943-955(Part III).
4. Spross J, Beauregard J, Crockett M, et al. Institutionalizing pain management at an acute rehabilitation hospital: An institutional case study (Abstract). *Proceedings of the 16th Annual Meeting of the American Pain Society*. New Orleans, LA: 1997.
5. Spross J. Management of cancer pain: Commentary 2. *Abstracts of Clinical Care Guidelines*. 1994;6(5):4–6.
6. Dalton J, Blau W. Changing the practice of pain management: An examination of the theoretical basis of change. *Pain Forum*. 1996;5(4):266–272.
7. Ferrell BR, Dean GE, Grant M, Coluzzi P. An institutional commitment to pain management. *Journal of Clinical Oncology*. 1995;13:2158–2165.
8. Ferrell BR, Eberts MT, McCaffery M, Grant M. Clinical decision making and pain. *Cancer Nursing*. 1991;14(6):289–297.
9. Spross J. Using principles of change and a technical assistance protocol to improve pain management in institutions. *New England Pain Association Newsletter*. 2000;5(3):8–14.
10. Jacox A, Carr DB, Payne R, et al. *Management of Cancer Pain. Clinical Practice Guideline No. 9*. Agency for Health Care Policy and Research, Public Health Service, U.S. Department of Health and Human Services. Rockville, MD: US Government Printing Office, 1994.
11. Weissman DE, Griffie J, Gordon DB, Dahl JL. A role model program to promote institutional changes for management of acute and cancer pain. *Journal of Pain and Symptom Management*. 1997;14(5):274–279.
12. Acute Pain Management Guideline Panel. *Acute Pain Management: Operative or Medical Procedures and Trauma*. Agency for Health Care Policy and Research, Public

Health Service, U.S. Department of Health and Human Services. Rockville, MD: U.S. Government Printing Office, 1992.

13. Donovan M, Evers K, Jacobs P, Mandleblatt S. When there is no benchmark: Designing a primary care-based chronic pain management program from the scientific basis up. *Journal of Pain and Symptom Management.* 1999;18(1):38-48.

14. Fagerhaugh SY, Strauss A. *Politics of Pain Management: Staff-Patient Interaction.* Menlo Park, CA: Addison-Wesley Publishing Company, 1977.

15. Oncology Nursing Society. Position statement: Cancer pain management. *Oncology Nursing Forum.* 1998;25(5):817-818.

16. Max M. Improving outcomes of analgesic treatment: Is education enough? *Annals of Internal Medicine.* 1990;113:885-889.

17. Jackson J. *Camp Pain: Talking with Chronic Pain Patients.* Philadelphia: University of Pennsylvania Press, 2000.

18. Ahmed A, Sims R. Demographic characteristics of US nursing homes and their residents: Highlights of the National Nursing Home Survey, 1995. *Annals of Long-Term Care.* 2000;8(1):62-67.

19. American Geriatric Society Panel on Chronic Pain in Older Persons. The management of chronic pain in older persons. *Journal of the American Geriatrics Society.* 1998;46:635-651.

20. Bernabei R, Gambassi G, Lapane K, Landi F, Gatsonis C, Dunlop, R, Lipsitz L, Steel K, Mor V. for the SAGE Study Group. Management of pain in elderly patients with cancer. *Journal of the American Medical Association.* 1998;279(23):1877-1882.

21. Cramer G, Galer B, Mandelson M, Thompson G. A drug use evaluation of selected opioid and nonopioid analgesics in the nursing facility setting. *Journal of the American Geriatrics Society.* 2000;48:398-404.

22. Ferrell BA, Ferrell BR, Rivera L. Pain in cognitively impaired nursing home patients. *Journal of Pain Symptom and Management.* 1995;10(8):591-598.

23. Ferrell B, Stein W, Beck J. The Geriatric Pain Measure: Validity, reliability and factor analysis. *Journal of the American Geriatrics Society.* 2000;48:1669-2000.

24. McCaffery M, Pasero C. *Pain: Clinical Manual*, 2d ed. St. Louis: C.V. Mosby, Inc., 1999.

25. Ferrell BR, Grant M, Ritchey KJ, Ropchan R, Rivera LM. The Pain Resource Nurse Training Program: A unique approach to pain management. *Journal of Pain Symptom Management.* 1993;8(8):549-556.

26. Gordon DB, Dahl JL, Stevenson, K. *Building an Institutional Commitment to Pain Management: The Wisconsin Resource Manual*, 2d ed. Madison, WI: University of Wisconsin, Board of Regents, 2000.

27. Benoliel JQ. Multiple meanings of pain and complexities of pain management. *Nursing Clinics of North America.* 1995;30(4):583-596.

28. Bookbinder M, Coyle N, Kiss M, Goldstein ML, Gianella A, Derby S, Brown M, Racolin A, Ho MN, Portenoy RK. Implementing national standards for cancer pain management: Program model and evaluation. *Journal of Pain and Symptom Management.* 1996;12(6):334-347.

29. Brockopp D, Brockopp G, Warden S, Barriers to change: A pain management project. *International Journal of Nursing Studies.* 1998;35:226-232.

30. Weissman D, Abram S, Haddox JD, Janjan NA, Hopwood MB, Howser D. Educational role of cancer pain rounds. *Journal of Cancer Education.* 1989;4:113-116.

31. Weissman, D. Cancer pain education for physicians in practice: Establishing a new paradigm. *Journal of Pain and Symptom Management.* 1996;12(6):364-371.

32. Chichin E, Schulman E, Harrington M, Norwood J, Olson E. End-of-life treatment decisions in the nursing home: Ethics and the nursing assistant. In *Quality Care in Geriatric Settings: Focus on Ethical Issues,* P Katz, R Kane, and M Mezey, (eds.). New York: Springer Publishing Co., 1995.

33. Joint Commission on Accreditation of Healthcare Organizations. *Pain Assessment and Management: An Organizational Approach.* Chicago: Joint Commission on Accreditation of Healthcare Organizations, 2000, 52–56.

34. Rogers EM. *Diffusion of Innovations,* 4th ed. New York: Free Press, 1995.

35. Bero L, Grilli R, Grimshaw J, Harvey E, Oxman A, Thomson M. Closing the gap between research and practice: An overview of systematic reviews of interventions to promote the implementation of research findings. *British Medical Journal.* 1998;317:456–468.

36. University of York NHS Centre for Reviews and Dissemination. Getting evidence into practice. *Effective Health Care.* 1999;5(1):1–16.

37. Wood M, Ferlie E, Fitzgerald L. Achieving clinical behaviour change: A case of becoming indeterminate. *Social Science and Medicine.* 1998;47(11):1729–1738.

38. Sayers M, Maranda R, et al. No need for pain. *Journal of Healthcare Quality.* 2000;22(3):10–15.

39. Miaskowski C. Improving cancer pain management: Should we continue the evolution or begin a revolution? In *Proceedings of the 19th Annual Scientific Meeting of the American Pain Society.* Atlanta, GA: American Pain Society, November 2000.

Improving Pain Management in Long-Term Care Facilities

DAVID E. WEISSMAN, MD, JULIE GRIFFIE, RN, MSN, CS, AOCN,
CHPN, SANDRA MUCHKA, RN, MS, CS, CHPN,
and SANDRA MATSON, BSN, MA, RN, C

*The Palliative Care Program of the Medical College of Wisconsin,
Milwaukee, Wisconsin*

*Improving pain management in long-term care facilities has several
unique barriers in comparison to the acute hospital setting. To address
these barriers, the Medical College of Wisconsin Palliative Care Program
began a project in 1996, initially working with 87 long-term care facilities, to improve pain management practices through a series of educational and quality improvement steps. This paper will review the overall
structure, results, strengths, and weaknesses of this approach to improving pain management in this important site of clinical care.*

We have been working to improve community pain management practices in Wisconsin since the late 1980s in partnership with the Wisconsin Cancer Pain Initiative. In 1990 and again in 1992, we held our first *Cancer Pain Role Model* programs, an educational effort designed to break down the common barriers to
cancer pain management.[1,2] The educational plan for the Role Model Program focused on bringing together teams of clinicians, nurses, and their physician clinical partners at a one-day conference, training them in the principles of cancer
pain management, and giving them suggestions for how to make changes in basic care practices in their clinical practice settings. These early programs were
partially successful at helping individuals to make change, but we quickly came
to recognize that additional work was needed to help individual clinicians to fully
change the practice of pain management in their practice settings.

INSTITUTIONS AS THE LOCUS OF CHANGE

To this end, in 1994 we began a new project focusing on health care institutions,
rather than individual clinicians, as the locus of change. This change represented
a fundamental shift by our project team in thinking about how to improve pain
management practices. Health care institutions, whether they be hospitals, long-

term care facilities (LTCFs), home health agencies, or hospice agencies, each have their own distinct culture, which can either support or hinder effective pain management. The elements of institutional culture that affect pain management include the knowledge, skills, and attitudes toward pain of the professional staff; the presence or absence of standards, policies, or clinical guidelines; and quality monitoring programs regarding pain management. Perhaps most important is the overall institutional commitment to providing excellent pain management services. Although it is true that through their daily practice physicians and nurses largely control the assessment and treatment of pain, it is also true that institutional aspects of care, for example, the presence of a standardized, facility-wide pain assessment tool or facility analgesic standards, can help to guide clinicians to do the right thing.[3-7]

To accommodate this new institutional focus, we expanded the educational content of the original Role Model Program to all pain management practices (not just cancer pain) and increased the educational contact time from one conference to two, thus including new topics of institutional change theory, hospital standards, and quality improvement. The decision to expand our focus to *all* pain, rather than just cancer pain, came after the realization that cancer pain typically affects a minority of the pain problems within a given health care institution and that just focusing on cancer pain, when similar institutional barriers exist for all aspects of pain management practice, would waste an opportunity for greater institutional impact. Furthermore, the attitudes, knowledge, and skills needed to improve acute, traumatic, postoperative, and much of chronic pain are nearly identical to those for managing cancer pain.

SPECIAL BARRIERS IN LONG-TERM CARE SETTINGS NEED TO BE ADDRESSED

Participants from LTCFs enrolled in an earlier role model project specifically told us that their issues for institutional change were different from acute care. These participants were unable to use the information and asked the project team to design a new intervention project specific to the needs of long-term care.[8] It is important to understand some of the unique barriers to good pain management practice in the LTCF.[9-13] First, as a heavily regulated industry, especially concerning the use of psychoactive medication, LTCF nurses and physicians are hesitant to use scheduled analgesics for chronic pain out of fear of regulatory scrutiny by state or federal surveyors. Second, most pain experienced by LTCF residents is nonmalignant and to date there has been little acceptance by physicians of routinely scheduled opioid therapy for chronic nonmalignant pain, although increasing evidence points to the relative safety and efficacy of opioids for this indication.[14] Third, physician involvement in the day-to-day care of LTCF residents is far less than for hospitalized patients. Contact typically occurs only once every 30 days. Fourth, the bulk of actual patient contact in the LTCF is via certified nursing assistants, who have little to no training in pain assessment. Thus, in the typical LTCF there are physician, nursing, institutional, and regulatory barriers that impede pain management above and beyond the already familiar barriers to pain management in hospitalized patients.

NEW PROGRAM DESIGNED SPECIFICALLY FOR LONG-TERM CARE SETTINGS

To address the special needs of pain in LTCFs, we designed a new educational intervention, building from our prior experiences with hospitals, in collaboration with the Wisconsin Bureau of Quality Compliance and the Wisconsin Division of Health, which are the regulatory agencies that monitor long-term care in Wisconsin.[15] Recruitment to the project was on a first-come, first-serve basis, with a target goal of 90 facilities. Letters of invitation were mailed to the directors of nursing and facility administrator of all long-term care facilities in eastern Wisconsin. In all, 87 facilities enrolled, divided into three training cohorts. To ensure top-level buy-in, each facility's administrator and director of nursing were required to sign a letter of commitment. Facilities were not required to pay any fee for participation; funding for the project came from local private foundations.

The educational plan included the following features:

- A site visit to the facility by a project team member, during which time a facility needs assessment was completed.*
- A series of four educational workshops, evenly spaced over one year, attended by a team of two to four facility staff, including middle and senior management in a position to make changes. Topics included pain assessment, treatment, standards development, quality improvement, staff education, and staff competencies. Teaching methods included lectures, small-group workshops, role-play exercises, and case studies.
- Completion by participants of a facility-specific Action Plan, a detailed blueprint for proposed changes.
- Chart reviews of pain assessment documentation performed by each facility team.

TARGET INDICATORS

To help facility staff to keep the goals in mind, a list of 14 target indicators of good pain management (Figure 3) was developed from existing national standards.[15] Indicators included elements of pain assessment, pain treatment, quality improvement, staff education, and facility commitment. The facility needs assessment catalogued the presence or absence of these indicators at the start of the project and again one year later at the project's conclusion.

---

*See Appendix B, pp. 378–379, for the Facility Needs Assessment, or download this form from the archived issue "Promoting Better Pain Management in Long-Term Care Facilities" of *Innovations in End-of-Life Care*, Vol. 3, No. 1, 2001, at <www.edc.org/lastacts>.

1. Standardized facility assessment tool for cognitively intact residents
2. Standardized facility assessment tool for cognitively impaired residents
3. Standardized facility pain scale(s)
4. Standardized pain documentation flow sheet
5. Explicit pain assessment/management policies
6. Interdisciplinary pain management team
7. Explicit facility plan for assessing resident/family satisfaction
8. Pain management quality improvement process in place
9. Explicit education program for residents and families
10. Education plan for new facility RNs
11. Education plan for new facility LPNs
12. Education plan for new facility nurse assistants
13. Education plan for new facility rehabilitation staff
14. Education plan for all new facility staff

Figure 3.   Target Indicators for Institutionalization of Pain Management Practice[15]

Copyright ©2000, US Cancer Pain Relief Committee. Reprinted with permission of Elsevier Science.

At the project's inception, only 12 facilities (14 percent) had more than half of the 14 indicators in place, compared to 64 facilities (74 percent) post-project. On average, each facility had only 3.4 of the 14 indicators in place at project inception, compared to 8.8 at project completion.[17] The most common indicators established during the year-long project included pain assessment tools for cognitively intact and cognitively impaired residents, development of a standardized facility pain scale, specific pain management policies and protocols, and training in pain management for new nursing staff. Pain documentation significantly improved over the course of the year, as evidenced by the chart review project. Overall, we were pleased with these results, feeling that this project had provided an excellent foundation for facilities hoping to improve their pain management practice.

EMPOWERING NURSES

From the perspective of project design, there were several factors that led to an overall positive impact. First, although not designed as such, this project to improve pain management was just as much a nurse empowerment project. Nurses, by far the largest group of participants at the teaching conferences, came away from each conference with new knowledge about and confidence in their own practices. When these teams first came together, there was a strong feeling of anger and frustration—frustration because they *knew* they were not doing a good job, frustration because they did not understand how to do it better, and anger,

focused on physicians, about basic conflicts in nurse–physician communication
that impede good pain management.[16]

What we heard over and over again from
participants was that we had empowered
them to go home and do things differently;
we gave them, in a sense, the building
blocks to initiate change. We gave them
the knowledge, skills, and a kind of esprit
de corps to say, "This is the way it ought
to be done." Essentially, this happened be-

> *What we heard over and over again from participants was that we had empowered them to go home and do things differently; we gave them, in a sense, the building blocks to initiate change.*

cause the new information was congruent with what they thought ought to be
done; we did not have to spend a lot of time convincing them that what we were
telling them was the right thing.

ASSESSING PAIN AND DESIGNING A TREATMENT PLAN

Foremost among the new information acquired by nurses was the ability to perform an accurate assessment, design a treatment plan, and then contact the physician for new orders.[†] To effect this empowerment we used case studies and
role-playing exercises.[‡19,20] In particular, participants all had the opportunity to
role play a pain assessment with a simulated patient and develop an analgesic
plan. Participants frequently commented about how powerless they felt prior to
this instruction and how they were often frustrated by physicians' seeming in-
difference to their requests for new analgesic orders. Following the instruction,
nurses reported greater self-confidence and outright success at achieving the desired interaction with physicians. Ultimately, nurses bought into the idea that
they could perform a credible pain assessment and that the time that they spent
on pain assessment and treatment planning would pay off. They could save time
by being proactive and thus avoid dealing with inevitable consequences of unrelieved pain.

WINNING ADMINISTRATIVE COMMITMENT

Another element of our success was that we stressed strong facility buy-in to
the project from the outset. We were emphatic about the need for commitment from the top, not just on the part of the director of nursing, but also
from the facility administrator. We encouraged the facility teams to meet on
a regular basis with their director of nursing and administrator so that they
could convey the information about project status and work collaboratively to

---

[†]See Appendix B, pp. 379–380, for the Guidelines for Analgesic Drug Orders.
[‡]Appendix B, pp. 381–383, for the Three-Person Pain Assessment Role-Playing Exercise.

overcome the inevitable barriers to change. We asked the administrators to assist teams by finding a regular monthly meeting time that teams could work on their project.

GENERATING FACILITY STAFF AND RESIDENT SUPPORT

We worked to have the facility teams obtain buy-in from other facility staff and from facility residents. In this way, we encouraged teams to transfer the locus of control of the project from the project faculty back onto the end users—the facility staff and residents. We asked them to take the issues that they were dealing with to the Residents' Council, a forum for residents to speak out on issues of concern, which is required for all LTCFs in Wisconsin.

We emphasized local creativity to solve local problems. For example, we did not mandate use of one specific pain assessment tool; we provided teams with several examples and asked them to try different and creative approaches with their residents. One team developed a pain assessment stick, a two-foot length of wood, with tactile markers for different pain levels for use with visually impaired residents.

LISTENING TO THE NEEDS OF PARTICIPANTS

We tried hard to be flexible in response to the needs of the facility teams. Two key domains of care that were not included in the original project design were added mid-course at the request of participants. The first was education about pain assessment in the cognitively impaired resident. For this topic we enlisted the support of Christine Kovach, RN, PhD, a nurse researcher with expertise in dementia care. Dr. Kovach met with the project teams, presented didactic information, and introduced participants to a novel treatment algorithm for pain in the cognitively impaired resident.[19,20] The second domain was education for nursing assistants. Many project teams requested specific educational material and strategies to use with these important staff members. This led to the development of teaching modules for nursing assistants and separate modules for all staff and licensed nursing staff, which were disseminated to all teams.[16]

TIMING OF WORKSHOPS AND MENTORING CHANGE

We designed the spacing of the educational workshops to occur every three months so as to allow project teams sufficient time to digest new information and then to work together toward change. At the conclusion of each workshop, the project teams were given time to map out an implementation strategy.

The project faculty's role was one of coaching: we would walk around the room during each education workshop, meet with each project team, discuss their tentative plans, challenge them to go a bit further in the planning than they thought possible, and together brainstorm strategies to overcome barriers. Between workshops, project faculty periodically contacted teams to assess the need for assistance and to give encouragement. We feel the relationship between the faculty and the project teams that we established, that of coaches and mentors rather than lecturers and experts, was crucial to success, in that it helped build the strong sense of trust needed to keep the teams moving forward.

INVITING REGULATORS AS PARTNERS IN CHANGE

From the inception of the project, we brought our state's long-term care regulators into the project design. We invited a regulatory representative to speak to the project teams on three key issues of concern to facility staff regarding how the state regulators would evaluate the following:

1. Adequacy of pain assessment documentation
2. Use of chronic opioids for nonmalignant pain
3. Manner of different prescription orders, for example, prn versus scheduled pain medication for a chronic painful condition

Of note, since this project began, a number of LTCFs in Wisconsin have been cited by state regulators for failure to adequately assess and treat pain. Thus, we feel that there was bidirectional learning in this project. Not only did the project teams learn how surveyors would conduct their business, but the surveyors learned key facts about pain assessment and treatment that could be used to raise the general level of pain management through the surveying process.

BARRIERS TO PROGRESS: TURNOVER, LACK OF "CHAMPION," TIME

Although this project helped many facilities to move forward, some facilities clearly had a hard time getting started and made little progress. The most important factor in project success was a *stable facility staff*; nothing dampened project momentum faster for a given facility than the turnover of the director of nursing, facility administrator, or project team members who attended early workshops. Even though new facility team members would attend subsequent workshops, it was virtually impossible for them to get up to speed. Conversely, when we look at those facilities that *were* able to make substantial and sustainable progress, we can always identify a core group of senior and middle management staff with a long tenure at that facility.

A second factor that impeded facility progress was the absence of a *champion*, i.e., an individual who recognized the problem of poor pain management and made a highly personal commitment to seek change through cheerleading and advocacy. Mentoring champions is not difficult once they are identified, and this project clearly had many. However, if no champion from a particular facility emerged, it was not possible for the project faculty to manufacture one, as champions must have a combination of strong internal motivation, personal energy, and excellent people skills.

The third impediment to project success was *time*. LTCFs are typically stretched very thin just to provide routine care; the addition of a new project, requiring considerable staff time for implementation, was clearly a burden for many facilities. Those facilities that needed to devote time to other new projects that came forward during the project year, projects such as a state regulatory survey, were doubly pressured for time, leading some to scale back or completely abandon their project goals.

> *Staff turnover, lack of a champion, and time—all relate to one core element needed for successful change: facility buy-in.*

Staff turnover, lack of a champion, and time—all relate to one core element needed for successful change: facility buy-in. In one sense, if the commitment is strong enough from senior leadership, then any or all of the three identified problems are potentially surmountable. Without strong commitment, the presence of any one of these three problems is enough to scuttle significant progress.

FOLLOW-UP

Since completing the one-year project with the initial 87 facilities, we have continued this work, revising project elements and developing new educational tools. A measure of the strong bond between the participating facilities and project faculty occurred at the final conference. In an open forum discussion with participants, project faculty asked, "How can the faculty continue to support you? What do you need?" The response was emphatically, "We want to keep working with you on this project, our work is not done!" The project faculty made a commitment to continue the project.

We now hold quarterly meetings with the same facility teams, discussing topics of interest and developing new resources through work groups comprised of project faculty and team members. Projects have included development of pain algorithms[§] for all facilities and a workbook of educational resources, *Pain 101*, for facility staff.[17] The most recent request by teams has been to expand the pain project to include other aspects of end-of-life care, advance care planning, communication skills, and non-pain symptom control. Plans are now being formulated and funding sought for a LTCF end-of-life project, similar in concept to the pain project.

Subsequent to working with the 87 facilities described, we have worked with other LTCFs—individual facilities, a group of nine facilities that come together for educational and staff development programs, and one large national LTC organization with more than 200 facilities. Most recently, we participated in a project, using the same design principles, for a consortium of different health care facilities (hospitals, hospices, LTCFs) working together in Missoula, Montana. The project organizers in Missoula were interested in improving both interfacility and intrafacility communication and coordination of pain care. This project has proven quite successful at breaking down some of the interagency barriers to pain management. As a consequence of this work, one Missoula hospital was cited by the

Joint Commission on Accreditation of Healthcare Organizations (JCAHO) for its exemplary pain management work.

We have added two new elements to the original project. First, following the pain assessment role play and development of an analgesic plan, nurses role play contacting the physician for new orders, based on the analgesic plan that they develop. This exercise provides nurses with an explicit opportunity to practice and receive feedback on the skill of communicating a pain assessment and treatment plan to a physician. A second element that we have added is the use of a project storyboard. We ask each participating facility to design a poster that graphically displays their work toward improving pain management, new assessment tools, analgesic guidelines, non-pharmacological treatment approaches, and the like. Participants from each facility bring their storyboard to the final project workshop to share with other participants; they are then encouraged to display the storyboard prominently in their facility for all staff and nursing home residents to see. This new feature has been popular with project participants; they feel a tremendous sense of accomplishment after their year of hard work and want to share their success with others.

Improving pain management practice in long-term care facilities is hard work; it takes an amazing amount of time, resources, and commitment to effect positive change. However, once the process is started, once small tasks have been successfully completed, the next task does not seem quite so insurmountable. We always encourage teams to start with the easy tasks first, the "low-hanging fruit," then build from success. The challenge is to take that first step.

ACKNOWLEDGMENT

The project was funded by grants from the Faye McBeath Foundation and the Eastern Wisconsin Area Health Education Center, Inc., under agreement No. STC-M 5U76 PE00234-04, with the Division of Medicine, Bureau of Health Professions, Health Resources and Services Administration, US Department of Health and Human Services. Additional funding was provided by Ortho-McNeil Pharmaceutical, Purdue Frederick Co., and Roxane Laboratories, Inc.

REFERENCES

1. Weissman DE, Dahl JL, Beasly J. Cancer Pain Role Model Program of the Wisconsin Cancer Pain Initiative. *Journal of Pain and Symptom Management*. 1993;8:29–35.
2. Weissman DE, Dahl, JL. Update on the Cancer Pain Role Model Education Program. *Journal of Pain and Symptom Management*. 1995;10:292–297.
3. Gordon DB, Dahl JL, Stevenson KK (eds.). *Building an Institutional Commitment to Pain Management*. Madison, WI: Wisconsin Cancer Pain Initiative, 1996.
4. Gordon DB. Critical pathways: A road to institutionalizing pain management. *Journal of Pain and Symptom Management*. 1996;11:252–259.

---

§See Appendix B, pp. 383–386, for these three pain algorithms.

5. Gordon DB, Stewart JA, Dahl JL, Ward S, Pellino T, Backonja M, Broad JE. Institutionalizing pain management. *Journal of Pharmaceutical Care in Pain & Symptom Control.* 1999;7:3–16.

6. Ferrell BR, Dean GE, Grant M, Coluzzi P. An institutional commitment to pain management. *Journal of Clinical Oncology.* 1995;13:2158–2165.

7. Bookbinder M, Coyle N, Kiss M, Goldstein ML, Holritz K, Thaler H, Gianella A, Derby S, Brown M, Racolin A, Ho MN, Portenoy RK. Implementing national standards for cancer pain management: Program model and evaluation. *Journal of Pain & Symptom Management.* 1996;12:334–347.

8. Weissman DE, Griffie J, Gordon DB, Dahl JL. A role model program to promote institutional changes for management of acute and cancer pain. *Journal of Pain & Symptom Management.* 1997;14:274–279.

9. Ferrell BA. Pain evaluation and management in the nursing home. *Annals of Internal Medicine.* 1995;123:681–687.

10. Ferrell BA, Ferrell BR, Osterwald D. Pain in the nursing home. *Journal of the American Geriatrics Society.* 1990;38:409–414.

11. Roy R, Michael T. A survey of chronic pain in an elderly population. *Canadian Family Physician.* 1986;32:513–516.

12. Mobily PR, Herr KA, Clark MK, Wallace RB. An epidemiologic analysis of pain in the elderly: The Iowa 65+ Rural Health Study. *Journal of Aging Health.* 1994;6:139–145.

13. Matson, Sandra. Improving Pain Management in Long-Term Care. Master's thesis, Medical College of Wisconsin, 1996.

14. Portenoy RK. Chronic opioid therapy in nonmalignant pain. *Journal of Pain and Symptom Management.* 1990;5:S46–S62.

15. Weissman DE, Griffie, J, Muchka S, Matson S. Building an institutional commitment to pain management in long-term care facilities. *Journal of Pain and Symptom Management.* 2000;20(1):35–43.

16. Weissman, DE. Doctors, nurses and storytelling. *Journal of Palliative Medicine.* 2000;3:251–252.

17. Griffie J, Matson, S, Muchka S, Weissman DE. *Improving Pain Management in Long-Term Care Settings: A Resource Guide for Institutional Change.* Milwaukee: Medical College of Wisconsin, 1998.

18. Griffie J, Weissman DE. *Nursing Staff Education Resource Manual: A Six-Session Inservice Education Program in Pain Management for Long-term Care Facilities.* Milwaukee: Medical College of Wisconsin, 2000.

19. Kovach CR, Weissman DE, Griffie J, Matson S, Muchka S. Assessment and treatment of discomfort for people with late-stage dementia. *Journal of Pain & Symptom Management.* 1999;18:412–419.

20. Kovach CR, Griffie J, Muchka S, Noonan PE, Weissman, DE. Nurses perception of pain assessment and treatment in the cognitively impaired elderly. *Clinical Nurse Specialist.* 2000;14:215–220.

Featured Innovation: Part II

Changing Pain Management Practice at Franciscan Woods

An Interview with MARY ARATA, BSN, RN, OCN

Franciscan Woods
Brookfield, Wisconsin

In 1995, Franciscan Woods, a transitional and extended care facility in Brookfield, Wisconsin, took part in the effort led by Weissman et al. to improve pain assessment and pain management in long-term care facilities.* Teams of two to four people from each institution took part in a series of four one-day training modules spread evenly over a one-year period. Trainings were comprised of didactic lectures, small group discussions, and focused role plays. After the first day of directed training, participants were charged with the task of creating an action plan to improve pain management within their respective institutions, structured around the adoption of 14 national practice indicators of an institutional commitment to pain management in long-term care facilities. In this interview with Samantha Libby Sodickson, Mary Arata, BSN, RN, OCN, team leader and oncology nurse at Franciscan Woods, discusses her experience of the year-long educational intervention, her institution's subsequent progress, and the ongoing challenges involved in implementing best practices in pain management in a long-term care facility.

Samantha Libby Sodickson: *Please describe the facility in which you work.*

Mary Arata: Franciscan Woods is a 120-bed facility for transitional and extended care, which is licensed as a skilled nursing facility. We have six nursing units. Three units are for long-term care and three are transitional-care nursing units. Two of the skilled units are medical–surgery rehabilitation units, and the third is our oncology unit. I am a team leader on the oncology unit. Each unit has 20 beds, and over the years our unit has cared for as few as 14 to 16 patients, but more typically we have 18 to 20 patients per unit.

The facility opened in December 1993, and the oncology unit opened in March 1994. I began on the oncology unit in July 1994. The unit was initially staffed by

---

*See Featured Innovation: Part I, Improving Pain Management in Long-Term Care Facilities, David Weissman et al., pp. 265–274.

one nurse. In 1997, as our census grew, the position of case manager was added. The case manager coordinates care with the other disciplines, does the required assessments for state and Medicare reimbursement, coordinates the family conferences, and communicates with physicians. The floor is staffed with a team leader and two certified nursing assistants (CNAs) per unit.

SLS: *How did you become involved in the Medical College of Wisconsin (MCW) pain management program for long-term care?*

MA: I have worked in oncology/hospice units since 1981. One year after I became part of the oncology unit at Franciscan Woods, we were invited to participate in Dr. Weissman and his colleagues' program. I think there were 20 or 30 long-term facilities that were asked to take part. Administrators at our facility were very excited to have us participate. When we got there, however, we were a little overwhelmed by the program because they laid out a full outline of expectations.

SLS: *Can you tell me what the policies were, in terms of pain management,* before *you started the program?*

MA: Pain was assessed routinely on admission. There were no policies in place for continued assessments or guidelines for the treatment of pain with pharmacological or non-pharmacological interventions. The prn sheet provided space to chart the reason that the medicine was given. No guidance was present for consistent assessment or reevaluation of pain. Since we were a new facility, it was a wonderful time to develop a structure for pain assessment and management.

SLS: *Who else from your institution was involved in the training?*

MA: Initially, we were all nurses. When appropriate, the social worker or a pharmacist would attend, depending on the topic. We participated for a whole year in the initial cohort program. This is the second year that we have been invited back for a follow-up program of four presentations on different topics in pain management, offered over the course of one year.

PRINCIPLES OF PAIN ASSESSMENT AND MANAGEMENT

SLS: *What did the initial training sessions include?*

MA: In the first all-day session, we were presented with information on how to do appropriate pain assessment and all the things it would involve, in detail. Case studies were presented and discussion followed. Another very helpful presentation was on pain assessment of the elderly. Pain is one of the most frequent complaints of the elderly, but it is rarely addressed in medical or nursing literature. Some of the barriers to the assessment of pain in the long-term care setting are multiple diagnoses, multiple pain sites, multiple medications, atypical presentations, visual and hearing impairments, the myth that pain is a normal part of aging, stoicism, lack of on-site physician assessment, and CNAs filling the role as the primary caregiver.

We also had a presentation on the importance of non-pharmacological methods of pain management combined with pharmacological interventions. As a result of this session, we made it an expectation at our facility that with each pharmacological intervention a non-pharmacological intervention also would be undertaken and documented. Some of the non-pharmacological interventions suggested were changes in positioning, reassurance from the staff, education about a condition, listening to music, applying heat or cold, transcutaneous electrical neuromuscular stimulation, and distraction.

Additionally, we had presentations on the action and side effects of the various classes of pain relievers, as well as the recommended steps for their usage by a pharmacist. Someone from the state regulatory board talked to us about state regulations and what the state was looking for in terms of documentation and practice. They covered a wide variety of topics in depth.

SLS: *I understand that you had to come up with an action plan. How did that go?*

MA: The steps of the action plan were outlined by the program. Figuring out how to implement the steps was up to us. Our first task was to develop an interdisciplinary work group. We pulled in a pharmacist, a social worker, a physical therapist, a CNA, and our chaplain. We used them as resources on an as-needed basis to assist with the development of policy, procedures, documentation vehicles, and education plans. Two RNs led the group, and our medical director was available to us for recommendations and approval.

Because all the steps of the plan were linked with each other, we found ourselves working on several steps at a time. For instance, we needed to develop the uniform measures for pain assessment so that we could include them in our policy and procedures. At the same time, we found that we had to develop our pain flow sheet[†] so that we could also address its specific components in the procedures. In this way, one activity fed another.

STAFF EDUCATION

SLS: *What was the biggest initial challenge when you returned to Franciscan Woods?*

MA: Once we had a program ready to present, we faced numerous challenges, most significantly the need to educate staff about the theory of pain management, assessment, our institution's principles of pain management, and phar-

---

[†]The pain flow sheet can be found online in Vol. 3, No. 1 of *Innovations in End-of-Life Care* at <www.edc.org/lastacts> under Archived Issues.

macology. The staff also needed to become familiar with our new paperwork and methods of documentation. We had to teach them how to document what they assessed, how they intervened, and what the outcome was. Because the material presented was extensive, many people had to put in extra time by attending the training before or after their shifts, or covering shifts for other staff so that they could attend.

One ongoing challenge is to keep re-educating new staff as they come on board and to continue educating current members of the staff beyond the basics. We have developed a section that includes the basics of pain management and our expectations, which is presented in orienting new staff. But there are many more topics to be presented based on the needs that we have assessed in the staff. Our goal is to continue to have two in-services a year on pain-related topics, and to address areas of need as identified by quality improvement audits.

The training program also focused on the importance of developing a way to inform the residents and resident council of the facility's commitment to pain management. So, we had to develop a plan to teach the residents how to communicate about pain and outline what the residents should expect, as far as our response to their reports of pain. We also developed quality assurance surveys and audits for ongoing internal assessments of how we were doing. So, it was a long plan, one that involved a lot of development and education.

We have also had in-service training sessions on pain for the therapy department. They have responded very well; the occupational and physical therapists are good at talking with the nurses about pain interfering with therapies. People with uncontrolled postoperative pain cannot take part in their rehabilitation programs. If they cannot participate, they will not get stronger. Therapists know that patients cannot meet their rehabilitation goals unless their pain is controlled.

SLS: *Did you find that there were misconceptions about pain among the staff before you did the in-service training?*

MA: Oh, there were a lot of misconceptions! I think it's an ongoing process to re-educate and to remind people that pain is real. The patient labeled as "difficult" might reinforce misconceptions about pain. We need to believe the patient's report of pain, and remember that most people do not get addicted to pain medicine. If patients are reporting pain, we need to take care of it; we need to listen, and we need to look at more than just pharmacological interventions for pain relief.

> *We need to believe the patient's report of pain, and remember that most people do not get addicted to pain medicine.*

SLS: *Tell me about the training of your certified nursing assistants (CNAs).*

MA: We have two CNAs per unit and we do a hands-on CNA in-service. We talk about the importance of their conveying patients' reports of pain or any nonverbal signs of pain that they observe while providing care. We emphasize that they are our second set of eyes. What was wonderful in this program was that the MCW faculty provided educational models for us to use with CNAs. We then adapted them to our needs.

SLS: *How did you adapt the models you got from the MCW training?*

MA: We basically followed their outline for the general information. Then we developed handouts for our CNAs that included the main points of what we discussed. For example, one handout showed positioning techniques. We then did a training exercise in which we had a CNA get into a bed and the other CNAs took turns repositioning her. We spelled out the ABCs of pain control for the CNAs, gave them a copy of our pain scale, and taught them how to use it.

SLS: *How much time, generally, is spent training CNAs on the units?*

MA: They're all certified and trained before they come to us. After general facility orientation, they share an assignment for several days with another CNA. Then they are teamed with a CNA who serves as a mentor on their unit as they take on the responsibility of their own assignment. We also have CNA II positions. These are certified nursing assistants who show interest in learning additional skills. We teach them to do finger stick blood glucose monitoring and G-tube flushing.

ROUTINE PAIN ASSESSMENT

SLS: *What is your day-to-day pain assessment and management system? How often do you evaluate residents' pain?*

MA: Our protocol is to assess people for pain on admission. If they come in with pain medicines already ordered or if they are exhibiting signs of pain, as sometimes happens with non-verbal patients, then they are put on the pain management protocol, and the pain flow sheet is added to the medication book. People are to be assessed *at least* once per shift for the first three days and more often if needed. If they're put on a long-acting pain medicine, they are to be evaluated—depending on whether it is an oral or an IV route—within one to two hours of having received the medication to assess its effectiveness. So, our intervention is evaluated on an ongoing basis to see if it is working. Additionally, the CNAs report observations of pain to the nurses.

SLS: *If the CNAs report an observation of pain to you, what generally happens after that?*

MA: The CNAs' observations are very important to me. They observe and report something as painful, and then the nurses do the more detailed assessment. CNAs are expected to report any patient's complaint of pain or any signs of pain that they observe during care. If I know of a patient that is having trouble with pain, I will ask the CNA for their observations so I can include them with my assessment.

Because we deal with complex pain issues on a daily basis, the staff knows that the nurses on my unit are always available for consultation. We have two nurse managers in the facility, and they know to recommend that the nurses call us if they are having trouble controlling or treating a patient's pain. I think it's important to get nurses to look at the big picture, to look at the pain in the landscape of everything that's going on with the patient, and to call us when they have a question. Because we're asked to do so many things, sometimes it's hard to step back and look at the big picture.

REGULATIONS AND STANDARDS

SLS: *Can you speak about the role of regulatory constraints in long-term care and their effect on pain management?*

MA: We try to work within the guidelines, both of the Joint Commission for Accreditation of Healthcare Organizations (JCAHO) and the state. We learned through talks with state regulators that they were looking to see that our patients were functioning at their optimal level. Specifically, they want to know that pain would not be interfering with patients' ability to function at their individual best, which could mean anything from tolerating being able to sit up in a wheelchair, to being repositioned, to walking.

Much of the pain experienced in the long-term care setting is chronic. One issue that came up was the scheduling of prn pain medicine. We held many discussions on that topic with state representatives. As a result of these talks, it became part of our assessment and re-evaluation to understand that a patient did best if he or she had pain medicines on a scheduled basis. A pain medication that is ordered every four hours prn can be administered every four hours at the discretion of the nurse. So, a patient whose pain interferes with his or her ability to do activities of daily living (ADLs), such as eating or dressing, should have a pain pill scheduled an hour before these activities. For example, a patient who has trouble tolerating sitting in a chair for meals should be medicated before meals. Routinely, we will write nursing care orders to schedule medications to prevent pain from interfering with patients' ability to function or to prevent pain from diminishing their quality of life. We need to control the pain, not have the pain control the patient.

I am currently a member of a system-wide pain team. Our pain flow sheets have made it convenient to document most of the indicators that we are looking for in our measurement of patient satisfaction with pain control. Being a small facility, we were easily able to develop a new flow sheet to meet our needs.

In addition, we prepare a written summary weekly that addresses the specific issues of each patient and his or her condition. We added space for an entry that reports on pain management, because we decided that we wanted a weekly summary of how the patient's functioning was affected by pain. By creating a system that routinely documents pain control and delivers prn medications on a scheduled basis, we are better able to reach our goals of pain control.

JCAHO has accredited our facility twice since we opened. We had developed most of the program by the time of the second survey. One regulator complimented our project by saying that it was marketable.

SLS: *Are you in the process of making any further changes to comply with the new JCAHO pain standards?*

MA: I think we have all the tools in place. What we have to work on is a more consistent use of what we have developed. However, we are currently developing an audit tool within our system to look at assessment, intervention, and patient satisfaction. Analyzing these audits will lead us to further changes.

THE IMPACT OF TRAINING ON NURSE–PHYSICIAN INTERACTIONS

SLS: *The MCW faculty describes their training as having a core function of nurse empowerment. What was your experience?*

MA: The program really broadened my base of knowledge, from the simple pharmacological intervention to the more complex, and at our facility we've had very complex cases. It has given us knowledge that has empowered us to be proactive for the patient, to continually seek out whatever it is that the patient needs. As you know, doctors don't make visits very often. They come every 30 days, so we do a lot of telephone consultation with them.

As a result of the training, we now have a form that we can use to gather information, so we have a formalized way of presenting what we see to the doctors. It includes the assessment, the response to the current interventions, and a place where we can document what we think would be best for the patient. We've also talked about ways to present this information to physicians most effectively. Now that we use these strategies, we have had wonderful responses from doctors and have found them to be very accepting of our recommendations and requests. Over these few years, we have earned the respect of many physicians because of our expertise in pain management.

FAMILY AND PATIENT EDUCATION

SLS: *What kind of family participation do you have in the day-to-day pain assessment and management?*

MA: Some families are active participants in setting the goals for their family members. The nurses explain what's involved in pain management and discuss what the family's goals are. Is the goal comfort? Is it alertness? We talk about what getting the patient to a level of comfort might mean in terms of side effects. For example, say we can get their loved one comfortable, but then the patient is going to be sleepy. We ask, "Do you want your loved one awake?" So, we actively involve the family on an ongoing basis, as the patient's needs change.

SLS: *How have you educated your patients about assessing their own pain?*

MA: We have developed a card that has three different pain scales on it. It has word descriptors, numbers, and faces. On all three scales, the numbers coincide: the low numbers coincide with mild pain, and the middle numbers coincide with moderate pain, and so forth. We post these cards in each bedroom, and in the initial assessment on admission, we ask patients what their pain level is. Most hospitals in the area use the zero to ten scale. If the person comes to us using the zero to five scale, we stay with that scale. We find that by putting the face scale card in front of patients the graphic image of the face makes the pain scale more understandable to them. For some patients it's easier to use the word descriptors scale (mild, moderate, severe), and for other patients, the numbers are more meaningful. Whatever scale the patient picks at that time, we put that scale on their pain flow sheets, as well as what that patient's acceptable level of pain is. We keep the card in each patient's room so that we can use it repeatedly.

SLS: *How do you handle pain assessment in cognitively impaired patients?*

MA: That's an ongoing challenge. The key is educating the nurses and the CNAs to behavioral changes. The simplest changes in behavior can be signs of pain. We have a section on our pain flow sheets that specifically addresses all the different behaviors that we might observe that would be indicators of pain, such as increase in body movement, changes in daily activity pattern, or aggressive behavior. The ideal is to have staff that's familiar with the patient to note the changes in the patient's behavior and then to see if the behavior changes with a trial change in medication. This involves knowing your patients, performing repeated assessments, and then trying other pharmacological and nonpharmacological approaches to see what works.

SLS: *What kind of role does hospice play in your facility?*

MA: We usually have several hospice patients on our unit. The number has fluctuated from one to seven. We have two hospice organizations that admit our eligible patients to their programs. What hospice brings to our patients is terminal care expertise, extra staff, and extra psychosocial support for the patient and family. It brings another nurse into the picture for care planning. The extra time that the hospice nurse, social worker, and chaplain can spend with the patient and family is a real benefit. However, we do provide comfort-oriented care to those patients who are not eligible for or do not elect the hospice benefit.

ADOPTING NATIONAL PRACTICE INDICATORS

SLS: *One goal of the educational program was the adoption of 14 national practice indicators for an institutional commitment to pain management. What do you think is the relationship between having these target indicators in place and actual patient outcomes?*

MA: I think having the target indicators in place is very important. They provide the road map; they are the guideposts for us for the development of the policies and procedures. The pain flow sheets, the assessment tools, all these things make it easier for us to follow a plan.

You need to have a plan to take all the steps to improve pain management. Once you set things in place, you need to reassess how you're doing. Unless you are auditing, you do not know how you are doing. In the three or four years that we have been working through this process, we have already revised our initial tools. Our initial audit was primarily of our documentation. Our next step will include looking at patient satisfaction.

SLS: *In closing, is there some advice you could give others working in long-term care that you feel would make a significant difference in the day-to-day lives of patients?*

MA: Work together as a team. Bring all the people who interact with the patients together to work on pain management. Pain leaders need to educate the CNAs, the therapists, the nursing staff, the chaplains, and the social workers. Pain management is many faceted. Educating all the members of the care team increases the chances of recognizing and treating pain most effectively and in that way improves the day-to-day lives of patients.

Selected Bibliography

Part Five

Selected references by contributors to this part:

Griffie J. Palliative medicine nurse preceptorship at the Medical College of Wisconsin. *Journal of Pain and Symptom Management.* 1996;12(6):360–363.

Kovach CR, Weissman DE, Griffie J, Matson S, Muchka S. Assessment and treatment of discomfort for people with late-stage dementia. *Journal of Pain and Symptom Management.* 1999;18(6):412–419.

Spross J. Using principles of change and a technical assistance protocol to improve pain management in institutions. *New England Pain Association Newsletter.* 2000;5(3):8–14.

Spross, Judith A. The Influence of Selected Societal, Institutional, and Individual Factors on Nurses' and Physicians' Pain Management Knowledge. PhD diss., Boston College School of Nursing, 1999.

Spross J. Management of cancer pain: Commentary 2. *Abstracts of Clinical Care Guidelines.* 1994;6(5):4–6.

Spross JA. Pain, suffering and spiritual well-being: Assessment and interventions. *Quality of Life: A Nursing Challenge.* 1993;2(3):71–79.

Spross JA. Cancer pain relief: An international perspective. *Oncology Nursing Forum.* 1992;19(7):5.

Spross JA. Pain management: Issues in the hospital setting. *Sixth National Conference on Cancer Nursing.* Seattle, WA: American Cancer Society, 1991.

Spross JA. Unrelieved cancer pain: Selections from the literature. *Dimensions in Oncology Nursing.* 1990;4(4):4–9.

Spross JA. Cancer pain and suffering: Clinical lessons from life, literature, and legend. *Oncology Nursing Forum.* 1985;13(4):24–31.

Spross JA, Clarke, EB, Beauregard J. Expert coaching and guidance. In *Advanced Nursing Practice: An Integrative Approach*, 2nd ed. AB Hamric, JA Spross, CM Hanson (eds.). Philadelphia: W.B. Saunders Company, 2000:183–216.

Spross JA, Wolff M. Nonpharmacological management of cancer pain. In *Cancer Pain Management*, 2d ed. DB McGuire, CH Yarbro, BR Ferrell (eds.). Boston: Jones & Bartlett, 1995:159–206.

Spross JA, McGuire DB, Schmitt R. Oncology nursing position paper on cancer pain. *Oncology Nursing Forum.* 1990;17:595–614(Part I); 751–760(Part II); 943–955 (Part III).

Weissman DE. Cancer pain education for physicians in practice: Establishing a new paradigm. *Journal of Pain and Symptom Management.* 1996;12(6): 364–371.

Weissman DE, Griffie J, Muchka S, Matson M. Building an institutional commitment to pain management in long-term care facilities. *Journal of Pain and Symptom Management.* 2000;20(1):35–43.

Weissman DE, Matson S. Pain assessment and management in the long-term care setting. *Theoretical Medicine.* 1999;20:31–43.

Weissman DE, Griffie J, Gordon DB, Dahl JL. A role model program to promote institutional changes for management of acute and cancer pain. *Journal of Pain and Symptom Management.* 1997;14(5):274-279.

Weissman DE, Dahl JL. Update on the cancer pain role model education program. *Journal of Pain and Symptom Management.* 1995;10(4):292-297.

Weissman DE, Griffie J. The palliative care consultation service of the Medical College of Wisconsin. *Journal of Pain and Symptom Management.* 1994;9(7):474-479.

Weissman DE, Dahl JL, Beasley JW. The cancer pain role model program of the Wisconsin cancer pain initiative. *Journal of Pain and Symptom Management.* 1993;8(1):29-35.

Other selected references:

AGS Panel on Chronic Pain in Older Persons. The management of chronic pain in older persons. *Journal of the American Geriatrics Society.* 1998;46(5):635-651.

American Medical Directors Association. *Clinical Practice Guideline: Chronic Pain Management in the Long-Term Care Setting.* Columbia, MD: American Medical Directors Association, 1999.

Bookbinder M, Coyle N, Kiss M, Goldstein ML, Holritz K, Thaler H, Gianella A, Derby S, Brown M, Racolin A, Ho MN, Portenoy RK. Implementing national standards for cancer pain management: Program model and evaluation. *Journal of Pain and Symptom Management.* 1996;12(6):334-347.

Castle NG, Banaszak-Holl J. Top management team characteristics and innovation in nursing homes. *Gerontologist.* 1997;37(5):572-580.

Colleau S. Pain in the elderly with cancer. *Cancer Pain Release.* 2000;13(2). <www.whocancerpain.wisc.edu/WHOcancerpain/eng/13_2/pain.html> (accessed 29 Jul. 2002).

Dahl JL, Berry P, Stevenson KM, Gordon DB, Ward S. Institutionalizing pain management: Making pain assessment and treatment an integral part of the nation's healthcare system. *American Pain Society Bulletin.* July/August 1998:19.

ECHO Long Term Care Task Force, California Coalition for Compassionate Care. *ECHO Nursing Facility Recommendations: Recommendations for Improving End-of-Life Care for Persons Residing in California Skilled Nursing and Intermediate Care Facilities.* Sacramento, CA: Coalition for Compassionate Care, January 2000.

Ellison NM, McPherson L, McGuire L. *Dannemiller Memorial Education Foundation Pain Report: An Update on Issues, Research and Treatment Trends.* New York: Enhanced Marketing, Ltd. 2000.

Feldt KS. Improving assessment and treatment of pain in cognitively impaired nursing home residents. *Annals of Long-Term Care.* 2000;8(9):36-41.

Ferrell BA. Pain evaluation and management in the nursing home. *Annals of Internal Medicine.* 1995;123(9):681-687.

Ferrell BA, Ferrell BR, Rivera L. Pain in cognitively impaired nursing home patients. *Journal of Pain and Symptom Management.* 1995;10(8):591-598.

Ferrell BA, Ferrell BR. The Sepulveda GRECC Method No. 40. *Geriatric Medicine Today*. 1989;8(5):123–134.

Ferrell BR, Virani R. Institutional commitment to improved pain management: Sustaining the effort. *Journal of Pharmaceutical Care in Pain and Symptom Control*. 1998;6(2)43–45.

Ferrell BR, Ferrell BA. (eds.). *Pain in the Elderly*. Seattle, WA: IASP Press, 1996.

Ferrell BR, Dean GE, Grant M, Coluzzi P. An institutional commitment to pain management. *Journal of Clinical Oncology*. 1995;13:2158–2165.

Ferrell BR, McGuire DB, Donovan MI. Knowledge and beliefs regarding pain in a sample of nursing faculty. *Journal of Professional Nursing*. 1993;9(2):79–88.

Ferrell BR, Eberts MT, McCaffery M, Grant M. Clinical decision making and pain. *Cancer Nursing*. 1991;14(6):289–297.

Fox PL, Raina P, Jada AR. Prevalence and treatment of pain in older adults in nursing homes and other long-term care institutions: A systematic review. *Canadian Medical Association Journal*. 1999;160(3):329–333.

Fredey M. Doing something positive about pain: Palliative care at Sherrill House. *On Call*. October 2000:17–19.

Gordon DB. Critical pathways: A road to institutionalizing pain management. *Journal of Pain and Symptom Management*. 1996;11(4):252–259.

Gordon DB, Dahl JL, Stevenson KK. *Building an Institutional Commitment to Pain Management*. Madison: University of Wisconsin, Board of Regents, 1996.

Herr KA, Mobily PR. Complexities of pain assessment in the elderly: Clinical considerations. *Journal of Gerontological Nursing*. 1991;17(4):12–19.

Jette AM, Soreff S, Capriole CM. An advanced CAN education program: Meeting the need. *Annals of Long-Term Care*. 2000;8(3):47–51.

Kane RL, Kane RA. Assessment in long-term care. *Annual Review of Public Health*. 2000;21(21):659–686.

Loeb JL. Pain management in long-term care. *American Journal of Nursing*. 1999;99(2):48–52.

Loeb J, Pasero C. JCAHO standards in long-term care. *American Journal of Nursing*. 2000;100(5):22–23.

Oncology Nursing Society. Position Statement: Cancer pain management. *Oncology Nursing Forum*. 1998;25(5):817–818.

Rutman DJ. Palliative care needs of residents, families, and staff in long-term care facilitites. *Journal of Palliative Care*. 1992;8(2):23–29.

Won A, Lapane K, Gambassi G, Bernabei R, Mor Z, Lipsitz LA. Correlates and management of nonmalignant pain in the nursing home. *Journal of the American Geriatrics Society*. 1999;47(8):936–942.

Part Six

Quality of Life

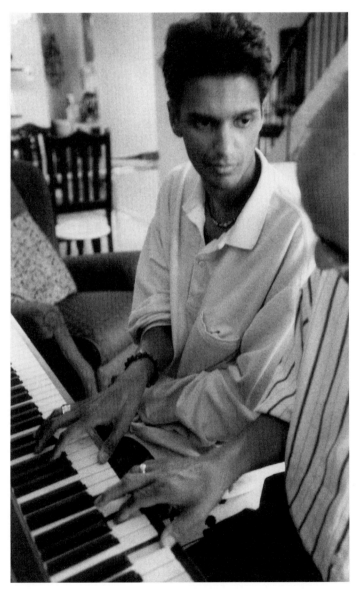

©1998 Roger Lemoyne and Living Lessons.

Assessment of Quality of Life in Palliative Care

STEIN KAASA, MD, PhD

Trondheim University Hospital
Trondheim, Norway

Most clinicians and researchers agree that improvement of the patient's quality of life is the ultimate goal in palliative care. A similar approach is taken by the World Health Organization (WHO), defining palliative care as "the active total care of patients whose disease is not responsive to curative treatment. Control of pain, of other symptoms, and of psychological, social, and spiritual problems is paramount. The goal of palliative care is achievement of the best quality of life for patients and their families. Many aspects of palliative care are also applicable earlier in the course of the illness in conjunction with anti-cancer treatment."[1] As early as 1948, the WHO included subjectivity in the definition of health, as follows: "Health is not only the absence of infirmity and disease, but also a state of complete physical, mental, and social well-being."[2,3]

There are challenges related to both of these WHO definitions. What is the meaning or the definition of the term "quality of life"? Do patients and their families have distinct understandings of this concept? Applying this framework to clinical practice is a challenge. For example, many clinicians ask, "What is the mandate of professional health care providers? How and how much should we, as professionals, intervene in the patients' social and spiritual life?" Another challenge is related to measuring quality of life in patient-focused palliative care and in research. Is it possible to measure quality of life? Should it be measured? If one decides to measure it, should it be done using a questionnaire or a more open-ended format?

DEFINITION OF QUALITY OF LIFE

Definitions are important. They can serve as an impetus for changing practice, introducing new programs, and working toward the allocation of more resources for palliative care. Moreover, the understanding of these concepts influences how medicine is practiced. The understanding of the concept of quality of life is affected by several factors, such as profession (i.e., doctor, nurse, chaplain, social worker), clinical specialty and experience (i.e., oncology vs. palliative care and hospice vs. palliative medicine), the stage of disease trajectory (i.e., last day of life vs. month of palliative treatment), culture, and the context/use of the concept (research vs. clinic).

In this part, Dr. Robin Fainsinger and Carleen Brenneis, RN, describe the Edmonton Palliative Care Program. Dr. Fainsinger defines quality of life as maximizing patient and family comfort across four broad domains: physical, psychological, spiritual, and existential. A similar approach is taken by Mariela Bertolino, MD, who is working in palliative care in Buenos Aires, Argentina. She mentions physical symptoms, psychological distress, social and financial issues, and spiritual or existential problems as the core elements affecting quality of life. From a practical, clinical point of view, Carleen Brenneis focuses on what is important day-to-day for the patient and the family. From her experience, clinicians need to meet people's physical and social needs before they can focus on their emotional and spiritual needs.

Most clinicians' experience with patients and families would confirm her observations. Without sufficient symptom control, communication with patients and their families will be focused on symptoms and not on family relationships and the process of saying farewell. What guidelines should be followed to provide optimal care to patients and families? In addition to calling on past experience and the particular information obtained from each patient and family, case by case, doctors should use evidence-based medicine.

To this end, a systematic, prospective collection of information about patients' (and families') subjective health is paramount. In summary, the approach to quality of life described so far is clinically focused and closely related (or identical) with the concept called "health-related quality of life" (HRQOL). The development of HRQOL was guided by the need to have subjective outcomes in clinical studies and measures intended to assess physical, social, and emotional domains.[4-7]

The concept of health-related quality of life has been challenged in reviews in general medicine and by comments from many clinicians in the field of palliative care. Gill and Feinstein take a philosophical position, arguing that quality of life can only be suitably measured by targeting the opinions of patients and by supplementing or replacing the existing instruments developed by experts.[8]

Others have agreed that there is clear evidence of a variety of factors influencing an individual's perception of both suffering and quality of life. Meaning and transcendence are important.[9] Furthermore, it has been acknowledged that the experience of terminally ill patients can only be understood as a dynamic phenomenon at two levels—the surface level, where language is literal, and the deep level, where the mode of knowing is intuitive.[10] These researchers argue that quality of life can only be assessed from an individual perspective without imposing a predetermined external value system. This stance implies that the patients themselves should be given the opportunity to choose the domains that are important to their quality of life, at a given point in time. According to this approach, quality of life is defined as a global, overall perspective, that includes in its scope one's philosophical perspectives on life. It challenges the health-related orientation and draws attention toward asking the patients not only to rate their symptoms or worries, but also to give relative value to them. Is such an approach too much to ask of staff working in a clinical setting?

ASSESSMENT OF HEALTH-RELATED QUALITY OF LIFE

Quality of life has practical implications for health care—one can measure changes in subjective health brought about by a medical intervention. Additionally, it may be regarded as a spiritual concept related to meaning and transcendence. In research and daily clinical practice, one can use HRQOL instruments that focus on subjective symptoms and function, such as the European Organization for Research and Treatment of Cancer questionnaire developed to assess the quality of life of cancer patients (EORTC-QLQ-C30),[5,11] and checklists specifically developed for palliative care, such as the Edmonton Symptom Assessment Schedule (ESAS).[12] This concrete, practical approach can improve symptom control and thereby improve patients' quality of life. Such instruments can also be used to accumulate knowledge about patient populations. For example, collecting data on symptoms and how well they are treated within a health care program can allow for comparisons of effectiveness across programs using these measures. However, as clinicians caring for patients as individual human beings, one must recognize their spirituality, individual suffering, and/or emotional distress as integral to their care. By talking to patients and families, we will learn more about these domains and so be able to address the meaning of quality of life in a more complete way.

The techniques for collecting information about subjective domains of life quality might include interviews or questionnaires. To assess health-related quality of life, standardized questionnaires are most often used. In palliative care, especially during the end of life, patients may not be able to complete an instrument that requires self-report. Under such circumstances, a proxy or health professional will need to rate the patient's experience.

During the last two decades, many tools have been developed and used, making comparisons between samples difficult. Most of these quality of life assessment tools were developed in oncology or for nonmalignant chronic disease, such as chronic pain, rheumatoid arthritis, heart failure, headache, and diabetes. Few instruments have been developed specifically for assessing quality of life in patients near the end of life. The heterogeneity of purpose and scales in these measures further complicates the question of cross-study comparisons.

In selecting measures for use in clinical research, quality assurance programs, or for individual patients, the content of the measure is of crucial importance. Additionally, standardization and the repetitive use of the same instrument build a shared clinical understanding of the meaning of a particular score on a specific scale or item. The clinical significance of a fatigue score of 60 on a zero to 100 scale for example, must be understood if that score is to be used in the clinical decision-making process. The score must resonate with shared meaning and provide an impetus to action for clinicians, in the same way that a hemoglobin of 7.8 suggests the possible need for a blood transfusion or some other type of intervention to adjust the hemoglobin level. One problem with all existing scales and measures of quality of life is that a 60 in one domain does not necessarily mean the same as 60 in another domain or, to put it another way, the metric is not similar between scales and single items.

Even without any gold standard for assessment of health-related quality of life in palliative care, some recommendations are possible. In a daily clinical setting, instruments that can be applied directly without any computation are most appropriate. A good example is the ESAS. However, one must be aware of the limitations of using single items covering complex domains with regard to both reliability and validity. For use in clinical research, more comprehensive HRQOL instruments such as the EORTC-QLQ-C30 can be used. Another instrument to consider is the McGill Quality of Life questionnaire (MQOL), which also includes existential domains, in contrast to the EORTC-QLQ-C30.[13] Specific instruments have been developed to assess quality of life from a more individual perspective, for example, the Schedule for the Evaluation of Individual QOL (SEIQoL) and the Schedule for the Evaluation for Individual QoL, Direct Weighting (SEIQoL-DW), a brief measure derived from the SEIQoL.[14,15] Designers of this instrument claim that by allowing the respondent to define the areas to be measured, the tool offers a more relevant and accurate measure of quality of life than forced choice questionnaires. The SEIQoL-DW might be well suited for individual consultations, but poses problems as an outcome measure for assessing quality of life among patients across palliative care services or in research aimed at detecting an effect of a specific intervention. Its strength—the capacity to capture individualized data—would become its weakness, because these individually chosen domains are statistically incomparable. Therefore, this instrument does not seem appropriate for population-based use.

There are few reliable and valid tools for use in measuring quality of life during end-of-life care. At the final stages of an illness, interviews and/or observations must be used as the method to collect information. Until new and better instruments are developed, a pragmatic approach to assessment is necessary. One of the simple tools, for example, the ESAS, or one of the HRQOL instruments, such as the EORTC-QLQ-C30, can be used in interview-based and/or observation-based situations. It is, however, important to underline that neither of these instruments has been developed nor validated for use during the final stage of a patient's life. Furthermore, there is much evidence that considerable differences often exist between proxy rating and patient rating of subjective outcomes.[16,17] At present, for use in research, one of the internationally validated questionnaires, such as the EORTC-QLQ-C30, is most promising. In daily clinical practice, a simpler tool, such as the ESAS, should be used.

. . . by systemizing the collection of information on patient symptoms and distress, appropriate interventions can be implemented and patient quality of life can be improved.

In summary, by systemizing the collection of information on patient symptoms and distress, appropriate interventions can be implemented and patient quality of life can be improved. A dynamic approach in clinical practice is needed to combine systematic assessment with individual patient information and communication.

REFERENCES

1. World Health Organization. *Cancer Pain Relief and Palliative Care: Report of a WHO Expert Committee*, Technical Report # 804. Geneva: World Health Organization, 1990.
2. World Health Organization. The Constitution of the World Health Organization. *WHO Chronicle*, 1947:29.
3. Doyle D, GWC Hanks, MacDonald N (eds.). *Oxford Textbook of Palliative Medicine*, 2d ed. New York: Oxford University Press, 1998, 3.
4. Cella DF, Tulsky DS, Gray G, Sarafian B, Linn E, Bonomi A, Silberman M, Yellen SB, Winicour P, Brannon J, et al. The functional assessment of cancer therapy scale: Development and validation of the general measure. *Journal of Clinical Oncology*. 1993;11:570–579.
5. Aaronson NK, Ahmedzai S, Bergman B, Bullinger M, Cull A, Duez NJ, Filiberti A, Flechtner H, Fleishman SB, de Haes JC, et al. The European Organization for Research and Treatment of Cancer QLQ-C30: A quality of life instrument for use in international clinical trials in oncology. *Journal of the National Cancer Institute*. 1993;85:365–376.
6. Priestman TJ, Baum M. Evaluation of quality of life in patients receiving treatment for advanced breast cancer. *Lancet*. 1993;1:899–901.
7. Ware JE. The status of health assessment 1994. *Annual Review of Public Health*. 1995;16:327–354.
8. Gill TM, Feinstein AR. A critical appraisal of the quality of life measurements. *Journal of the American Medical Association*. 1994;272:619–626.
9. Cohen SR, Balfour MM. Quality of life in terminal illness: Defining and measuring subjective well-being in the dying. *Journal of Palliative Care*. 1992;8(3):40–45.
10. O'Boyle CA, Waldron D. Quality of life issues in palliative medicine. *Journal of Neurology*. 1997; 244[Suppl 4]:S18–S25.
11. Kaasa S, Bjordal K, Aaronson N, Moum T, Wist E, Hagen S, Kvikstad A. The EORTC Core Quality of Life Questionnaire QLQ-C30: Validity and reliability when analyzed with patients treated with palliative radiotherapy. *European Journal of Cancer*. 1995;31A:2260–2263.
12. Bruera E, Kuehn N, Miller MJ, Selmser P, Macmillan K. The Edmonton Symptom Assessment System (ESAS): A simple method for the assessment of palliative care patients. *Journal of Palliative Care*. 1991;7(2):6–9.
13. Cohen SR, Mount BM, Strobel MG, Bui F. The McGill Quality of Life Questionnaire: A measure of quality of life appropriate for people with advanced disease. A preliminary study of validity and acceptability. *Palliative Medicine*. 1995;9:207–219.
14. O'Boyle CA, McGee H, Joyce CRB. Quality of life: assessing the individual. *Advances in Medical Sociology*. 1994;5:159–180.
15. Hickey AM, Bury G, O'Boyle CA, Bradley F, O'Kelly FD, Shannon W. A new short form individual quality of life measure (SEIQoL-DW): Application in a cohort of individuals with HIV/AIDS. *British Medical Journal*. 1996;313:29–33.
16. Spitzer WO, Dobson AJ, Hall J, Chesterman E, Levi J, Shepherd R, Battista RN, Catchlove BR. Measuring quality of life of cancer patients: A concise QL-index for use by physicians. *Journal of Chronic Diseases*. 1981;34:585–597.
17. Presant CA. Quality of life in cancer patients: Who measures what? *American Journal of Clinical Oncology*. 1984;7:571–573.

Addressing Quality of Life at the Edmonton Palliative Care Program

An Interview with ROBIN L. FAINSINGER, MBchB, CCFP

Edmonton Palliative Care Program
Edmonton, Alberta, Canada

The idea for an integrated palliative care program in Edmonton, Alberta, in Canada was conceived in 1992 by Drs. Eduardo Bruera and Neil Mac-Donald and other colleagues in the area. Three-and-a-half years later, the Edmonton Palliative Care Program was born. The existence of an integrated national health system undoubtedly helped these leaders to create an entity defined by cooperation across different settings, staff, and systems. Eighty-five to 90 percent of the patients seen by staff affiliated with this program are suffering from cancer, although the program is not restricted to those with cancer diagnoses.

The Edmonton Palliative Care Program is the name of an integrated web of services housed across a number of different institutions that are now available to patients and families in greater Edmonton, a catchment area of approximately 840,000 people. In 1999, there were 1,400 cancer deaths in this region. Five different facilities have inpatient palliative care beds. Specifically, specialist palliative care physicians admit and care for patients with the most intractable physical and/or psychosocial symptoms at a 14-bed tertiary palliative care unit at Grey Nuns Hospital. Fifty percent of the patients at Grey Nuns die there, with the remainder discharged to other settings, including the 57 hospice beds that exist in four other facilities with continuing palliative care units. Family physicians are able to continue to look after their patients with the support of an interdisciplinary palliative care team in these inpatient hospice units. Most of these patients can no longer manage at home, and remain in these units for the rest of their lives. All these palliative care beds are usually at 95 to 98 percent capacity.

In addition to these designated inpatient beds, the program boasts three palliative care consult services: two at acute care hospitals, the University of Alberta and the Royal Alexandra, and another at the Cross Cancer Institute, a freestanding building for outpatient and inpatient cancer services. The Edmonton Regional Palliative Care Program is the name given to the administrative structure for these efforts, which include a roving team made up of four palliative care physicians and four specialized nurses who consult to family doctors and their at-home patients as well as to patients in nursing homes, on the continuing palliative care units, and in smaller hospitals in the area. The Edmonton Regional Palliative Care Program provides clinical leadership, teaching, and research standards to staff in all the different settings in which palliative care is available.

In Canada, the terms "hospice" and "palliative care" are used interchangeably, with no time restrictions on access to either. In contrast, in the United States, the term "hospice" refers to the Medicare Hospice Benefit, which requires physicians to certify that a patient is likely to die within six months in order to gain access to a specific set of end-of-life services and benefits. Physicians in Edmonton make referrals to these inpatient beds based on severity of symptoms and the availability of family caregivers at home. In general, patients who wish to die at home do so, if they have a family member able to provide care or can afford to hire round-the-clock care.

In spite of its decentralized makeup, the physicians in all these settings know one another and one another's programs very well. They participate in the activities of the Division of Palliative Care Medicine at the University of Alberta Medical School and work together in the postgraduate training program in palliative care, which draws international leaders who wish to develop programs in their own settings. Financed by one payer, the Canadian national health system, but administered independently by each province, the Edmonton Palliative Care Program provides a unique example in North America of an integrated community-based program that aims to meet the palliative care needs of patients seamlessly across all possible settings, as well as being an internationally acclaimed center for research and teaching in this field.

Innovations *turned to Robin Fainsinger, MD, clinical director of the Edmonton Palliative Care Program, and to Carleen Brenneis, RN, administrative director of the Edmonton Regional Palliative Care Program, to learn about how this integrated program addresses the question of quality of life. In the following interview with Anna L. Romer, EdD, Dr. Robin Fainsinger describes his understanding of quality of life and the four purposes (clinical, teaching, research, and administrative) for which this concept can be useful. He focuses primarily on the uses of this concept at the bedside and in tracking access to palliative care as a global marker of patients' quality of life. In the Featured Innovation: Part I, Dr. Fainsinger describes the genesis and use of some key tools designed by the Edmonton team.*

Anna L. Romer: *How do you define "quality of life"?*

Robin L. Fainsinger: That is a question I think about a lot. Essentially, we have come up with the same broad domains as others: the physical, psychosocial, spiritual, and existential. When we define quality of life in palliative care, we are talking about maximizing patient *and* family comfort across these domains. Quality of life is a complex mix of these elements, with many nuances in that broad framework.

The patient and family are always the unit of care. With respect to quality of life of the patient and family, we talk about function and autonomy—the sense of control that people require. We talk about advance care planning. We talk about patient and family satisfaction, well-being, and the perception of care received. We talk about the family burden and the need to relieve that burden, while at the same time strengthening relationships among family members. In addition, we need to remember bereavement. On the health care provider side, we talk about provider continuity and skill, which the health care system needs to provide. Quality of life includes all these elements.

It has been suggested that we need to be careful about our definitions because when we, as health care professionals, talk about these domains, we can get stuck with a narrow interpretation that perhaps serves our administrative or financial purposes. What families and patients define as quality of life may not necessarily be the

> *What families and patients define as quality of life may not necessarily be the same sorts of things that we are attempting to measure to justify our existence to administrators and the people that finance our programs.*

same sorts of things that we are attempting to measure to justify our existence to administrators and the people that finance our programs. These multiple perspectives complicate the definition of quality of life.

DIFFERING DEFINITIONS FOR DIFFERENT AUDIENCES

The thing that bothers me most about how we define this concept is this: What we measure in numbers to report to the people to whom we justify the existence of our palliative care programs is relatively simple, compared to what we would need to measure to prove to ourselves that we really *are* providing quality of life to patients and families. One factor that disturbs me and makes this question complex is timing. When should we measure quality of life? Do we measure it at the point of entry to the program? Do we measure it at some defined midpoint? How do we measure it toward the end of life, when patients may no longer be able to report on their quality of life? We certainly cannot get any measurements from patients after death.

We can get quality of life measurements from families, but their perceptions are, by definition, colored by their experience: "I'm worn out. My relative's going to pass away in the next few days, and this has been a horribly exhausting experience for me." The fact that we may have provided exemplary 24-hour physical and psychosocial support will not necessarily change the fact that the caregiver is exhausted.

So then, if you ask a family member a week into bereavement, he or she may still be exhausted. If you ask the person three months or six months later, he or she may be feeling a lot better about things. Or, at that point, the memory of the relative's death may have focused on the fact that, although you provided exemplary care for six months, in the last six hours of life a phone call was missed or a physician or nurse did not show up at the right time. So, deciding what makes up this concept becomes complex. How to measure quality of life accurately is very troubling. And for whom are we measuring it?

Things become more complicated with defining and measuring quality of life when we care for patients who die at home. We would certainly do this with the motivation to improve the quality of life for our patients. However, we need to examine how we measure the financial, physical, and psychological cost to the quality of life of the families who provide this care, often in difficult circumstances.

IMPLEMENTING THIS CONCEPT IN PRACTICE

At the end of the day, I think we do what we can. And we do it at different levels for different purposes. There are clinical, teaching, research, and administrative purposes for measuring the concept of quality of life. We look at the clinical aspects so as to ensure that we are providing the best quality of life to patients. We look at quality of life for teaching purposes, because we learn things that help us to teach some of the aspects of physical and psychosocial support for patients and families. In terms of our administrative purposes, it becomes easier to measure quality of life in a more global way in order to prove that the program is meeting its goals.

INITIAL GOALS OF THE EDMONTON PROGRAM

Let me review what the initial goals of the program were. Dr. Eduardo Bruera designed the Edmonton program with the vision of developing a comprehensive program to increase the access of patients with terminal cancer to palliative care services. That was key, as well as being what we were interested in. But the second key goal was to decrease the number of cancer patients who die in acute care facilities. Dr. Bruera and others focused particularly on cancer-related deaths simply because, for many of us, this is the largest population that we look after. In addition, from a statistical point of view, it is easier to measure and report on this group because it is a little easier to define. This second goal gave us a financial rationale for the program. If our program could generate cost savings, we could justify both why the health care system needed us and why we needed the funds to develop the hospices and provide community palliative care. The third goal of the program was to increase participation of family physicians in the care of terminally ill patients.

IMPROVED ACCESS TO PALLIATIVE CARE:
A GLOBAL MARKER OF SUCCESS

An example of an administrative use of the concept of quality of life is that ever since the program was established, we have been able to show that we've met these goals. The number of patients with cancer-related deaths who had access to the palliative care program has gone from about 20 to 25 percent of patients before the program to about 85 percent of advanced cancer patients who now see a palliative care consult team at some point in their final illness. If patients were in the tertiary unit, this contact would be a lot more intensive. If the patient's care had been relatively straightforward—that is, the patient was seen in an acute care hospital, went home, and was seen by the family physician—the contact would have been shorter. But the bottom line is that more patients suffering from cancer now have access to palliative care.

By measuring the number of inpatient days for cancer-related deaths both before the program was instituted and then afterward, we were able to show that we decreased the number of inpatient days for cancer-related deaths from around 25,000 to 7,000. When you calculate this cost savings, depending on what you pick as the cost of an acute hospital bed, it is a considerable amount of money.

ALR: *Let's use a patient example to illustrate how the program works. Take Mrs. Smith. She's at home, suffering from advanced emphysema, on oxygen, and not getting out of bed. She's got a weak heart. In the United States, if she had a family caregiver and an astute physician, she'd be a candidate for the Medicare Hospice Benefit. Without a family caregiver, she would need to be able to afford supplemental home care to stay at home. What would be available to Mrs. Smith in Edmonton, if she did not have someone who could care for her 24 hours a day, but she wanted to remain at home?*

RLF: No program is perfect, and you have just hit upon our Achilles' heel. Patients in Mrs. Smith's situation have very little chance of remaining at home for the rest of their lives, unless they have enough money to pay for a 24-hour caregiver. Home care can provide a lot of services in the home, and we, the palliative care program, can provide all the symptomatic and supportive advice possible. But if there is no one to provide physical care to a bedridden, confused patient, it is impossible for that person to remain at home in most circumstances. Home care can provide about four to five hours of a personal care attendant in the home, which means there's still another 19 or 20 hours a day that the family must fill in or pay for those services. In this regard, the situation is quite similar to that in the United States. There are exceptional circumstances; if someone clearly looks like he or she will pass away in the next couple of days, *sometimes* the home care services are able to put in 24-hour care for that short period. But for the person who has become bedridden for a number of days or weeks at the end of his or her life, the services do not exist. This is why we have the hospices.

ALR: *So that person would be a candidate for the inpatient hospice?*

RLF: That person would absolutely be a candidate for hospice. The reality is that from a simply administrative, economic point of view it makes more sense to have that person in an inpatient hospice unit where you have one nurse looking after six or seven patients, rather than the six or seven nurses that would be required if those patients were each at home.

FINANCING AN INTEGRATED SYSTEM OF CARE

ALR: *Is the Edmonton Palliative Care Program financed through the Canadian national health system?*

RLF: All the services I've described, including the home care services, although limited, are covered. There is a nominal charge of $15 a day for being in one of the continuing palliative care units, which for most people is far less than they would receive in pension money. So, for most people, this nominal cost is not a hardship.

There are some gaps in any system. For example, although it is a nominal cost, if the patient is relatively young—not in the seniors group—and has a family and a mortgage, then that nominal cost can be a burden. Also, there are hidden costs with being at home, in terms of some dressings, or the tubing of pain pumps, or perhaps some sort of technical thing that may not be covered 100 percent by insurance.

ALR: *It sounds as though the hospitals and/or hospices are not in financial competition with one another. Is that correct?*

RLF: There is absolutely no financial competition among any of these institutions. All the hospices have plenty of work. There's no financial or profit margin that one must prove to justify the institution's existence. What we have to prove to justify our existence is that we are doing what we say we are doing. Patients across the region have access to palliative care, and we are looking after them in the most appropriate setting for their *needs*, which relates to patients' and families' quality of life.

INTEGRATED INFRASTRUCTURE MAKES WEB OF CARE POSSIBLE

ALR: *Can you say more about the communication across the different places in which patients are cared for, so that as patients move across settings, the staff in each is aware of what health care providers in other settings are doing?*

RLF: The programs are interconnected so that we could attempt to have a seamless flow of patients from one place to another. The physicians are part of the same structure. We meet in the same places. We have the same common educational rounds and sit on the same administrative committees. We answer to the same authority within this complex web. So, if the patient goes from the Royal Alexandra Hospital to the tertiary palliative care unit, or to a hospice, to the home, or to the Cross Cancer Institute, we know whom we need to contact to ensure that the palliative care services we started continue. In addition, we use the same assessment tools to measure symptoms, cognition, and pain syndromes. This gives us a common language in the transfer of information.

QUALITY OF LIFE AT THE PATIENT AND FAMILY LEVEL

ALR: *How do you take this amorphous and multifaceted term "quality of life" and apply it in practice at the bedside?*

RLF: From a bedside point of view, we have a number of outcome measures that we use throughout the city, either on a daily basis or two or three times a week, depending on the patient's setting. Probably, the most useful tool I would point to is the Edmonton Symptom Assessments Scale (ESAS),* which is a scale with two versions: a numerical scale and a visual analogue scale on a number of domains, from the physical to the psychosocial. The domains that it assesses are pain, tiredness, nausea, depression, anxiety, drowsiness, appetite, feeling of well-being, and shortness of breath. There is also a space for "other problems" elicited from the patient. In the numerical version, on a scale from 0 to 10, the person indicates how much of a problem that item is at this point in time, with 0 being no problem, and 10 being the worst possible. In the visual analogue, the patient sees a linear continuum and makes a mark on this line to indicate how much of a problem the domain is.

Now, there are many quality of life scales. There is a confusing array of different ways that we can measure symptoms. What I like about the ESAS is that it is extremely short. It takes the least time of any scale of which I am aware. It's the most straightforward and simple way for people to tell you how they're feeling right now, on a repetitive basis. Using this same scale over time, we have a way of following the progress of people's symptoms.

Some of the so-called physical symptoms are perhaps the easiest to track. People have sometimes asked, "What do you mean by *depression*? And what do you mean by *best feeling of well-being*?" I would point to some of the research where, for example, people like Harvey Chochinov have shown that one of the best screening tools for depression is a single question: "Are you depressed?"[1] And, essentially, that's what we are doing with this question. Robin Cohen showed that asking people many questions about quality of life also correlated with a single question that essentially was a global question about their well-being:[2] for example, on the feeling of well-being visual analogue scale: "How are you, given all these problems? Tell me how you're feeling right now." That's essentially what we ask people when we say, "How are you?" Most of the time when we do that in a polite social situation we do not take the time to listen to the answer. But

---

*Readers can download this tool and others from the Edmonton Palliative Care Program's Clinical Assessment page at <www.palliative.org/pc_assess.html>, where tools are listed with hotlinks to each. The homepage for the Edmonton program is <www.palliative.org>.

we are being serious when we ask this question of our patients. So, it is a simple tool, and it is easy to administer. We use it as a standard across the city, in *all* settings. *All* this information goes into an extremely large database of information collected in the home, in hospices, in the consulting services, and in the tertiary unit.

In this way, we *do* have a simple, clinical quality of life measurement that we can follow over time, both to assess the result of our interventions and to use clinically with patients. We use this tool to open a conversation with patients about their current assessment of their quality of life. When a patient indicates, for example, that his or her anxiety is 8 out of 10, and yet we had not realized that this person was anxious, the ESAS gives us a wonderful clinical opportunity to say, "Well, I noticed that you assessed your anxiety in this way. Let's talk about that a little bit more; what *are* you anxious about?" So, from a bedside point of view, it is clinically useful.

From a teaching point of view, it is also a useful learning tool. We can show students how we picked up that a patient is experiencing pain, intervene to address the pain, and then observe with gratification as the pain visual analogue disappears, down to close to zero with appropriate treatment. We also use other assessment tools, including a staging system for cancer pain. We follow measures of cognition, and we use screening questions for past history of alcohol abuse.

By using quality of life assessments to identify the patients with the most problematic issues, we then want to ensure that we look after these patients in the component of our program most suited to their needs. For example, the comprehensive, well-resourced tertiary palliative care unit would obviously be the best setting for patients with the most complex physical and psychosocial issues. Use of these quality of life assessments helps us to identify these patients and then track the impact that we are having on them as we continue to treat them and monitor their progress. At the same time, if administrators were to challenge us to demonstrate that we are using our resources appropriately, we can use this information for that purpose as well.

ALR: *Are you able to use the information you get from these tools, to alleviate symptoms or problems other than pain?*

RLF: From a day-to-day clinical point of view, we find the tool very useful in terms of picking up things that we may otherwise have missed. It allows us to respond—to ask patients and families to clarify what it is they are trying to tell us and to monitor things on a day-to-day basis. We have also used these tools in many research publications. And we use them on a monthly basis with the administrative authorities to demonstrate that we are doing what we set out to do.

ALR: *How do you address the needs of families, in terms of quality of life?*

RLF: We don't have a quality of life tool that we use on a regular basis to measure what we are doing for families, which is probably an area we should be looking at, in fact. One practical problem of measuring quality of life is that even some of the simple things I have talked about are difficult to do. Many programs balk at the idea of measuring anything. It's seen as being intrusive at a time when patients and families are having some difficulty.

RESISTANCE TO QUALITY OF LIFE MEASUREMENT

ALR: *How do you respond to those who feel that assessment is burdensome to dying patients: "I don't want you doing any assessments. This patient is dying. I just want you to care for this patient's clinical symptoms and psychosocial needs, but no tools, assessment, or research"?*

RLF: Our answer is to call attention to the paradox here. Just for a moment, think about the fact that one of the criticisms of pain and other symptom management is that health care providers do not ask about the patient's experience. What we're doing is, we are asking. And we are asking a lot of questions. As a result, most people appreciate the fact that they are being assessed and that staff members are taking the time to ask them about these symptoms. But we have a wide, diverse world of patients and families, and not everyone tolerates a lot of questions.

One way to respond to this resistance is to explain *what* it is that we are attempting to do and *why* we are asking patients questions about their ability to concentrate and remember things. We explain our concern about how medications may affect the person and our need to understand a wide range of different symptoms so that we can discuss these symptoms with the patient and attempt to respond to the symptoms. Most people who have some initial negative reaction will then understand the value of the tool. So, the vast majority of people will then either be happy because it wasn't a problem in the beginning or because they have understood the explanation. There will be the rare individuals that just refuse, and we have to respect people's right to be cared for the way that they want and accept that we will not have measurement outcomes in a few situations.

GAPS IN FAMILY AND CLINICIAN PERSPECTIVES ON QUALITY OF LIFE

One problem with the ESAS is that, ideally, it's meant to be filled in by the patients. But as patients deteriorate, it becomes more and more difficult to have them complete it, and we then end up doing proxy assessments with staff or families completing it. We noticed that when families complete the ESAS as proxies for patients they report *pain* as being the most difficult problem, often in a patient in whom the pain had been previously well controlled. The family is reporting that the pain is a horrible problem now that the patient is semicomatose and unresponsive. So we ask the family to explain what they are seeing that makes them believe that the patient is in pain.

What we found is that people see many things—including agitated confusion, or the fact that the patient appears to be breathing relatively fast, or that the patient is not eating—and whatever the family observes, they have a huge tendency to label these observations as *pain*.

This observation on our part has been a great learning opportunity about the gap in the care that we're providing to families. We perhaps have not explained well enough to families how we understand the symptoms that they are observing. What is significant is that we *thought* we were doing it, but, obviously, for some families, not well enough. We would meet family members weeks or perhaps months after their relative had died, and we would remember that the relative became unresponsive and *appeared* to pass away with no discomfort. But the family members tell us, "Oh, it was awful! My mother had a horrible time." And yet we hadn't recollected the passing in at all the same way. It was this dissonance between staff and family perspectives that led to the development of another tool, the Edmonton Comfort Assessment Form (ECAF).[†]

Part of this perspective gap is due to the distress that families experience when a loved one dies, no matter how good the care is. Some of my frustration about measuring quality of life derives from this tension. At the end of someone's life, I think we have to be realistic. We have to remember that, at the end of the day, death is a traumatic experience for families. If we were to tell families, "You have the good luck to be part of our palliative care program, and we are just a wonderful palliative care program. We are so wonderful, we are going to grant you one wish. What would your wish be?" Many people, if they honestly searched in their hearts, would say, "If you are that wonderful, my wish is that you make my relative not die." And *that's* what we have to remember when we try to show outcomes in quality of life.

> *We need to be realistic about what it is that we are trying to do. The global dimensions . . . are easier to measure. The micro, day-to-day assessments of quality of life for patients who are dying are shifting sands. We have to be rather humble about our ability to accurately measure and represent these day-to-day changes.*

ALR: *Do you have any other thoughts on addressing quality of life in an integrated palliative care program?*

RLF: To a large extent, it is confusing, complicated, and difficult. We need to be realistic about what it is that we are trying to do. The global dimensions—for example, access to palliative care and the right location for the right patient—are easier to measure. The micro, day-to-day assessments of quality of life for patients who are dying are shifting sands. We have to be rather humble about our ability to accurately measure and represent these day-to-day changes.

REFERENCES

1. Chochinov HM, Wilson KG, Enns M, Lander S. Are you depressed? Screening for depression in the terminally ill. *American Journal of Psychiatry.* 1997;154:674–676.
2. Cohen SR, Mount BM, Strobel MG, Bui F. The McGill quality of life questionnaire: A measure of quality of life appropriate for people with advanced disease. A preliminary study of validity and acceptability. *Palliative Medicine.* 1995;9(3):207–219.

[†]Readers can download this tool and others from the Edmonton Palliative Care Program's Clinical Assessment page at <www.palliative.org/pc_assess.html>.

Featured Innovation: Part II

Addressing Quality of Life at the Edmonton Palliative Care Program

An Interview with CARLEEN BRENNEIS, RN, MHSA

Edmonton Palliative Care Program
Edmonton, Alberta, Canada

In the Featured Innovation: Part II, Carleen Brenneis, RN, MHSA, program director of the Edmonton Regional Palliative Care Program, comments on how patients' quality of life is assessed and promoted through an integrated program of palliative care services in Edmonton, Alberta, Canada. A thorough historical summary of the Edmonton Regional Palliative Care Program is given before Part One of this Featured Innovation. In this interview with Karen S. Heller, PhD, Ms. Brenneis describes the services currently provided and the barriers to improving quality of life for patients and families that she and her colleagues still need to overcome.

Karen S. Heller: *How would you define "quality of life"?*

Carleen Brenneis: Quality of life is a fairly complex construct. The term itself is really a middle-class term, and I don't find it commonly used by our patients. When we started to develop the Edmonton Symptom Assessment Scale (ESAS), we had quality of life as one of our indicators.* This indicator was hard to explain to patients because quality of life really involves all the components of your life: how you are doing physically, socially, emotionally, spiritually, and so forth. So it was very hard for people to answer. We then moved toward asking them about their feeling of wellness or well-being, and people seemed to understand that better. So, I think quality of life is a health care term, which we health care providers use in talking among ourselves, but we don't tend to use that language when talking to patients or clients.[†]

---

*Readers can download this tool and others from the Edmonton Palliative Care Program's Clinical Assessment page at <www.palliative.org/pc_assess.html>.

[†]In the Edmonton Palliative Care Program, people who are treated in acute care facilities or hospice facilities as inpatients or outpatients are referred to as "patients," whereas those who receive home care services are referred to as "clients." For the purposes of this interview, we refer to all recipients of care from the program as patients.

In our program, we use "well-being" to refer to the individual's overall comfort, both physical and psychosocial. When people truthfully respond to the question "How are you?", they are describing their well-being. We ask patients to describe how they are doing as a whole person: body, mind, and spirit. This begins to answer the question with respect to some of the components of quality of life. But it seems to be better understood than saying, "How is your quality of life today?"

One of the most important components of our program is that we expect that asking about a patient's well-being will be a regular part of our discussions with patients. We operationalize the concept of "quality of life" by expecting clinicians working in any palliative care setting in the Edmonton area to ask the questions on the ESAS. These questions open up the opportunity for people to tell us how they are doing. Quality of life is really a temporal question as well: "How are you doing at the moment?" Yesterday, one of our staff told me, "You know, I just asked one of my patients that question and he said, 'I just had the most wonderful bath, it was great.'" He might answer the question differently with respect to different time frames—that moment, that day, or the rest of his life.

KSH: *How frequently do you ask patients these kinds of questions?*

CB: Patient control and choice are very important in all our philosophies of palliative care. The most effective way you can give patients control is by asking them how they are doing and by asking them what is important to them. Our expectation is that when a nurse goes into a patient's room in the morning she says, "I'm with you for the day. What's important to you? What do you need today? How can I help you?" The same expectation applies when the occupational therapist and physical therapist go in. We are beginning to look at what each specific discipline has to offer in palliative care. Palliative care is really driven by the patients' wants and needs, more so probably than in most areas of health care.

KSH: *How do you assess well-being and address quality of life needs for home care patients?*

CB: We use the same tool, the ESAS, in the home, in hospice, and in the Grey Nuns tertiary acute care unit. Thus, when we are referred to patients, we all use the same language and we have the same expectations. Interdisciplinary staff provides palliative care in each setting. Each profession (physicians, nurses, occupational and physical therapists, social workers, chaplains) addresses different components of quality of life. We conduct family conferences to ensure that all members of the health care team, which includes the patient and his or her family members, agree on the goals of treatment. Family conferences involve the patient, family,

> *When the family is part of the unit of care, it is very important to know how family members are doing, particularly in the home, where they are the primary caregivers. Part of our assessment includes finding out how the family is doing.*

and appropriate staff, such as the family physician, social worker, and, if preparing for discharge, home care staff. The patient and family are the unit of care, so we try to address the family's quality of life at a given point in time.

KSH: *How do you assess the family's well-being and life quality when a loved one is dying?*

CB: When the family is part of the unit of care, it is very important to know how family members are doing, particularly in the home, where they are the primary caregivers. Part of our assessment includes finding out how the family is doing. We do not have a set of assessment questions for the caregiver, per se. We have tried different ways of gathering this information, but have not yet found the right mix of questions. In the home, however, it is critically important that you ask the caregiver the same questions as the patient. We also talk to families about what their goal is—are they thinking about a home death? We know through some of the research we have done that if you are going to have a home death, the caregiver and the patient need to agree; if one or the other does not want a home death, of course, it is not going to work.

KSH: *What kinds of concerns do families bring up when asked about quality of life?*

CB: The Palliative Care Association of Alberta, of which I am a member, recently wrote a caregiver guide that is responsive to the needs identified by people in our province. We did it by asking the home care nurses of the province, as well as patients and families, "What is important, what do we need in this manual?" By and large, their comments reinforced the importance of meeting patients' physical needs first. This is consistent with Abraham Maslow's hierarchy of needs, which posits that you need to meet people's physical and social needs before they can focus on their emotional and spiritual needs.[1] We hear that time and again from the families, patients, and our own staff. We hear from patients, "You need to deal with my pain, with my physical discomfort." This may not be the most important thing for their quality of life, but in order for them to deal with their emotional and psychosocial issues, you first have to deal with these physical issues.

We also hear repeatedly that family caregivers want information to enable them to help with the patient's physical and psychosocial needs. They want to know, for example, "How do I help turn the patient? How do I help in other ways? Whom do I call if I need help?" Safety is so important in the home. Families need to feel that help is a phone call away. All these pieces are part of quality of life.

KSH: *Have you defined the concept of quality of life for your program? Do you feel that you are all speaking the same language when you talk about it?*

CB: I think the core dimensions of quality of life (physical, psychosocial, existential, and spiritual) are explicit in our mission and objectives. We still have tremendous work to do, particularly in the psychosocial area. Research in the psychosocial area is difficult. We've done some work on hope, and we regularly review the literature in this area.[2]

KSH: *Do you think that increasing access to palliative care services contributes to improved quality of life near the end of life?*

CB: Access to palliative care services is one indicator of quality of life, because it is a component of a person's social situation. If patients feel that their needs are being met, if they have options in terms of location of care, if they feel that they have choices that they understand—all this adds to quality of life because people then feel that they have some control.

We measure and record "access" at a consultant's level. So, when we say we have 91 percent access this year to palliative care services, we mean that 91 percent of the cancer patient population has received a palliative care consultation. The consultation involves a full palliative assessment, which includes asking about all the different areas of quality of life.

KSH: *Is one assumption underlying your program that quality of life in the acute care setting would not be as good for dying patients as it would be in hospice or at home?*

CB: Yes, although care in acute care settings can be excellent, the focus there is to meet acute care needs and discharge patients when they no longer need that level of care. We assume that people would prefer to be at home or in a community setting, such as inpatient hospice, rather than in an acute care hospital. Patients need acute care when they need the diagnosticians and enhanced nursing care. For basic palliative care, however, 90 percent of care can be provided in the home, according to Derek Doyle.[3] We believe that patients can receive excellent palliative care in a community setting or at home and therefore, we need to provide these services in such settings.

One goal of our program was to decrease the number of cancer patients dying in acute care settings. In fact, 87 percent of patients suffering from cancer were dying in acute care settings in Edmonton before this program began. Presently, 40 to 45 percent of patients with cancer are dying in acute care settings. More patients in the final phase of life are being cared for in hospices and at home.

One thing that we emphasized was that, if we were moving care to the community, we needed to transfer resources there. Behind this transfer of resources is the belief that you cannot simply move people out of acute care and call it palliative care; you need to provide the resources to do this care. These resources consist primarily of nursing, with access to medical and interdisciplinary teams. So we enhanced our home care service and created an enhanced service system in hospice. Continuing care facilities were funded for enhanced nursing, interdisciplinary care, and medication, so they are really more like institutional hospice settings.

KSH: *How are hospice and palliative care funded in Canada?*

CB: All our funding is centralized. We are a regional program within the province of Alberta, and so the community and acute care funding are all combined. Service is need based, so if you need home care, hospice, tertiary, or acute level care, provision of a given level of service is based on the assessment of the consultants and nurses in the program for what level of care you need. Our criteria for entry to inpatient hospice care is based on an expected two-month length of stay, but if someone needs it for longer, there is not any cutoff point. It is not funded that way at all.

KSH: *What kind of help are people getting through the Edmonton Palliative Care Program overall?*

CB: As people come into the program, they may receive a few hours of care a week, which increases as the patients' needs require. A person can get 24-hour care in the home near the end of life, but we would not provide 24-hour care for weeks and weeks on end. There is an expectation that the family caregivers are helping out; however, we do have to watch for caregiver burnout. If someone has absolutely no family, it is very difficult to provide home care. Lack of a family caregiver is a common indication for people to come into a hospice setting. In Canada, acute care services are all under Medicare; home care is not. Home care is organized in various ways throughout the country. It can be different from province to province, even region to region, at this point. In our region, palliative care professionals work within home care, which is part of our overall health care system. The nursing and interdisciplinary services are part of the home care program, and we have other agencies we contract with for licensed practical nurses and palliative personal care attendants.

KSH: *What is the size of the population in your catchment area?*

CB: In the region served by our program—Edmonton and the surrounding suburbs, including some rural areas—there are 840,000 people. To drive from one end to the other of this region would probably take two and one-half hours in one direction and an hour and one-half in the other. The visiting team covers quite a distance, so we broke the team up to cover quadrants of the city. The visiting team includes four physicians and four nurses. Part of our community team (at least one nurse and one to one and one-half physicians) provides consultation to the hospices. When a person is admitted to the continuing care unit hospices, there is an automatic consultation to the team, following which we are only involved as required. But we do provide advice and attend conferences on a weekly basis.

KSH: *What kinds of diagnoses do your patients have?*

CB: Of all the patients seen last year, 92 percent had a primary diagnosis of cancer. Like most palliative care programs, we started out based on an oncology model, and then slowly we have begun to bring in patients with other diagnoses. In 1999, there were 1,400 cancer deaths in the Edmonton region. The palliative care program provided care to 91 percent of those patients.

A hospice is not necessarily the right setting all the time for patients with other diagnoses; however, some patients with congestive heart failure, chronic obstructive pulmonary disease, and amyelotrophic lateral sclerosis fit very well in the hospice model. But it's not the right setting for *all* patients; some need to remain under the care of their specialist. If you look at the "mixed" model that Linda Kristjanson talks about,[4] sometimes it is most appropriate for patients with a particular diagnosis to be seen by palliative consultants in that particular specialty area. In a setting that serves a small number of patients suffering from AIDS, for example, it might be very fitting to do that. So we tend to visit patients with AIDS or with kidney disease wherever they happen to be. We have good relationships with other disciplines; they come to our city-wide palliative rounds and describe what they are doing in palliative care. We talk with one another about what are their needs and ours, and how we can work together, so we are building those bridges over time.

KSH: *Could you give me an example of how somebody would move from one palliative care setting to another?*

CB: No matter where you are in the region, you should be able to access a consultant. If a patient is at home and the home care team and the physician feel that the patient needs higher-level care, they'll call in a regional palliative care team, and a nurse or physician will go out and visit the patient and gather all the information. We always do it with the approval of the family physician or attending physician because, as consultants, we are not providing the primary medical care. The family physician is the primary physician and we come in and consult to that person. We want to make sure that the primary physicians are supporting whatever we are doing. If we do visit a patient in the home and suggest some changes of medication, somebody has to provide orders. So we work very closely with the family physicians, or the attending physicians wherever they are, to make sure that they know we are coming in and agree.

In our latest satisfaction survey of the family physicians, we learned that this approach is working. Once we go into the home and assess what level of care that the patient needs (usually it fits exactly with what the family physician and the home care nurses are telling us), we would then triage the needs. We have centralized access to our 57 hospice beds, so the consultant provides information to a hospice triage nurse (one of our four nurse consultants), who decides what level of care is appropriate. If a patient is at home and requires an inpatient hospice bed, this person would get the available bed before someone who is already in acute care, because the person in the hospital is already safe. So we always are triaging based on the greatest need. If we go in and we see that the person needs tertiary-level care, we would talk to the physicians on the tertiary unit, and if the family physician agrees, we would move the patient to that site. So, the consultant who assesses the patient, be it in acute care, at the tertiary level, in the home, or in the hospice, also accesses the other levels of care.

KSH: *When the patient is dying at home, who does the family or patient call if they have questions—their own family physician or someone on your palliative care team?*

CB: Families and patients would call their own physician or a palliative home care phone number. When a patient is served by home care, the patient can call a centralized number for all home care patients. This number has 24-hour coverage, with a palliative nurse and physician consultants on call at all times. It is extremely important that patients feel safe at home. Persons, particularly near the end of life, need constant assessment, they need to feel they can call anytime and get expert answers.

KSH: *If the family caregivers start to burn out, do you have respite care?*

CB: We do some respite care in the hospices. Generally, there is some respite care available in the region, although access to it depends on the level of care that the patient needs. Home care does most of our respite care. If the family needs a break, for example, if they have a big event to attend, we will try to provide respite care in the home, rather than move the client out of the setting. Again, access to this service is need based.

KSH: *What aspects of quality of life do you feel you do best in addressing and which would you like to work on more?*

CB: I think what is really important is the balance. Like most programs, we are very good at talking to the patients about where they are at and what is important for them. Our program is known to be fairly strong at addressing the physical needs of patients, and we are able to monitor how we are doing in that area through all the ESAS assessments that we use throughout the program. We enter the ESAS scores into a database, so we can complete audits and monitor how well we are meeting patients' needs. We did an audit of our home care services, in which we looked at whether anything was done if the ESAS score was greater than 5 out of 10. [Higher scores indicate worse symptoms.] If so, was the family physician aware of this problem? Was the family physician treating the problem? Were there changes in the medications? Our audit demonstrated that we do well at talking to people and assessing their concerns.

It is harder to address quality of life when you are looking at what we call a "black" ESAS, which means that you are not looking at the scores on specific symptoms, such as pain and nausea, but rather across the board at *all* the symptoms, and the scores are *all* high, so that the bar graph looks black. If someone is not doing well on many of the ESAS indicators, for example, the person has depression, anxiety, and drowsiness, is missing that feeling of well-being, and is experiencing pain, then that person is probably suffering. When you are dealing with these multidimensional components, this is when the consultants are called in and we talk about possibly moving the patient to the tertiary palliative care setting and providing further support.

KSH: *What improvements are you still seeking to make in the services that you provide to address quality of life?*

CB: We would like to have a psychologist available in the community. Right now, to have a psychologist available at home or in the local community, people need to pay for the service. We have access to the psychologists at the Cross Cancer Institute, who are excellent, but they don't leave the building, so if we need help in the home and people are really ill, we have a bit of a gap. This is one area in which I think we can improve.

I think there is always work to be done to improve the area of psychosocial assessment. Although we report psychosocial indicators on the ESAS, it's going to be years before we really understand how to interpret them completely. For example, we looked at the areas of depression and anxiety; these indicators need to be reported to the physician and they need to be discussed. It is harder to audit the follow-up on these measures objectively using a chart review process. We did look at whether things were being done or not, and we found that in the psychosocial area it is harder to determine. You can treat and talk with people who have depression, but you may not change it. If someone is depressed coming into his or her situation of life-threatening illness, you may not be able to change that. So, it's a little bit tougher to know what impact we may be having in this area.

Considering ways to improve more broadly, we need to look ahead. Right now, our model and our care work well, but it is not going to look this way two, three, or five years down the road. We have an older population and we are expecting a 56 percent increase in the number of people needing palliative care in the next decade,[‡] so we need to plan now for how we are going to deal with the workload. So this is our biggest challenge. We have good options for patients now, but how do you meet the growing needs of an aging population?

KSH: *When people are unable to report how they are feeling and you need to turn to someone else to speak for them, do you feel as confident of the kinds of assessments that you are making, or that you are able to meet their needs?*

CB: You do not know exactly how the patient is feeling, but we still will do an assessment based on the caregiver and the staff's input. We try to deal with cognitive impairment by regular assessment, really watching for delirium and treating when appropriate. If you want people to make choices and to be involved in their care, they have to be awake and aware to do this. You need to listen to what the person tells you. When a person cannot tell you how they are doing, we do ask the caregiver and staff to assess, and we may use an assessment tool called the Edmonton Comfort Assessment Form (ECAF),[§] which asks a caregiver and staff

---

[‡]Alberta Cancer Board, Division of Epidemiology, Prevention & Screening, August 1999.
[§]Readers can download this tool and others from the Edmonton Palliative Care Program's Clinical Assessment page at <www.palliative.org/pc_assess.html>.

to assess comfort. This tool was initially named the Edmonton Discomfort Assessment Form, but has recently been renamed.

KSH: *Are appropriate community-based services available everywhere in the region for people to access? For example, for spiritual support, are the churches involved? Are there community volunteers?*

CB: We have pastoral care and chaplains in hospices, acute care settings, and the tertiary unit, and we count on the community to provide this kind of support. We encourage people to be involved in their own support systems, religious or not. I think there are different levels of access and certain families are more connected with the community than others. We create a bereavement resource list every year, and we connect with families by telephone after the patient's death to make sure that, if they want further information, we can provide it to them. We try to identify families who are not well connected in their communities ahead of time.

KSH: *How does the Edmonton program delimit the scope of its responsibility for ensuring patients' and families' quality of life?*

CB: You usually can only bring someone back to where they were before they had a particular symptom, if you are able to control it. We do not get a score of less than 5 out of 10 using the ESAS tool on every patient. We do the best we can. You are not going to fix everything. Particularly on the tertiary unit, where we have some very difficult situations, we talk to the staff about the fact that we can only do so much and then, when we have done everything that we can, we journey with the patient. We don't desert them; we provide support wherever the person is, whether it is in the home or the tertiary care unit.

Patient autonomy plays a role, too. A patient may choose not to be connected with services or not to take a particular medication, particularly when in the home. We need to provide information and support, but a person has a right to choose to follow our suggestions or not.

KSH: *How do you see that the nursing role contributes to the patients' quality of life, as distinct from the physician's role on this team?*

CB: There are tremendous nursing needs when people become physically debilitated and emotionally stressed; the nurses need to be in there completing the whole nursing process, coordinating care, bringing in the other disciplines, or filling in for them when they are not there 24 hours a day. So palliative care requires the full nursing process, from assessment, coordination and collaboration, direct nursing care, and ongoing evaluation with the patient and family of the care provided. Advocacy is a well-established nursing role and very important in palliative care. The nurses conduct the ESAS. From a nursing perspective, it's a very fulfilling, very rewarding area to work in because you need to use all your skills.

KSH: *How do you promote cooperation and a sense of common mission across care settings?*

CB: Insofar as we are not funded per patient in Canada, there is no competition for patients among care settings. With respect to working collaboratively and making sure that patients are in the right setting, this is the role of the regional program office. We have a philosophy of care that says people need to be at the right setting at the right time, and we have criteria for admissions for all the different areas. And when patients are at the wrong place at the wrong time, we talk with everyone about how we could do better the next time. So, we have a strong common goal and vision, and because we are a regional program, I have access to acute care hospitals, to the community, to hospice, and to the continuing care community. We cross all the borders, which makes a huge difference in our ability to meet patients' needs. The goals and visions are shared and agreed on at the top levels of acute care, continuing care, and home care. In addition, this shared vision is reinforced by matrix reporting. In our setting, everybody does not report to this office; home care personnel report to the home care office, hospice staff report through their continuing care management, and acute care staff report to hospital management, but they have a responsibility to this office for their outcomes, their quality of care, and their standards of care. Another aspect of this is that, if I wished to advocate for increased funding or more staff in a certain area, I would identify the needs, communicate them to the people who make these kinds of decisions in this particular setting, and if approved, they would then hire staff. So it is a constant balance. This is why we do look at where patients are over time, for example, how many patients are dying in acute care settings versus at home and so forth, because it is all part of the picture of how we are doing as a palliative care program. So we try to collect this information and share it with the administrators in the different areas to help them to understand the big picture.

KSH: *What kinds of barriers have you faced in getting things accomplished?*

CB: I think the biggest barrier for any palliative care program is to make sure that you are all talking about the same thing and this comes through developing and refining your goals, your vision, and your language. For us, probably one of the hardest barriers is coming up with a common language and agreeing to do things alike in all the settings in which we provide care. Getting staff to do the ESAS everywhere entailed tremendous work in the beginning. All our staff members think that they ask these questions and that they provide palliative care; but if the staff is not assessing symptoms in a constant way and in a way in which we can all communicate

> *I think the biggest barrier for any palliative care program is to make sure that you are all talking about the same thing and this comes through developing and refining your goals, your vision, and your language.*

with one another, the team may not be helping the patient over time. Palliative care specialists need to communicate the information to the family physician in ways that help him or her to make a difference for the patient. So, in the beginning and still, in areas of acute care the greatest barrier that we face is finding a good common language, common definitions, and common philosophy. We need to find this language to move ahead and be able to describe palliative care to other health professionals, and to communicate with our clients and the public so as to improve their understanding of what palliative care is.

Right now, many people have a lot of questions: What does hospice versus palliative care mean? Are they different? The public understands hospice care better than palliative care, but what do they understand about hospice care? Is hospice care tertiary-level care? Is it care in the home? Does the word "hospice" imply a setting? My personal belief is that hospice is a philosophy, but more, it is a setting of care. Now in the United States you have a different answer. I believe that we need to find a term, be it palliative care or end-of-life care, that describes it all in a language that is uncomplicated and clear to the public. We need to present a clear, concise vision of hospice/palliative care. If the end-of-life community does not begin to present a common picture to administrators and to the public, how are we ever going to move this field ahead? It is crucial within our own community, let alone internationally, that we begin to articulate what palliative care is in plain language to the public and to other health professionals.

In Canada, palliative care recently became a subspecialty within medicine and we are heading in that direction now in nursing, as well. It is probably at least five years away yet, but it is coming. The Canadian Palliative Care Association is doing very powerful work by articulating 13 basic principles of palliative care.[5] We are just finishing this consensus work over the next year. I think this will be very helpful in beginning to articulate what hospice and palliative care really are. In 1995, a special Canadian Senate report was issued entitled "Of Life and Death," which was primarily driven by euthanasia and assisted suicide.[6] The report concluded that before you can address euthanasia and assisted suicide, you need to ensure that the principal elements of palliative care have been offered to patients and families. They did a review this year, spearheaded by Senator Sharon Carstairs, and the unanimous recommendation was that palliative care needs to be offered throughout Canada.[7] This senate report, issued in June 2000, is really increasing the focus again on palliative care and increasing pressure on all levels of government to do more. They are talking a lot about quality of life issues within that framework.

KSH: *Have you faced any barriers in terms of getting palliative care on the health care agenda in Edmonton?*

CB: Another big barrier most programs face today is getting buy-in from the people who control the resources. There are such multiple needs in health care. Palliative care competes with heart transplants and MRIs. So one needs to understand what is happening in the community and be able to articulate those needs to the administrators, so that they are able to carry the palliative care agenda forward to a table with many players. You cannot expect administrators to finance palliative care just because it sounds like a good thing. There is tremendous work in program planning that needs to happen in order to create a viable program.

> *You cannot expect administrators to finance palliative care just because it sounds like a good thing.*

Simply knowing the number and location of cancer deaths in your area is incredibly powerful information. Administrators want this information. In addition, you need a champion in your region, hospital, or other setting to begin to discuss it. We had a very strong tertiary unit before the Edmonton Palliative Care Program began, but we knew that only 21 percent of patients with cancer had access to palliative care, because there were limited beds on that unit. So we needed information about the entire population. It is useful to research how your community is planning to meet the needs of its aging population. There are many ways of doing this planning. We have one model and it worked for our community because we brought in all the stakeholders—the administrators, the family physicians, the consultants and specialists, the community—and said, "How do you think we can make this work? Here's what we think would work, do you agree?" To get that level of buy-in, we had to provide the information to them to act on. So, I think another major barrier is a lack of time and expertise to pull all that information together.

KSH: *What message would you like to leave with our readers about how quality of life should best be promoted in practice?*

CB: I think the core palliative care program has got to respond to what the patient wants and needs, which implies finding out what is important to each individual patient. This concept should be part of the philosophy and goals of a palliative care program.

REFERENCES

1. Maslow A. *Motivation and Personality*, 3d ed. New York: Harper & Row, 1987.
2. Nekolaichuk CL, Bruera E. Forum: On the nature of hope in palliative care. *Journal of Palliative Care*. 1998;14(1):36–42.
3. Doyle D. The provision of palliative care. In *Oxford Textbook of Palliative Medicine*, 2d ed., D Doyle, G Hanks, N MacDonald (eds.). New York: Oxford University Press, 1998, 41–53.
4. Kristjanson L. *Generic versus Specific Palliative Care Services*. Ottawa: Health Care & Issues Division, Health Canada, 1997.
5. Ferris FD, Cummings I (eds.). *Palliative Care: Toward a Consensus in Standardized Principles of Practice*. Ottawa: Canadian Palliative Care Association, 1995.
6. Canada Senate. *Of Life and Death*. Ottawa: Report of the Special Senate Committee on Euthanasia and Assisted Suicide, 1995.
7. Canada Senate. *Quality End-of-Life Care: The Right of Every Canadian*, subcommittee to update *Of Life and Death*. Ottawa: Standing Senate Committee on Social Affairs, Science, and Technology, 2000.

Promoting Quality of Life Near the End of Life in Argentina

An Interview with MARIELA BERTOLINO, MD

Tornú Hospital–FEMEBA Foundation
Buenos Aires, Argentina

In the following interview, Mariela Bertolino, MD, discusses the current status of palliative care in Buenos Aires, Argentina, and ongoing efforts to improve this care in her country. She comments on the use of the Edmonton Symptom Assessment Scale for measuring quality of life in her palliative care program, which is based in Tornú Hospital–FEMEBA Foundation, a public hospital in Buenos Aires. Her program serves approximately 350 patients a year on an outpatient basis and has six inpatient beds, which are the first and, thus far, only specifically designated palliative care beds in a country of 30 million people. The interview was conducted by Karen S. Heller, PhD.

CONCEPTUALIZING QUALITY OF LIFE

Karen S. Heller: *How would you define the concept "quality of life" for patients in your program in Buenos Aires?*

Mariela Bertolino: The idea of life quality is very meaningful for us and for all those working in palliative care. We are trying to help people in the advanced stages of different diseases. Most of our patients have cancer, and some have difficulties with physical symptoms, psychological distress, social and financial issues, as well as spiritual or existential problems.

For us, quality of life is a concept that tries to put all these issues together, and it has inspired our program's policies regarding patients and families. But sometimes, even when we try to make this construct of quality of life reflect the realistic problems, needs, or concerns of the people who are ill and their families, we find that it is difficult to use a tool to measure it on a regular basis. In talking with pa-

> *. . . the concept of "well-being" includes all the things that give the patient some satisfaction or happiness, or its absence is indicated by what is disturbing to the patient.*

tients and families in our clinic, we are probably more familiar with the term "well-being" than "quality of life." For us, the concept of "well-being" includes all the things that give the patient some satisfaction or happiness, or its absence is indicated by what is disturbing to the patient. In general, we try to allow people to lead the best possible lives at the end of life and to find the best possible well-being, which varies a lot from person to person.

When we do our assessments, during the patient interview, we talk first about physical and psychological symptoms; after that, we address psychosocial problems and, sometimes, existential difficulties. Then, at the end of the interview, we ask the patient, "With all of that, how would you say you are feeling?" The answer tells us about the patient's well-being. Thus, the idea of "well-being" integrates how the patient feels, physically, emotionally, and spiritually, all together.

> . . ."well-being" integrates how the patient feels, physically, emotionally, and spiritually . . .

KSH: *It sounds as though you ask the same kind of questions that are on the Edmonton Symptom Assessment Scale.* Do you use that tool?*

MB: We do the Edmonton Symptom Assessment Scale (ESAS) with patients on a regular basis, although we made one modification by adding insomnia as an item. Also, the ESAS has the well-being item in the middle, and sometimes, for practical reasons, I ask about well-being after having done all the other items. At the end of the interview, I try to get the number on a scale of 0 to 10 that would best describe how the patient is feeling overall.

KSH: *To what extent do you focus on the family caregivers? Do you also assess their well-being in any way?*

MB: We do, but not with that tool. Although we include the family in the interview and ask many questions concerning the problems of the family, we do not have anything structured to measure what is happening with them.

PALLIATIVE CARE IN ARGENTINA

KSH: *Since you did some of your training in Canada, you have a good perspective on the ways in which palliative care is delivered in both countries. What differences or similarities do you see?*

MB: We have many differences, some of which are very important. I would say that there are organizational differences. I work in a public hospital, which is

---

*Readers can download this tool and others from the Edmonton Palliative Care Program's Clinical Assessment page at <www.palliative.org/pc_assess.html>, where tools are listed with hotlinks to each. The homepage for the Edmonton program is <www.palliative.org/>.

supported by the government and an external foundation: Federación Médica de la Provincia de Buenos Aires (FEMEBA). However, unlike Canada, Argentina does not have a national health insurance program. We have many payment systems, including some private social insurance, but more than half of the people who come to our hospital for palliative care have no insurance and are in a very delicate economic situation. They may not have money to pay for medications or sometimes even for transportation to the hospital. So, although our goals are probably the same as those of our colleagues in Canada, our possibilities for delivering care are sometimes limited by the financial problems of the family and the patient.

KSH: *How do you structure the care provided in your program?*

MB: We provide both inpatient and outpatient care. We have a small inpatient palliative care unit with six beds. In addition, we have two beds for outpatient palliative day care, where people come to the hospital for several hours a day, but then return home. We have an outpatient clinic, where we do consultations five days a week, Monday through Friday. We also deliver a little home care within the hospital's catchment area. The greater metropolitan area of Buenos Aires is huge—approximately 13 million people—with many hospitals. Each hospital has a catchment area, which designates the region from which people can come to that hospital. So we provide palliative care to people in our area of the city. We do not go to the homes of people who are living beyond our area. Other inpatient palliative care units are being planned elsewhere.

KSH: *Does health insurance pay for home care?*

MB: It all depends. Home care here in Argentina is not generalized yet, so this is a type of care that is not really offered to everyone. That's a very big problem.

KSH: *Do you have hospice care in Argentina?*

MB: No, we don't. We have been running this program since 1996, but we just put in the six-bed inpatient unit in the fall of 2000, and it is the only unit where you can specifically deliver inpatient palliative care in Argentina, a country of 30 million people.

KSH: *How many people does your program serve every year?*

MB: We have 250 new patients a year, and we have 300 to 350 patients continuously in treatment, because some patients enter one year and continue into the next year. We try to treat patients from the earliest stage possible, so oncology may refer patients still in active cancer treatment to us if they are having any physical or psychological symptoms. We try to do what we call "continuous care," providing both supportive and palliative care, not only at the very end of peoples' lives but, if possible, before they get to that.

KSH: *How is this kind of care presented to oncology patients?*

MB: The other physicians (oncologists or internal medicine physicians) that refer patients to us present palliative care as a discipline that helps people to feel better. Many of them put the accent on the care that we can deliver together with the oncologists and internists. So, if patients can have cancer treatment, they will have it, while we address their symptoms; and if they cannot benefit from cancer treatment, we address more of the problematic issues that may arise at the end of life.

KSH: *Do you work with the family physician?*

MB: Fewer than 5 percent of our patients have a family physician. This is a big problem, which means that when we assume the care of a patient sometimes we end up being a kind of family physician. That's not our idea, but often the patient cannot afford a family physician.

KSH: *How is the care that you provide paid for?*

MB: If a patient has insurance, the insurance provider pays the hospital. If people do not have insurance, this hospital pays for their care. If someone seen as an outpatient cannot afford to pay for consultations with our team, the assessment and treatment can be absolutely free of charge, but in many cases the patient must buy any medication that is needed after the consultation.

KSH: *How much free care do you provide, overall?*

MB: We provide free care to more than half of our patients. Even the patient who has prepaid health insurance may not be able to buy all the medications. Sometimes patients can afford a little bit and the rest we have to give them.

TREATING PAIN

Because most of our patients cannot afford the medication, we implemented a program with the hospital pharmacy, whereby the pharmacy prepares opioid medications, which are provided free for outpatients. This medication is not commercially prepared by a pharmaceutical company. Rather, it is compounded in the pharmacy, for example, by mixing morphine powder and water. In this way, we are able to make medication available to outpatients in a way that is more economical for the hospital and is free of charge to the patients.

KSH: *Is the financial burden on poor people such that they may not fill prescriptions for medicines or they may not take the medicine in the prescribed doses, but rather will try to take less to stretch it out?*

MB: Yes, that happens. In our institution, we are able to alleviate this a little bit because of the wonderful job that is done by our pharmacy. But if you go to some other hospitals, which also are providing palliative care on an outpatient basis, they do not have morphine to give to the patients, and although they prescribe it, afterward, all the possibilities that you just mentioned may happen.

KSH: *Can you be sure that your patients are taking the medicine?*

MB: Most of them, yes. The most important medicines are the opioids and their adjuvants (antiemetics, laxatives, etc.) and we can deliver these. Sometimes, when we use up the amount of medication that we have in the hospital, we have a hard time getting more, but I cannot complain. I'm happy about what we can get in this hospital. But our situation is not universal in Buenos Aires.

We did a survey two months ago, asking every pharmacy in the 33 hospitals of Buenos Aires about their medications. There are 23 hospitals that deliver oncology treatment. Of these 23 hospitals, two do not have morphine at all, and five do not have any oral formulation of morphine. Only five hospitals have some alternatives to morphine, let's say oxycodone, methadone, or hydromorphone. This is astonishing because you know that you have to have a strong opioid alternative to morphine in order to treat cancer patients and to deal with the side effects of morphine. As you can see, cancer pain treatment is not very well organized in the city of Buenos Aires.

KSH: *Why is pain medication so hard to come by?*

MB: The problem exists at different levels. If we analyze the cancer pain management recommendations of the World Health Organization, we could say that the barrier is insufficient health care provider education. There are many doctors that do not know how to prescribe strong opioids. We do not get thematic, systematic education on this topic in the universities. Until now, we have lacked a clear political policy and directives concerning the treatment of cancer pain from the Argentinean Minister of Health. Also, the cost of the different opioid medications is very high in Argentina. Morphine prices are higher here than in Canada or in the United States, because we have very high taxes on this kind of medication. So, with high prices, hospitals do not buy the medication.

PALLIATIVE CARE TEAMS

Last year the Argentinean Palliative Care Association did a survey and found only 25 supportive care or palliative care teams for all of Argentina, and most of these teams are in Buenos Aires. A team is defined as being made up of at least two different professionals; usually it is a physician and a nurse, or a physician and a psychologist, or a physician and a social worker. Many of these people are not paid for delivering this kind of care. They do it for free. They come to the hospital and volunteer from 10 to 20 hours per week in a palliative care program. The physicians work in different hospitals, and even if they do not have beds of their own, they provide palliative care to patients on the various hospital wards.

KSH: *How is your palliative care program staffed?*

MB: We have seven physicians, most of them working part-time, from 10 to 20 hours per week. Two physicians, including myself, work full-time, 40 hours per week. We have six or seven nurses working with us, one on each shift (there are three shifts on Monday through Friday and two shifts on Saturday and Sunday). In addition, a psychologist comes here 10 hours per week. The social worker is from the hospital, and she attends some of the team meetings and sees patients or the family when we refer them to her. A hospital chaplain works very closely with us. He comes to our team meeting weekly and sees patients two or three times per week.

KSH: *How long do people stay on your inpatient palliative care unit?*

MB: In general, not very long. We try to do a short period of hospitalization, between three and seven days. But, sometimes, we can have people here for two or three weeks. We also care for other people in the different wards at the other hospitals in the city throughout the year. The length of stay in the wards is sometimes longer, generally because of social reasons. By this I mean that people could be at home if someone could be there to take care of them, but home care may not be available and the family may have to work, so they are at the hospital because of social and economic reasons, not medical ones.

KSH: *Where do people die, mostly at home or in the hospital?*

MB: In Buenos Aires, they mainly die in the hospital. This is primarily because, even if you would like to be at home, if you cannot get medication or you cannot have the professionals supervise your treatment at home, people have to come to the hospital. This is not the same in other areas of Argentina. In the provinces and in smaller cities, such as San Nicolas, where Dr. Roberto Wenk has run a palliative care program for many years and where there is some delivery of home care, approximately 70 percent of people die at home. This is exactly the opposite of what happens in Buenos Aires. Here in Buenos Aires, approximately 30 percent of our patients die at home and 70 percent die in the hospital.

ADDITIONAL FACTORS AFFECTING QUALITY OF LIFE

KSH: *What other kinds of changes are needed in order to improve patients' quality of life?*

MB: First, improving access to palliative care. This means increasing the number of teams, the number of specific beds, and access to treatment and strong opioids, provided at a very low cost. Also, we need to develop the home care program further. In the general hospitals that do not have specific palliative care teams, we need policies that could allow people to be cared for in a more homey environment. We need policies that acknowledge that the family is part of the unit of care and that encourage involvement of the family in setting the goals of treatment.

In our inpatient palliative care program, patients have no visitation limits. However, in many hospitals in Argentina, there are still restrictions on visits and other kinds of things like that. For example, in many acute care hospitals, children are not allowed to go and see their parents. So, this is another area that needs improvement.

ETHICAL ISSUES

One more thing that is very important is to continue to work toward preventing what we would describe as "overtreatment"—delivering treatment that is clearly too aggressive or futile, including the admission of some patients to intensive care units who would not receive any benefit from that type of care.

KSH: *In Argentina, are there ethical and legal concerns about withdrawing or withholding treatment from dying patients that affect decision making near the end of life?*

MB: Yes. Mostly these concerns are raised because of presumed legal reasons or some ethical reasons, but the reasons are not discussed in a very deep way. Many physicians are afraid of legal consequences if they do not continue to treat a patient who is clearly at the end of his or her life.

MEASURING SUCCESS

KSH: *How do you measure your success in helping people to have good quality of life, even as they approach death?*

MB: We do not measure it in a structured way. We do a lot of different things, such as assess satisfaction with care from a certain period of time, but we do not do this on a regular basis. We have not accumulated direct evidence of satisfaction, but indirectly and anecdotally we know we are having an impact. For example, more than 90 percent of the families of our patients return to the hospital some days after the patient dies. They come to return all the patient's leftover medication, and they come to tell us how important the palliative care was. Generally, they tell us how important it was to feel that they were supported and what they think about the care.

BEREAVEMENT SUPPORT

KSH: *What kind of bereavement support do you give to family members after a patient dies?*

MB: We offer them the possibility of bereavement interviews with a psychologist in our group, and we also send a letter one year after the death of the person. But, I would say, fewer than 5 percent of people continue with bereavement support after the death of the patient. One goal of treatment for the patient and family before death is to prevent complicated grief. The fact that so few family members return for bereavement support on a regular basis may be related to the effectiveness of our interventions. However, we also know that families find it hard to return to the same place where their loved one died. So, if they need specific bereavement support after the death, we believe families prefer to go to some other place. The problem with providing bereavement support in the same center where the patient died is that it is often difficult for the family to come back and relive all the memories in the place where they had been with the patient while he or she was still alive. It is one of the limits of what we offer; even if they felt good about the support we provided, it is hard for the family to accept bereavement support here.

> *The problem with providing bereavement support in the same center where the patient died is that it is often difficult for the family to come back and relive all the memories in the place where they had been with the patient while he or she was still alive.*

KSH: *Are there community-based bereavement resources where people can obtain support?*

MB: There are independent bereavement support groups now available, but they are not well known, even though some of them have been going on for more than five years. They are very good and very professional.

THE EDMONTON PROGRAM AS A MODEL FOR THE BUENOS AIRES PALLIATIVE CARE EFFORT

KSH: *As someone who is familiar with the Edmonton program, can you tell us how that model may have influenced the way you are providing palliative care in Buenos Aires?*

MB: It continues to be our inspiration in terms of organization and how they view palliative care, for example, in terms of providing care, doing research, and being very critical of their own results in order to try to improve different things.

We have implemented many of their assessment tools, not only the ESAS, but also another one called the Edmonton Comfort Assessment Form, which we use during the last days of life, when the patient can no longer communicate or provide any more information. We also use the Edmonton Functional Assessment Tool, and many of the tools that they have.[†] These tools have focused our assessments and have enabled us to analyze what we do on a regular basis.

KSH: *Is there anything about the Edmonton model that does not work as well in your own environment?*

MB: No, I would not say that. However, there may be cultural differences, for example, in relation to communication. In Argentina, people have more difficulty talking about their diagnosis of cancer and a poor prognosis, even though we are seeing a huge change in public attitudes about this in recent years. But in Canada, when one has a diagnosis of cancer, it is stated very clearly. Often there is a discussion with the patient and family about prognosis from the very beginning, in a very open way. Here, this probably takes a longer period of time to accomplish. In this hospital, more than 70 percent of our patients know their diagnosis at the first interview with us. This is a major change from the way it happened 10 years ago in Argentina. But you still have to be very careful in providing information about diagnosis and prognosis, to allow people time to cope with that and to accommodate the psychological and the cultural issues.

KSH: *Do patients prefer that you tell a member of the family rather than themselves?*

MB: Sometimes. Maybe 10 years ago, I would have answered, yes, 100 percent. Now we ask the patient, "Would you like to discuss all the test results with us and what we think about the illness, or would you prefer us to speak with your family?" Sometimes the family asks the physician to protect the patient and not tell the patient what is happening. In this situation, the team tries to spend some time obtaining the family's confidence, to show that we are respecting their ways of communicating, but also showing what we believe would be important for the patient to know. We try not to simply follow what the family orders us to do, but we would not want to directly oppose them at the outset by saying, "Well, we have another point of view, and we are going to tell the patient what we think he or she must know." So we usually take our time and go more slowly in these circumstances. Thus, the disclosure of the diagnosis and prognosis to the patient may take one or two weeks, which may be slower than at other places.

[†]See the Clinical Asseement page at <www.palliative.org/pc_assess.html> to read about and download these tools.

IMPROVING THE PALLIATIVE CARE PROGRAM

KSH: *How are you continuing to try to improve your program?*

MB: We are trying to get more financial support, both from the government and from private sources. We currently have substantial support from FEMEBA. It is thanks to FEMEBA that our program exists, really. FEMEBA is a foundation run by a federation of physicians who work in the province of Buenos Aires. These physicians decided to create a program to teach health care professionals in a variety of domains, including palliative care. They have a very important program for palliative care training called Programa Argentino de Medicina Paliativa, which included the creation of our palliative care unit at the Tornú Hospital as a clinical practice training center for health care professionals. Our unit was born through their support. In addition, government funding also supports our program because we are based in a public hospital. We also try to raise funds for items that the unit needs through the help of volunteers.

RESEARCH EFFORTS

Another important goal is raising funds for research. Sometimes it is not easy, but we know we cannot run an effective palliative care unit without being critical about the knowledge that we have, so we would like to obtain new data or new solutions by doing research. For example, we are doing some multicenter clinical research with Dr. Eduardo Bruera.[‡] We are doing some descriptive research using all the assessment we do on a regular basis, such as analyzing the symptoms that patients have, the consumption of different opioids, where and how people die, where they spend the last 24 hours of life, how frequently we have to use sedation for the last 24 hours, and so forth.

KSH: *Are you doing any research to learn more about the spiritual or psychological needs of patients or some of the other aspects of quality of life?*

MB: We are doing a pilot study looking at suffering and discomfort at the end of life, when the patient cannot talk. We are comparing the impression that the family had about the patient's suffering in the last days of life with the impression of suffering that the physician and the nurse who cared for the patient had. We don't yet have all the data, but based on preliminary findings, we have an idea about the family's impressions. It's really interesting, yet not surprising, that the family members still perceive a huge amount of suffering, even if they have had support and the patient had generally good symptom control, which may be related sometimes simply to the fact that the patient is dying.

[‡]Dr. Eduardo Bruera founded the Edmonton Palliative Care Program in Canada and is now based at Anderson Cancer Center at the University of Texas in Houston.

They usually say, "Well, I think she's suffering a lot," and when we ask why, the reason they give is "because she's dying." So there is probably a cultural aspect to their perceptions, a belief that if you are dying, you are suffering. In addition, although we did not ask family members about their own suffering, I think it may be one of the keys to the problem, because in describing a high amount of suffering of the patient, they may be describing their own suffering. In general, we are finding that the physicians think that patients are suffering less than the families think they are, which is not a surprise.

> *. . . although we did not ask family members about their own suffering, I think it may be one of the keys to the problem, because in describing a high amount of suffering of the patient, they may be describing their own suffering.*

KSH: *Do you try to address suffering in patients?*

MB: We try, a lot, with mixed results. Sometimes we think some situations are going well, and at other times we have the impression that, even if we put forth a lot of effort, the situation is not what we would like it to be. In some situations, we can feel a little frustrated and we must recognize the limits of the care provided. Sometimes there is a history of family and psychological problems that makes it very difficult for patients at the end of life.

STANDARDS OF PALLIATIVE CARE

KSH: *What is happening in Argentina right now to bring about improvements in palliative care?*

MB: All the people working in palliative care in Argentina have done a lot of work with the government, and, as a result, we began seeing change in the year 2000. The Minister of Health is going to create a set of standards for the function and organization of palliative care services. If these standards are accepted, this could mean that palliative care services would become generalized, and clinicians and programs providing palliative care would know what benchmarks they are supposed to be reaching.

The standards apply to three levels of palliative care. On the primary care level, the standards recommend that any professional who is working with a patient in an advanced stage of disease, and who can show that he is well-trained and experienced in providing palliative care, be paid for that kind of care and work in what we call a functional team. This means that he or she would work in a team created just for that patient, in liaison with different professionals. The second and third levels of care refer to the composition of palliative care teams. On the second level, the standards recommend that there be at least three specialties involved in patient care, for example, a nurse, physician, and psychologist or a nurse, physician, and social worker. The third level of care is the most intensive, defined by a complete team of caregivers and an inpatient palliative care unit.

PLANS FOR AN OBLIGATORY PROGRAM IN PALLIATIVE CARE

These new standards of palliative care, created with various medical and other health professional associations, led to the inclusion of palliative care in the obligatory medical program (PMO: Programa Medico Obligatorio) or the baseline level of medical assistance that all systems that provide care must meet. That is to say, palliative care would become a required program or service in health care institutions. This new requirement is going to be implemented soon. If this happens, it will be a big step forward. It would make the provision of palliative care obligatory at all levels of health care, including both private and public practice, and so insurance companies would be required to pay for it. This mandate would come from the Ministry of Health and would affect all Argentinean health care institutions, professional associations, and payers.

This new inclusion of palliative care in the PMO was accepted by all the health care professional associations, but the College of Pharmacies just made an amendment, putting in some details concerning their own practice. Initially, palliative care centers were defined in relation to the four basic disciplines working in palliative care: medicine, nursing, social work, and psychology. The pharmacists were considered as playing a supportive role in the program. The College of Pharmacies, however, has insisted that they are not a support, but are an integral and essential component—one of the basic disciplines that needs to be involved. I think this amendment is good; they are very necessary.

The standards were approved, and we have put forth this pharmacy amendment, which could be accepted soon. It is unclear whether the government will support these palliative care initiatives with funding, but it seems that they would be obliged to do so. I think we are overcoming a very difficult situation and this initiative will help in creating palliative care teams and putting money into palliative care.

KSH: *What encouraged the Ministry of Health to support the standards and an obligatory palliative care initiative?*

MB: The whole palliative care movement, the years of conferences and statements of people working in the different medical societies, has paved the way for this initiative. The Minister of Health finally said, "Well, yes, this is a problem. We have to think about it and improve what we are doing." They created a commission to advise the minister of health on all the scientific issues, which included representatives from different professional societies: nurses, physicians, social workers, psychologists, the Argentine Medical Association, Asociación Argentina de Medicina y Cuidados Paliativos, and so forth. This commission created the standards for palliative care after one year of work.

KSH: *In summary, what do you think would help to improve patients' quality of life near the end of life?*

MB: There are many things. First, I would say that we have to recognize the differences among patients and try to adapt treatment to the specific needs of each patient. To provide personalized care, we must continue to remember and respect patients' autonomy. We must do this, because in Argentina many practitioners still have a paternalistic attitude toward patients. In addition, we really need more education in palliative care for health care providers, and we have to do more to inform the public about palliative care, because strong public support would make it much easier to implement palliative care programs. All this would enable new palliative care programs to develop and deliver a high quality of care.

Health Policy and Education: Tools for Promoting Quality of Life

An Interview with VITTORIO VENTAFRIDDA, MD, PhD, MCRP

Milan, Italy

Professor Vittorio Ventafridda, MD, PhD, MCRP of Milan, Italy, trained in anesthesiology and worked for some time as a cancer pain specialist before making palliative care his central interest. Founder of the Italian palliative care movement, one of the authors of the WHO analgesic ladder, one of the founders of the International Association for the Study of Pain (IASP) and of the European Association for Palliative Care (EAPC), Professor Ventafridda has most recently focused on shaping national and international policies regarding palliative care. In this interview with Anna L. Romer, EdD, he speaks about the genesis of his interest in palliative care, and how policy and education can improve care of the dying, which includes most centrally the relief of suffering and cultivating an interest in the quality of patients' lives at the end of life.

Anna L. Romer: *Could you begin by describing how you became interested in palliative care?*

Vittorio Ventafridda: In the early 1970s I was working at the Istituto Nazionale Tumori, the largest cancer institution in Italy, where as an anesthesiologist I was devoted to performing pain blocks and other invasive procedures. After some years, I realized that treating pain with these modalities was different from treating the suffering of the whole person who was dying. I began to think that during my many years in this cancer institution we had only scratched the surface of the problem, that is, the problem of facing "total pain," which is quite different from applying a technical modality. There are still many pain experts who are far from understanding this problem of suffering. This realization changed my attitude and behavior completely.

I began working with dying patients, especially in their homes, with a home care service funded by the Floriani Foundation,* which allowed me to integrate

---

*The Floriani Foundation has sponsored nurses and doctors to create several palliative care groups scattered across Italy. The foundation also runs a school of palliative medicine and a bioethics committee and hosts a library and database of references.

my work at the hospital. As a result of this new work, I had the opportunity to discover a new world, and I became more aware of the patients' and families' experience of dying. In 1988, after a previous congress in Venice on cancer pain in the late 1970s, I held another one in Milan regarding end-of-life care, focusing on pain and symptom control, psychosocial issues, and the dying process. These congresses revealed a great interest, which led to the founding of the European Association for Palliative Care (EAPC) and then the Italian Association of Palliative Care [Associazione Italiana di cure palliative].

ALR: *It sounds as though you are defining pain more broadly than physical symptom management. Would it be fair to say that your central interest is in relieving suffering?*

VV: My understanding of pain has broadened. I see it differently from how I did when I founded the IASP. At the beginning, I found that oncologists, pain experts, and the medical establishment did not understand what I was doing. Some pain experts were against palliative care, because they thought it was not scientific enough and not doctor's work. In my efforts to convert others to the cause of palliative care, I met with great difficulty. Many of the barriers that I encountered, including the lack of financial resources allocated for palliative care, still exist in Europe.

ALR: *What inspired this wider understanding of pain?*

VV: First of all, following patients changed my understanding. I was very deeply involved in pain treatment in the 1970s; I was doing a lot of new studies of surgical and anesthesiological procedures. Patients were kissing my hands because their pain was fully relieved—and then they went home, the pain returned, and they became desperate because they thought that they were dying. When I was nearby and could observe the process of dying in these patients—the desperation, loneliness, and all the needs that we had ignored completely—I was quite shocked. I wanted to understand each patient's end-of-life experience. I am still quite interested in the last week, the last days, the last hours of life.

COMPONENTS OF QUALITY OF LIFE IN PALLIATIVE CARE

ALR: *As you think about quality of life in palliative care, in the Italian context, what do you think are the most important features of quality of life?*

VV: Quality of life is a broad term often used in politics, but it also refers to the subjective wishes of patients, which must be recognized. One first needs to address unpleasant physical perceptions. Pain and other symptoms are what you see right away. We do not yet offer adequate pain relief. Pain and symptoms reported by the patient are important because often they are the tip of the iceberg of suffering. Then you find lots of social and emotional problems, which should also be relieved. Unfortunately, in Italy, we often find that pain is considered to be a sign of a pathology that should be treated, but both scientifically and clinically, it is not regarded as very important. We do not give enough attention to pain management.

Right now, the Italian Ministry of Health has charged me with organizing a pain-free hospital. I will try even though I know it will be a difficult task. Our goal is to make assessing pain a fifth vital sign, similar to the U.S. effort.[†] This is a campaign to educate all the care providers in the hospital. Pain experts need to convey to nurses and doctors how to evaluate pain at least three times a day and then to track these assessments in the medical charts so that doctors will be aware of patients' pain and thus treat it more appropriately.

POLICY WORK

I found that we can make breakthroughs, not only through changing practice, but also by promoting changes in health policy. To this end, you have to involve politicians—people who have power in health policy. In order to do that, I worked closely with the European Community (EC) in Brussels and with the Council of Europe in Strasbourg.

ALR: *What was your main message to these policy makers?*

VV: I was striving to make clear the importance of cancer pain relief and palliative care to leaders involved in "Europe Against Cancer," a public health effort promoted by the European Community.[‡] I am also involved in another Ministry of Health project, which is working toward the full recognition of palliative care specialists and palliative medicine as a specialty.

Two years ago we reached the first step when the Italian government recognized the need for hospices in every single region of the country. But they did not provide for the staffing of these hospices. So, with my collaborators, I am trying to fill this gap. Currently, my work is for the most part only on this policy level, and I am no longer directly involved in patient care.

My main goal is to modify the focus of Italian official health policy to include palliative care. This is really difficult. I still believe that doctors are one of the main barriers to improving pain management and palliative care. I think the doctors sometimes forget that a simple touch and time spent listening can be as important as a shot of morphine. We need to change attitudes if we want to win the battle against suffering.

[†]The American Pain Society has created the phrase "Pain: The Fifth Vital Sign" to elevate awareness of pain treatment among health care professionals. For more information, see the American Pain Society website at <www.ampainsoc.org> and enter "fifth vital sign" in the search tool.

[‡]Information about the Europe Against Cancer program is available on the European Association for Palliative Care website at <www.eapcnet.org>.

ALR: *Since you are naming doctors as the primary barriers to addressing pain adequately, what is the key message you have for them?*

VV: I want doctors to understand that life has limits. These limits should be recognized as part of life. We have to attend to quality of life and human dignity at the end of life. One of the first things doctors need to recognize is that when we cannot cure, we must care as much as possible. We must offer all the resources available to our patients as human beings until the end of the life. When we die, the dying process often entails suffering, as we have seen in the results of the SUPPORT study.[1] We have read many other reports (some conducted in Italy) confirming how poorly we care for patients at the end of life. There is tremendous suffering, and especially in the society we live in now, where the denial of death, the rush for profit, and a lack of interest in terminally ill patients all contribute to this problem. We can do a lot to be close to the dying person, not only medically, but also in a holistic way. Care of dying persons requires a team approach as well as making sure that the people can stay at home or at least have a comfortable environment.

> *There is tremendous suffering, and especially in the society we live in now, where the denial of death, the rush for profit, and a lack of interest in terminally ill patients all contribute to this problem. We can do a lot to be close to the dying person, not only medically, but also in a holistic way.*

ALR: *Do you think that physicians are really the most suited to be providing this human contact?*

VV: No, I think the nurses are primary, as well as family. The nurse plays the most important role in providing palliative care. However, nurses need to be educated and so do families. I think of the doctor as a manager who knows a great deal about the problems and can work with the team. Certainly, the doctor's word has more charismatic power, but the entire team is important.

ALR: *Can you describe the attitude you would like doctors to have toward end-of-life care?*

VV: I believe it is important to have an attitude of interest. Doctors must be interested in caring for terminally ill patients. Some doctors may not be interested in doing this work themselves, but I would like them to recognize that care for the dying is very important work.

If you go into any pediatric unit, you see how nurseries are kept. You see how much interest there is in the beginning of life, interest not only in the well-being of babies, but also scientific interest. In contrast, attention is not focused on what happens in the last hours of life. A patient is losing consciousness, and losing the capacity to communicate before losing consciousness. We must have an interest in the few hours before dying. There is so much we have to study in order to make the exit from life better than it is now.

NEED FOR EDUCATION

We need education for medical students so that doctors come out of medical school with knowledge of care of the dying. We also need to educate children in the schools about death. What is death? How does death occur? How do we cope with death? We need to change attitudes about dying and we need to start from the beginning.

This is difficult, because we live in a society where we have values that are totally different. We value efficiency, money, reaching the top of a profession. When we focus on these things, it is easy to deny death completely.

ALR: *How do physicians speak about death with patients in this context?*

VV: Well, we have a great problem. In Italy, the family does not allow the doctor to say anything to the patient except that cure is possible. Families and doctors often give the patient any kind of possible treatment, which can lead to overtreatment. I have tried to convince my colleagues that such an approach increases patients' suffering. I think disclosure should be done gradually, because you have to have established some intimacy with the patient before telling this kind of news. This can be time-consuming. Today, doctors don't have time—they say, "You don't have anything, you will be cured, you will come out in a few days, few weeks, few months." But they don't take care to say, "You are dying." The patient will realize that he or she is dying, in my opinion, in a matter of a few weeks. Before death, the great majority of patients already know that they are dying.

> *. . . we have a great problem. In Italy, the family does not allow the doctor to say anything to the patient except that cure is possible.*

AREAS FOR IMPROVEMENT

So, disclosure is one of the areas in which we need to work. If physicians have been clear about the diagnosis, the path is easier. We can reach an intimacy with patients, and we can communicate a great deal during this last phase of life. Patients' quality of life will improve when communication is clear. But this question of disclosure is very difficult. I think we need to solve the problem of educating families in order to help these patients. Without education, most of these patients are often receiving futile treatment and dying in the intensive care unit.

ALR: *Do you think that patients and their families want death to occur in the intensive care unit?*

VV: A patient will do anything possible to save his or her life, not all patients, but the majority. Even if a patient doesn't want a certain treatment, the family may encourage the patient to accept a very difficult procedure with the hope of saving the patient's life. In my experience, many times the patients' relatives are unwittingly responsible for the suffering of the patient.

ALR: *It sounds as though disclosure and family expectations are, perhaps, two of the biggest barriers to quality of life in your setting.*

VV: Yes, that's right, as well as patients' expectations.

ALR: *Where do you feel that the most pressing need for progress and/or improvement is, given that scenario?*

VV: First, we need to correct the aspect of disclosure, not in a simple way, but by taking time to understand patients and tell them what they can hear. Second, we need people to understand that palliative care is important for the relief of suffering. I would like to hear people say, "If I am in that situation in my life, I would prefer palliative care." We need to change attitudes. I have already seen some changes since the late 1970s when I started this work. This work, to be continued by the next generation, is a slow and ongoing process.

ALR: *If you think of teaching medical students, i.e., the next generation of doctors, what would be the number one lesson about providing palliative care and enhancing patient and family quality of life?*

VV: Ethics of end-of-life care. What I mean is, teach students how to give correct treatment—treatment that is not futile. Teach students the correct way to speak with the patients; how to offer a great environment to patients, at home, in a hospice, or in the hospital; and how to work as a team in order to help patients at the end of life. There are many items in the curriculum of palliative care that should be taught to doctors in the last years of medical school.

> *. . . we must start from the beginning if we want to change attitudes. People should know that everyone goes through this moment of life. I believe that in this final moment, we should find no isolation.*

But also—and this is a dream—we need to start to teach about death and dying in grammar school, and not wait until college, because as I say, we must start from the beginning if we want to change attitudes. People should know that everyone goes through this moment of life. I believe that in this final moment, we should find no isolation. My dream is that we each will have someone who will take care of us and that there will be no possibility of futile surgical treatment or futile intensive care treatment at the end of life.

REFERENCE

1. SUPPORT Principal Investigators. The study to understand prognoses and preferences for outcomes and risks of treatments (SUPPORT): A controlled trial to improve care for seriously ill hospitalized patients. *Journal of the American Medical Association.* 1995;274:1591–1597.

Selected Bibliography

Part Six

Selected references by contributors to this part:

Aaronson NK, Ahmedzai S, Bergman B, Bullinger M, Cull A, Duez NJ, Filiberti A, Flechtner H, Fleishman SB, de Haes CJM, Kaasa S, Klee M, Osoba D, Razavi D, Rofe PB, Schraub S, Sneeuw K, Sullivan M, Takeda F, for the EORTC Study Group on Quality of Life. The European Organization for Research and Treatment of Cancer QLQ-C30: A quality-of-life instrument for use in international clinical trails in oncology. *Journal of the National Cancer Institute.* 1993;85:365-376.

Bertolino M, Tatangelo M. Servicios especializados en Cuidados Paliativos. Una necesidad? *Nuevas tendencias en Oncología.* 1998;7(3):285-286.

Bertolino M, Vinant P, Lassaunière JM. Les soins palliatifs chez les patients atteints de cancer digestif avancé. *Gastro Enterologie Pratique.* 1993;45:4-6.

Brenneis C. The interaction between family physicians and palliative care consultants in the delivery of palliative care: Clinical and educational issues. *Journal of Palliative Care.* 1998;14(3):58-61.

Bruera E, Neumann C, Brenneis C, Quan H. Frequency of symptom distress and poor prognostic indicators in palliative cancer patients admitted to a tertiary palliative care unit, hospices, and acute care hospitals. *Journal of Palliative Care.* 2000;16(3):16-21.

Bruera E, Neumann CM, Gagnon B, Brenneis C, Quan H, Hanson J. The impact of a regional palliative care program on the cost of palliative care delivery. *Journal of Palliative Medicine.* 2000;3(2):181-186.

Bruera E, Neumann CM, Gagnon B, Brenneis C, Kneisler P, Selmser P, Hanson J. Edmonton Regional Palliative Care Program: Impact on patterns of terminal cancer care. *Canadian Medical Association Journal.* 1999;161(3):290-293.

Bruera E, Moyano J, Siefert L, Fainsinger RL, Hanson J, Suarez-Almazor M. The frequency of alcoholism among patients with pain due to terminal cancer. *Journal of Pain and Symptom Management.* 1995;10:599-603.

Bruera E, Suarez-Almazor M, Velasco A, Bertolino M, MacDonald S, Hanson J. The assessment of constipation in terminal cancer patients admitted to a palliative care unit: A retrospective review. *Journal of Pain and Symptom Management.* 1994;9:515-519.

Fainsinger RL. Palliative care in Edmonton. *Supportive Care in Cancer.* 1995;3(2):91-92.

Fainsinger RL, Bruera E, MacMillan K. Innovative palliative care in Edmonton. *Canadian Family Physician.* 1997;43:1983-1991.

Fainsinger RL, Miller MJ, Bruera E, Hanson J, MacEachern T. Symptom control during the last week of life on a palliative care unit. *Journal of Palliative Care.* 1991;7:5-11.

Jørdhoy MS, Fayers P, Saltnes T, Ahlner-Elmqvist M, Jannert M, Kaasa S. A palliative-care intervention and death at home: A cluster randomised trial. *Lancet.* 2000;356:888-893.

Kaasa S, Malt U, Hagen S, Wist E, Moum T, Kvikstad A. Psychological distress in patients with advanced cancer. *Radiotherapy and Oncology.* 1993;27:193–197.

Lassaunière JM, Bertolino M. Soins palliatifs: Aspects généraux, traitement de la douleur de Métastases osseuses, aspects psychologiques. In *Métastases Osseuses,* D Bontoux, M Alcalay (eds.). Poitiers, France: Expansion Scientifique Française, 1997, 146–157.

Lassaunière JM, Hunnault M, Vespieren P, Moh-Klaren J, Bertolino M, Zittoun R, Colombat P. Platelet transfusions in advanced hematological malignancies: A position paper. *Journal of Palliative Care.* 1996;12(1):38–41.

Lawlor PG, Fainsinger RL, Bruera ED. Delirium at the end of life: Critical issues in clinical practice and research. *Journal of the American Medical Association.* 2000;284:2427–2429.

Louie K, Bertolino M, Fainsinger R. Management of intractable cough. *Journal of Palliative Care.* 1992; 8:4:46–48.

Wenk R, Bertolino M, Pusseto J. Direct medical costs of an Argentinean Domiciliary Palliative Care Model [letter]. *Journal of Pain and Symptom Management.* 2000;20(3):162–165.

Other references related to the Edmonton Palliative Care Program:

Bruera E, Kuehn N, Miller MJ, Selmser P, MacMillan K. The Edmonton symptom assessment system (ESAS): A simple method for the assessment of palliative care patients. *Journal of Palliative Care.* 1991;7:6–9.

Bruera E, MacMillan K, Hanson J, MacDonald RJ. The Edmonton staging system for cancer pain. Preliminary report. *Pain.* 1989;37:203–209.

Other selected references:

Axelsson B, Sjoden PO. Assessment of quality of life in palliative care—Psychometric properties of a short questionnaire. *Acta Oncologica.* 1999;38(2):229–237.

Axelsson B, Sjoden PO. Quality of life of cancer patients and their spouses in palliative home care. *Palliative Medicine.* 1998;12(1):29–39.

Bowling A. *Measuring Health: A Review of Quality of Life Measurement Scales,* 2d ed. Buckingham, England: Open University Press, 1997.

Bowling A. *Measuring Disease: A Review of Disease-Specific Quality of Life Measurement Scales.* Buckingham, England: Open University Press, 1995.

Boyd KJ. The role of specialist home care teams: Views of general practitioners in South London. *Palliative Medicine.* 1995;9:138–144.

Bruera E, Miller MJ, McCallion J, MacMillan K, Krefting L, Hanson J. Cognitive failure (CF) in patients with terminal cancer: A prospective study. *Journal of Pain and Symptom Management.* 1992;7:192–195.

Bruley DK. Beyond reliability and validity: Analysis of selected quality-of-life instruments for use in palliative care. *Journal of Palliative Medicine.* 1999;2(3):299–309.

Byock I. Hospice and palliative care: A parting of the ways or a path to the future? *Journal of Palliative Medicine.* 1998;1(2):165-176.

Byock IR, Merriman MP. Measuring quality of life for patients with terminal illness: The Missoula-VITAS quality of life index. *Palliative Medicine.* 1998;12(4): 231-244.

Campbell SM, Roland MO, Buetow SA. Defining quality of care. *Social Science and Medicine.* 2000;51:1611-1625.

De Graef A. *Quality of Life in Head and Neck Cancer.* Utrecht: University Medical Center, 1999.

Devery K, Lennie I, Cooney N. Health outcomes for people who use palliative care services. *Journal of Palliative Care.* 1999;14(2):5-12.

Dudgeon DJ, Harlos M, Clinch JJ. The Edmonton symptom assessment scale (ESAS) as an audit tool. *Journal of Palliative Care.* 1999;15(3):14-19.

Dudgeon DJ, Kristjanson L. Home vs. hospital death: Assessment of preferences and clinical challenges. *Canadian Medical Association Journal.* 1995;152:337-339.

Gomas J. Palliative care at home: A reality or "mission impossible"? *Palliative Medicine.* 1993;7:45-59.

Hickey AM, Bury G, O'Boyle CA, Bradley F, O'Kelly FD, Shannon W. A new short form individual quality of life measure (SEIQoL-DW): Application in a cohort of individuals with HIV/AIDS. *British Medical Journal.* 1996;313:29-33.

Kanji T, Hanson J, Bruera E. Community liaison for terminally ill patients discharged from a cancer center. *Supportive Care in Cancer.* 1996;4(3):240.

King CR, Hinds PS. *Quality of Life: From Nursing and Patient Perspectives.* Boston: Jones and Bartlett Publishers, 2000.

Koch T. Life quality vs. the "quality of life": Assumptions underlying prospective quality of life instruments in health care planning. *Social Science and Medicine.* 51:419-427.

Manfredi PL, Morrison RS, Morris J, Goldhirsch SL, Carter JM, Meier DE. Palliative care consultations: How do they impact the care of hospitalized patients? *Journal of Pain and Symptom Management.* 2000;20:166-173.

McMillan SC, Weitzner M. How problematic are various aspects of quality of life in patients with cancer at the end of life? *Oncology Nursing Forum.* 2000;27(5):817-823.

McMillan SC, Weitzner M. Quality of life in cancer patients: Use of a revised Hospice Index. *Cancer Practice.* 1998;6(5):282-288.

McWhinney IR, Bass MJ, Orr V. Factors associated with location of death (home or hospital) of patients referred to a palliative care team. *Canadian Medical Association Journal.* 1995;152:361-367.

McWhinney IR, Stewart MA. Home care of dying patients. Family physicians' experience with a palliative care support team. *Canadian Family Physician.* 1994;40:240-246.

Nekolaichuk CL, Bruera E, Spachynski K, MacEachern T, Hanson J, Maguire TO. A comparison of patient and proxy symptom assessments in advanced cancer patients. *Palliative Medicine.* 1999;13:311-323.

Nekolaichuk CL, Maguire TO, Suarez-Almazor M, Rogers WT, Bruera E. Assessing the reliability of patient, nurse, and family caregiver symptom ratings in hospitalized advanced cancer patients. *Journal of Clinical Oncology*. 1999;17(11): 3621–3630.

O'Boyle CA, Waldron D. Quality of life issues in palliative medicine. *Journal of Neurology*. 1997;244 [Suppl 4]:S18–S25.

Philip J, Smith WB, Craft P, Lickiss N. Concurrent validity of the modified Edmonton symptom assessment system with the Rotterdam symptom checklist and the brief pain inventory. *Supportive Care in Cancer*. 1998;6:539–541.

Portenoy RK, Thaler HT, Kornblith AB, Lepore JM, Friedlander-Klar H, Coyle N, et al. Symptom prevalence, characteristics and distress in a cancer population. *Quality of Life Research*. 1994;183–189.

Salander P, Bergenheim AT, Henriksson R. How was life after treatment of a malignant brain tumor? *Social Science and Medicine*. 2000;51:589–598.

Singer PA, Martin DK, Kelner M. Quality end-of-life care: Patients' perspectives. *Journal of the American Medical Association*. 1999;281(2):163–168.

Somogyi-Zalud E, Zhong Z, Lynn J, Hamel MB. Elderly persons' last six months of life: Findings from the Hospitalized Elderly Longitudinal Project. *Journal of the American Geriatrics Society*. 2000;48[Suppl 5]:S131–S139.

Stewart AL, Teno J, Patrick DL, Lynn J. The concept of quality of life of dying persons in the context of health care. *Journal of Pain and Symptom Management*. 1999;17:93–108.

Tierney RM, Horton SM, Hannan TJ, Tierney WM. Relationships between symptom relief, quality of life, and satisfaction with hospice care. *Palliative Medicine*. 1998;12(5):333–344.

Townsend J, Frank A, Fermont D, Dyer S, Karra O, Walgrove A, et al. Terminal cancer care and patients' preference for place of death: A prospective study. *British Medical Journal*. 1990;301:415–417.

Wood ML, McWilliam CL. Cancer in remission: Challenge in collaboration for family physicians and oncologists. *Canadian Family Physician*. 1996;42:899–910.

Zweibel NR. Measuring quality of life near the end of life. *Journal of the American Medical Association*. 1988;260(6):839–840.

Part Seven

Appendices

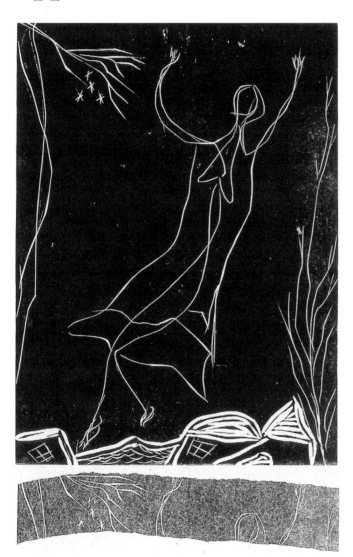

"Set Adrift"
©1992 Eleanor Rubin (woodcut).

Appendix A: Circle of Life Award

Celebrating Innovation in End-of-Life Care

The Circle of Life Award

On July 31, 2001, the American Hospital Association (AHA) recognized the efforts of nine programs in end-of-life care and announced three winners of its Circle of Life Award: Celebrating Innovation in End-of-Life Care at the AHA Health Forum Summit in San Diego, California. The Circle of Life Award focuses on recognizing and honoring innovative programs that improve the care that people receive near the end of life. The awards, supported by a grant from The Robert Wood Johnson Foundation, are sponsored by the AHA, the American Medical Association, the National Hospice and Palliative Care Organization, and the American Association of Homes and Services for the Aging.

The three 2001 award winning programs each received $25,000 to further their efforts to change the way that Americans view and experience care at the end of life. They are:

- Beth Israel's Department of Pain Medicine and Palliative Care (New York, New York)
- Palliative CareCenter and Hospice of the North Shore (Evanston, Illinois)
- St. Joseph's Manor (Trumbull, Connecticut)

Six other programs were recognized with a citation of honor. These are Balm of Gilead, Dana–Farber Cancer Institute, Hospice & Home Care of Juneau, Hospice of Napa Valley, MidPeninsula Pathways Hospice Foundation, and the VA Hospice Care Center at Palo Alto Veterans Affairs Health Care System.

Innovations in End-of-Life Care <www.edc.org/lastacts/> features the efforts of these award-winning programs in a series of thematic issues. This edited volume of *Innovations in End-of-Life Care* features two Circle of Life award winners from 2000 and 2001, respectively. The first, Franciscan Health System West, is featured in Part One and Beth Israel's Department of Pain Medicine and Palliative Care appears in Part Two.

For information on future Circle of Life Awards, visit the AHA website at <www.hospitalconnect.com/aha/awards-events/circle-of-life/index.html>. To read about the 2002 award winners, visit *Innovations in End-of-Life Care* online, Vol. 4, No. 4, 2002 at <www.edc.org/lastacts/>.

Appendix B: Targeted Resources and Tools

Part One: Building Bridges for Better Continuity of Care

A. ORIGINAL TOOLS FROM CONTRIBUTORS

1. Opening a Clinic Checklist

Copyright © 2000 by Franciscan Health Systems West. Reprinted with permission.

This tool is excerpted from Improving Care through the End of Life Training Manual authored by featured innovator Georganne Trandum. For further information about the training manual and tools to start an Improving Care through the End of Life program in your own clinic, please contact Georganne Trandum at georgannetrandum@chiwest.com.

Opening a Clinic Checklist

1. CLINIC IDENTIFICATION
   Clinic self-referral ☐
   Expansion plan ☐
   Identified specialty clinics _____ —

2. SITE READINESS
   Leadership commitment ☐
   Number of physicians —
   Number of eligible patients (include Medicare patients) —
   Financial commitment _____ ☐
   Space and equipment available ☐
   Capability of generating office visit lists on five diagnoses ☐
      (*Heart, Cancer, Lung, CVA, Dementia*) ☐
   Medical records commitment ☐
   Computer, software, modem, printer ☐

3. INITIAL PRESENTATION & PLANNING MEETINGS
   Improving Care through the End of Life   Mimi Pattison, MD
      Medical Director
   Improving Care through the End of   Georganne Trandum, RN, OCN
      Life Director
   Clinic Medical Director _____
   Clinic Administrator _____
   Physician Champion _____
   Initial presentation (__/__/__)
   Subsequent meetings   (__/__/__), (__/__/__), (__/__/__)

4. SECURE STAFFING
    Clinic Care Coordinator/Sponsor   _____
    Chaplain/Sponsor   _____
    Volunteer Coordinator/Sponsor   _____
    Volunteers (initial base of four)   (1) _____
        (2) _____
        (3) _____
        (4) _____

5. EDUCATION (Physicians, Nurses, PAs, ARNPs)

OUTCOME: 80% of providers will complete 5 hours of education 8 weeks from clinic startup

    1-hour introduction with "Supportive Care of the Dying" video ☐
    4 hours education (*one 4-hour segment or two 2-hour segments*) ☐
    Video: "Pain & Symptom Management & Hospice Referrals" ☐
    Booklets (*Hospice Teaching Tool*) ☐
    Pain and Symptom Management File ☐
    "Giving Bad News" ☐
    Advance Care Planning—How to complete forms ☐
    Education for Physicians on End of life Care (EPEC) curriculum ☐
    Resources ☐

6. EDUCATION/TRAINING (Clinical Care Coordinator)

    Computer Training   .... ☐
    • Word
    • Excel
    • PowerPoint
    • Access
    Referral Process   .... ☐
    • Criteria
    • How to generate lists
    Medical Records   .... ☐
    • Retrieval of charts
    • System to identify patients
    • Authorization to document end-of-life care in medical records
    Data Collecting   .... ☐
    • Referrals
    • ICD9 codes
    • Survey data
    • Access database (# of patients, deaths, LOS, support services etc.)
    • IHI methods
    Communication with Physician/Triage Nurses   .... ☐
    • Informal (hallways)
    • Formal (monthly written reports)
    • Weekly with Physician Champion
    • Documentation in medical record

Communication with Patients .... ☐
- Initial contact
- Home visits
- Office visits
- Ongoing intermittent calls in assessment of acute or chronic issues
- Monthly volunteer contact

Communication with Team Members .... ☐
- Chaplains
- Volunteers
- Other disciplines and health care professionals
- Public

Resources .... ☐
- System-wide
- Community
- Nurses in clinic
- Manual

Chaplain Training .... ☐
- Referral process
- Home visitation
- Communication/Documentation

Volunteer Training .... ☐
- Basic recruitment and interview
- Expectations/Contract
- Survey data training
- Support
- Ongoing education

Follow-up and Support from Director .... ☐
- Informal calls, contacts
- Formal, monthly reports
- Task force meetings
- Steering Committee meetings

7. EDUCATION/TRAINING OF VOLUNTEERS ☐

Orientation
Initial methodology
Monthly meetings/ongoing education
Support
Evaluation

8. EDUCATION/TRAINING OF CHAPLAIN ☐

Clinical pastoral education (CPE) as base
Initial methodology
Monthly meetings
Ongoing education (internal/external)
Support

9. FORMS □
    Opening a Clinic Checklist □
    Sample Note to Physicians/Providers □
    Referral Form □
    Nursing Assessment □
    Patient Information Flow Scheme □
    Referral Approval □
    Follow-up Introduction to Patients □
    Advance Care Planning Information Sheet □
    "This May Be the Greatest Gift You Can Give Your Family" □
    Advance Care Planning Form □
    Volunteer Job Description □
    Volunteer Application □
    Volunteer Contract □
    Welcome Memorandum □
    Volunteer Training □
    Initial Training Procedure □
    Patient Survey □
    Diagnosis Abbreviation List □
    Ideas for Questions □
    Volunteer Call Schedule □
    Help with Survey Questions □
    Developmental Landmarks and Tasks for the End of Life □
    Volunteer Information on Hospice □
    When a Patient Is Referred to Hospice □
    Tips on Listening □
    Tips on Total Listening □
    Listening Skills □
    Ongoing Education: Perspectives on Dying Questionnaire □
    What to Do with a Complaint □
    Bereavement Calls □
    Evaluation □
    Volunteer Evaluation □
    Improving Care through the End of Life Memorandum □
    Spiritual Care Counselor/Chaplain Time Journal □

B. WEBSITES RELATED TO CONTRIBUTORS

Center to Improve Care of the Dying (CICD)
⟨www.medicaring.org⟩

The MediCaring concept derives from the work of Dr. Joanne Lynn and others on a feasibility study to develop an alternative medical benefit that emphasizes comprehensive, supportive, home-based care for individuals enrolled in Medicare. This website is sponsored by the Center to Improve Care of the Dying (CICD), part of RAND Health, in collaboration with Americans for Better Care of the Dying (ABCD) and the Institute for Healthcare Improvement (IHI).

Centre for Bioethics at the Clinical Research Institute of Montreal
⟨www.ircm.qc.ca/bioethique/english/index.html⟩

The Centre for Bioethics exists to anticipate, identify, analyze, and resolve ethical issues arising in the organization and delivery of health care in clinical practice and in the design and conduct of biomedical research. David J. Roy has directed the Centre since its inception in 1976. Dr. Neil MacDonald directs the Cancer Ethics Program at the Centre.

Education for Physicians on End-of-Life Care (EPEC)
⟨www.epec.net⟩

EPEC is a project of the American Medical Association's Institute for Ethics and is supported by a grant from The Robert Wood Johnson Foundation. This initiative is designed to educate all US physicians on the essential clinical competencies required to provide quality end-of-life care. The website includes resources and information about the educational modules.

Institute for Healthcare Improvement (IHI)
⟨www.ihi.org/⟩

IHI is a Boston-based, independent, nonprofit organization working since 1991 to accelerate improvement in health care systems in the United States, Canada, and Europe by fostering collaboration, rather than competition, among health care organizations. IHI sponsors collaboratives on a variety of topics in health. Dr. Joanne Lynn chaired the "Improving Care at the End of Life" collaborative in 1997, in which featured innovators Dr. Mimi Pattison and Ms. Georganne Trandum participated to design the *Improving Care through the End of Life* program.

C. OTHER RELEVANT WEBSITES

Edmonton Palliative Care Program
⟨www.palliative.org/⟩

Offered jointly by the Division of Palliative Medicine, Department of Oncology at the University of Alberta, Edmonton, Canada, and the Edmonton Regional Palliative Care Program host an extensive palliative care site for both professional and non-professional audiences. The purpose of the site is to acquaint the visitor with the basic philosophy of palliative care and its workings in large or small centers. Content includes clinical information, patient assessment tools, cancer material, and links to related resources.

End-of-Life Nursing Education Consortium (ELNEC) ⟨www.aacn.nche.edu/elnec⟩

A comprehensive, national education project to improve end-of-life care by nurses. ELNEC is a partnership of the American Association of Colleges of Nursing (AACN) and the Los Angeles-based City of Hope Cancer Center, supported by The Robert Wood Johnson Foundation.

End-of-Life Physician Education Resource Center (EPERC) ⟨www.eperc.mcw.edu/⟩

The purpose of EPERC is to assist physician educators and others in locating high-quality, peer-reviewed training materials. This website supports the identification and dissemination of information on end-of-life training materials, publications, conferences, and other opportunities. EPERC is supported by The Robert Wood Johnson Foundation and located at the Medical College of Wisconsin.

On Our Own Terms: Moyers on Dying ⟨www.pbs.org/wnet/onourownterms/⟩

In a four-part, six-hour series, Bill Moyers crosses the country from hospitals to hospices to homes to capture stories and candid conversations from multiple perspectives on this topic. The website features end-of-life care resources and community action plans, as well as providing readers with the tools to engage in an ongoing dialogue about facing the end of life. Viewers can order videotapes of the series.

Partnership for Caring: America's Voices for the Dying ⟨www.partnershipforcaring.org⟩

Formerly "Choice in Dying," this is a national nonprofit organization devoted to raising consumer expectations and demand for excellent end-of-life care. The site offers resources for talking about end-of-life choices, the process of health care agency, and state-specific advance directives.

Toolkit of Instruments to Measure End-of-Life Care (TIME) ⟨www.chcr.brown.edu/pcoc/toolkit.htm⟩

Dr. Joan Teno has built a "toolkit" that provides a comprehensive list of tools and references, including measurement instruments related to palliative care. This site contains annotated bibliographies of tools for specific domains, including quality of life, pain and other symptoms, emotional and cognitive symptoms, functional status, survival time and aggressiveness of care, advance care planning, continuity of care, spirituality, grief and bereavement, and patient-centered reports and rankings (aka statisfaction) for the quality of care and caregiver well-being.

Part Two: Institutionalizing Palliative Care

A. ORIGINAL TOOLS FROM CONTRIBUTORS

1. Mini version of process audit tool: Variance Tracking: PCAD

Copyright © 2000 by Beth Israel Medical Center, Department of Pain Medicine and Palliative Care. Reprinted with permission.

Marilyn Bookbinder of Beth Israel Medical Center's Department of Pain Medicine and Palliative Care has provided this tool to track variations in practice as nurses implement the PCAD.

Mini Version of Process Audit Tool: Variance Tracking: PCAD

Patient Name: _____	PMR #: _____
Date:_____	

Repeat for each day on PCAD Care Path. If no, provide explanation in Comments section.

Y   N   N/A   Advance directives were discussed and patient/family preferences identified.
Comments:

Y   N   N/A   Goals of care were clarified with patient/family.
Comments:

Y   N   N/A   Pain and symptoms were adequately managed.
Comments:

Y   N   N/A   Supportive interventions and consults were enacted.
Comments:

Y   N   N/A   Unnecessary interventions were discontinued and none were ordered.
Comments:

Y   N   N/A   Patient/family psychosocial and spiritual support was provided.
Comments:

Y   N   N/A   Unnecessary regulations were eliminated.
Comments:

At discharge:

Y   N   N/A   Bereavement services/resources were provided.
Comments:

Y   N   N/A   Patient was transferred to alternate care setting (e.g., hospice, SNF, home care, etc.).
Comments:

B. WEBSITES RELATED TO CONTRIBUTORS

American Hospital Association (AHA)
⟨www.hospitalconnect.com/aha/awards-events/circle-of-life/index.html⟩

AHA is a key sponsor of the 2001 Circle of Life Award. Visit this site for more information about this year's award and/or to apply for next year's award.

Beth Israel Medical Center's *Stop Pain!* Website
⟨www.StopPain.Org⟩

This is an extensive site, addressing many topics in depth. Find resources for educators, physicians, nurses, patients, and caregivers. It highlights Beth Israel's extensive commitment to supporting patients and their families through the Department of Pain Medicine and Palliative Care. The *Palliative Care for Advanced Disease* (PCAD) pathway highlighted in the Featured Innovation, Part Two of this book, can be downloaded in PDF format from this site for free. You must register in order to gain access to these tools and instructions for their use. Follow this link to register and for the unit reference manual: ⟨www.stoppain.org/services_staff/pcad1.html⟩. For further references related to the PCAD, go to ⟨www.StopPain.org/services_staff/pcad5.html⟩.

European Association for Palliative Care (EAPC)
⟨www.eapcnet.org/⟩

The EAPC was founded with 40 individual members in 1988. It is now a federation of national and regional societies of palliative care, representing more than 25,000 individuals across Europe and other parts of the world. The website at present serves as an information source about the EAPC and its activities including descriptions of publications and congresses. The site also offers a directory of participating organizations around the world, including contact names and addresses. Many resources are available in French and English, and congresses offer simultaneous interpretation of all sessions. A number of *Innovations'* editorial board members play leadership roles in this organization, including Dr. Stein Kaasa, who serves as president of the EAPC.

Journal of Pain and Symptom Management
⟨www.elsevier.nl/locate/jpainsymman⟩

Edited by Dr. Russell K. Portenoy of Beth Israel Medical Center, the *Journal of Pain and Symptom Management* provides the professional with the results of important new research and clinical information related to pain management and palliative care. The journal boasts an international editorial board, including leading researchers and clinicians. Each board member is an active figure in pain or palliative care and a major contributor to the literature.

Marie Curie Cancer Care
⟨www.mariecurie.org.uk/⟩

Founded in 1948, Marie Curie Cancer Care is now the United Kingdom's largest and most comprehensive cancer care charity. The Marie Curie Nursing Service and Marie Curie Centres (hospices) care for people seriously ill with cancer, while the Marie Curie Research Institute investigates the causes and treatments of cancer.

United Hospital Fund (UHF)
⟨www.uhfnyc.org/⟩

UHF is a health services research and philanthropic organization that addresses critical issues affecting hospitals and health care in New York City. UHF originally funded the BIMC effort (see Featured Innovation, Part One) through its Hospital Palliative Care Initiative, designed to promote better end-of-life care practices in New York City hospitals.

C. OTHER RELEVANT WEBSITES

Australian Department of Veterans' Affairs Community Nursing: Clinical Pathways Manual
⟨www.dva.gov.au/health/provider/community%20nursing/pathways/pathindex.htm#pathways⟩

The Australian Department of Veterans' Affairs posts an extensive list of clinical pathways in PDF format at this site. Readers need Adobe Acrobat to access these tools. This series includes a Palliative Care Clinical Pathway dated July 2000.

Center to Advance Palliative Care (CAPC)
⟨www.capcmssn.org⟩

Established by The Robert Wood Johnson Foundation to promote wider access to excellent palliative care in hospitals and health systems in the United States, CAPC aims to provide assistance in the planning, development, and implementation of hospital and health-system-based palliative care programs. The site includes a variety of resources and materials.

Center to Improve Care of the Dying
⟨www.medicaring.org⟩

The Center to Improve Care of the Dying (CICD) is a unique, interdisciplinary team of committed individuals engaged in research, public advocacy, and education activities to improve the care of the dying and their families.

Edmonton Palliative Care Program
⟨www.palliative.org/⟩

An extensive palliative care site for both professional and nonprofessional audiences offered jointly by the Division of Palliative Medicine and Department of Oncology at the University of Alberta in Edmonton, Canada, and the Edmonton Regional Palliative Care Program. The purpose of the site is to acquaint the visitor with the basic philosophy of palliative care and its workings in centers large or small. Content includes clinical information, patient assessment tools, cancer material, and links to related resources.

Institute for Healthcare Improvement (IHI)
⟨www.ihi.org/⟩

IHI is a Boston-based, independent, nonprofit organization working since 1991 to accelerate improvement in health care systems in the United States, Canada, and Europe by fostering collaboration, rather than competition, among health care organizations. IHI sponsors collaboratives on a variety of topics in health.

International Association for Hospice & Palliative Care (IAHPC)
⟨www.hospicecare.com⟩

IAHPC is a nonprofit international organization dedicated to the development and improvement of palliative care worldwide by encouraging countries to develop their own model of palliative care provision rather than expecting them to copy models more appropriate to affluent countries. IAHPC is currently chaired by *Innovations* editorial board member Dr. Eduardo Bruera. Readers can join the IAHPC at this website, as well as access its many resources. These include "World Palliative Care Reports," which are short summaries of state-of-the-art palliative care in specific countries, a monthly newsletter, an extensive ethics page, updates on IAHPC activities, and links to key palliative care journals and organizations.

Toolkit of Instruments to Measure End-of-Life Care (TIME)
⟨www.chcr.brown.edu/pcoc/toolkit.htm⟩

Dr. Joan Teno has built a "toolkit" that provides a comprehensive list of tools and references, including measurement instruments related to palliative care. This site contains annotated bibliographies of tools for specific domains, including quality of life, pain and other symptoms, emotional and cognitive symptoms, functional status, survival time and aggressiveness of care, advance care planning, continuity of care, spirituality, grief and bereavement, and patient-centered reports and rankings (aka statisfaction) for the quality of care and caregiver well-being.

Part Three: Supporting Family Caregivers

A. ORIGINAL TOOLS FROM CONTRIBUTORS

1. Quick Tips for Working with the Doctors

From the Brooklyn Hospital Center and Wartburg Lutheran Home for the Aging Caregiving Initiative, funded by the United Hospital Fund. Quick Tips for Working with the Doctors, created by Beth-Ann Gillery, CSW. This tool provides tips for caregivers in preparing for, and getting the most out of interactions with their loved one's doctor.

QUICK TIPS FOR WORKING WITH THE DOCTORS

The First Visit
- Introduce yourself to the doctor, giving your name and relationship to the patient.
- Inform the doctor what he/she should know about the patient, his/her health, circumstances, and anything else you think the doctor needs to know.

Be Prepared
- Think about what you want to know from your doctor and prepare questions in advance.
- Write questions on an index card or in a notebook. Take notes when talking to your doctor.
- Ask for more explanations until you understand.
- Bring a friend to help you remember and understand. Ask your friend to take notes.

Phone Talk
- Become familiar with the doctor's secretary. Introduce yourself and find out her name. Use her name whenever you call.
- Be pleasant and greet her. She is your link to the doctor.
- Ask when is a good time to call to speak to the doctor.
- If you must leave a message, make sure you leave your name, the name of the patient, and your relationship to the patient.
- Leave a clear short message.
- Leave a telephone number and when YOU will be at this number. Be there!
- Leave two numbers if necessary.
- Have your questions ready when you do speak to the doctor.

IF YOU HAVE AN EMERGENCY, SAY SO: "THIS IS AN EMERGENCY!"

B. WEBSITES RELATED TO CONTRIBUTORS

Carers: Government Information for Carers
⟨www.carers.gov.uk⟩

A British governmental site with a great deal of information for family caregivers, called *carers* in the United Kingdom. This site posts the British *National Strategy for Carers*, a 1999 governmental policy on caregivers with a foreword by Prime Minister Tony Blair. This document is available in PDF format from the homepage. Readers may also find the *Quality Standards for Local Carer Support Services* at ⟨www.carers.gov.uk/qualitystan.htm⟩ in PDF format. You may also get to this page by clicking on the "Information Zones" button in the left margin and then the "Help for the Carer" button to find a list of documents of interest, including these quality standards. The King's Fund established a working group to develop these standards in response to the National Strategy for Carers. This working group included representatives from the Association of Directors of Social Services, Department of Health, National Health Service (NHS) Confederation, and National Carers' organizations and was chaired by Penny Banks of The King's Fund. In February 2000 the British government approved these standards.

Hospice Foundation of America
⟨www.hospicefoundation.org/⟩

Hospice Foundation of America is the nation's largest charity whose sole mission is to promote the hospice concept of care and is supported primarily by individual donations. Information about annual teleconferences is available from the homepage. For 2002, the initiative was "Living with Grief: Loss in Later Life." These teleconferences are available for purchase on video, dating back to 1996.

National Alliance for Caregiving
⟨www.caregiving.org/⟩

Special feature of this site: the *National Alliance for Caregiving's Family Care Resource Connection* at ⟨www.caregiving.org/content/fcrc.html⟩. Each entry in the *Family Care Resource Connection* has been reviewed and rated for its quality, usefulness to family members, timeliness, and accessibility. The resources are rated on a scale from four stars (the best) to one star. Reviews are prepared by experts in family caregiving and highlight the strengths and weaknesses of each item. Items include books, videos, websites, magazines, fact sheets, and other resources addressing the range of issues and questions faced by family caregivers.

Princess Royal Trust for Carers
⟨www.carers.org/⟩

This organization sponsors Carer Centres throughout the United Kingdom for the six million adult carers there (*carer* is the British term for an unpaid family caregiver). They estimate that there are also 50,000 young carers, or people under the age of 18 who are providing care for parents or siblings. The site offers an online carer discussion group and chat room, as well as an extensive list of links to sites based in the United Kingdom on a wide variety of related topics.

The TBI Help Desk for Caregivers: Jamaica Hospital Medical Center ⟨www.tbi-help.org⟩

Another project funded by the United Hospital Fund Families and Health Care Project, this website offers resources and tools for caregivers of patients with traumatic brain injury.

United Hospital Fund—Families and Health Care Project ⟨www.uhfnyc.org/⟩

Carol Levine's recent book, *Always on Call: When Illness Turns Families into Caregivers* is available from the homepage. To get to the *Families and Health Care Project*, directed by Carol Levine, click on the Research and Policy Initiatives button in the left margin of the home page. The *Families and Health Care Project* provides a wealth of resources and information for caregivers and families. Note the frequently asked questions (FAQ) about family caregiving page and the Resources/Links for family caregivers. Carol Levine also wrote the special report *Rough Crossings: Family Caregivers' Odysseys through the Health Care System* published by United Hospital Fund, 1998. Find the table of contents, executive summary, and ordering information at ⟨www.uhfnyc.org/pubs/books/bkrough.html⟩.

C. OTHER RELEVANT WEBSITES

Administration on Aging ⟨www.aoa.gov/⟩

This US Government agency website has many useful resources for older Americans and family caregivers. These include policy and legislation information, such as an overview of the Older Americans Act (OAA) Amendments of 2000, full text of the OAA Amendments of 2000 (amendments only) at ⟨www.aoa.gov/Oaa/2000/hr782.html⟩, and frequently asked questions (FAQ) about the OAA Amendments of 2000. This act was signed into law by President Clinton in November 2000. The National Family Caregiver Support Act is a key part of this new legislation. In addition, this site offers an array of resources specifically targeted to caregivers: notably Caregiver Resources and *Because We Care: A Guide for People Who Care*. For health care providers, a new guidebook is available in PDF format: *Achieving Cultural Competence: A Guidebook for Providers of Services to Older Americans and Their Families* (January 2001). Review article "Family Caregiving in an Aging Society" by Sharon Tennstedt, PhD, presented March 29, 1999, at the U.S. Administration on Aging Symposium available at ⟨www.aoa.gov/caregivers/FamCare.html⟩

AARP WebPlace: Caregiving
⟨www.aarp.org/indexes/health.html#caregiving⟩

American Association of Retired Person's WebPlace: Caregiving provides a wealth of information about the many services, publications, and support systems that are available to caregivers. Also see ⟨www.dsaapd.com/newpage4.htm⟩ for a list of books and publications related to caregiving.

American Society on Aging
⟨www.asaging.org/⟩

Offers educational programs, conferences, and publications. ASA recently sponsored a joint conference with the National Council on Aging, which included a preconference special program "Meeting the Needs of Family Caregivers."

AgeNet Eldercare Network
⟨www.agenet.com/⟩

AgeNet, Inc., operates a comprehensive, national eldercare network to meet the specific needs of the fast growing aging population and their adult caregiving children. Resources for caregivers include the business side of eldercare, bringing together suppliers of eldercare products and services with businesses such as nursing homes, assisted living facilities, home health care providers, health systems, and organizations or companies with employee assistance programs. A variety of links and information are available at this site, from how to handle home care and where to buy products to caregiver support.

Beth Israel Medical Center
Department of Pain and Palliative Care
⟨www.StopPain.org⟩

This site has extensive tools and resources for family caregivers. The index, at ⟨www.StopPain.org/caregivers/index.html⟩ includes Getting Started—Now You Are a Caregiver, Navigating "the System," Symptom Management at Home, Goals of Care in Progressive Illness, You Have Needs, Too, and Where to Find Help. Tools include checklists and suggestions for developing an action plan, articulating the patient's needs and how to assess one's interpersonal resources, information about particular symptoms, and many other items.

Caregiver.com
⟨www.caregiver.com⟩

Includes Alzheimer's Caregiver, with articles about dementia care and opportunities to chat with other Alzheimer's caregivers and experts in the field. Also offers weekly "Caretips" and poetry. Readers may subscribe to Caregiver Magazine, but may view the current weekly newsletter for caregivers for free online.

CaregiversCount
⟨www.caregiverscount.com⟩

This site is an online resource for nonpartisan information affecting caregivers and their families. Provides information about legislation and initiatives in Washington, D.C., that affect caregivers. This organization grew out of a white paper presented September 12, 2000, authored by Robert B. Blancato, former executive director of the 1995 White House Conference on Aging. Blancato has called for the development and passage of a Universal Caregivers Act in 2001. Readers may download Blancato's September 12, 2000, presentation, "The Future of Caregiving," in PDF format at ⟨www.caregiverscount.com/qa.html⟩.

Caregiving.com
⟨www.caregiving.com/⟩

This site offers tips, support, advice, and resources for caregivers and is run by Denise Brown, who operates the Center for Family Caregivers, a nonprofit organization dedicated to helping persons who care for chronically ill or disabled family members and is based in Park Ridge, Illinois. Ms. Brown also publishes Caregiving newsletter, which can be found at ⟨www.caregiving.com/caregiving/index.htm⟩.

Carers Online
⟨www.carersonline.org.uk⟩

A lobbying organization for carers (family caregivers) across the United Kingdom. This site has extensive links for organizations within the United Kingdom on policy development and research on carers, information, local and regional support groups, and publications on specific illnesses.

Chapter 11: Family Caregiving. Part of the Report of the Priority Expert Panel on Long-Term Care for Older Adults
⟨www.nih.gov/ninr/research/vol3/FamCare.html⟩

One of a series of expert panels constituted by the National Center for Nursing Research (NCNR) between FY 1988 and 1992, in conjunction with the development of the National Nursing Research Agenda (NNRA). Chapter 11 covers Family Caregiving; the entire report can be found here as well.

Crossroads—Caring for Carers
⟨www.crossroads.org.uk/⟩

Crossroads is the major charity in the United Kingdom providing practical support to carers (family caregivers) in the home. Their main service is providing short breaks for carers. This organization provides 3.7 million care hours to 28,600 carers in England and Wales.

Empowering Caregivers
⟨www.care-givers.com/pages/main.html⟩

Empowering Caregivers is an extensive online resource, full of information and opportunities for caregivers to find community and support. They offer message boards, information on local community support, journal exercises for caregivers to work through their experience, articles on healing music and alternative therapy techniques, and chats with experts.

Faith in Action
⟨www.interfaithcare.org⟩

Faith in Action is the national program office for an interfaith volunteer program that aims to better the lives of people with long-term health needs. Supported by The Robert Wood Johnson Foundation, this national program office has helped to build more than 1,100 interfaith volunteer programs across the United States. Faith in Action provides start-up grants as well as support and advice on how to develop successful, sustainable caregiving programs that serve their communities and has recently received a new infusion of funds. Grant applications are currently available.

Familycare America Newsletter: A Lifeline to Families Caring for Family Members
⟨www.familycareamerica.com/⟩

Substantive site with many resources some of which cost money ($), but many of which are free. It includes an interactive assessment tool ($), a search tool that uses U.S. zip codes to locate resources for local long-term care facilities, home health agencies, elder law attorneys, and the like, in the United States, products for sale, and a library with extensive resources. Library includes many useful checklists and forms, articles on caregiving basics, death and dying, resources for long-distance caregiving, and many other topics. The page about state and local long-term care ombudsmen includes tips for how to use these consumer watchdogs to get the latest information about long-term care facilities. A free monthly online newsletter with timely and wide-ranging articles is also available.

Family Caregiver Alliance
⟨www.caregiver.org/⟩

This site has many resources, current articles, and links to further information on caregiving, disease processes, and current events related to caregiving.

Home Care Companion: Resources for Caregivers
⟨www.homecarecompanion.com⟩

Books, videos, and training resources for instruction on basic caregiving procedures are available at this site.

Human Development and Family Life Bulletin: Caregiving for the Elderly
⟨www.hec.ohio-state.edu/famlife/bulletin/bullmain.htm>

The Human Development and Family Life Bulletin is a resource for professionals who work with children, youth, and families. It includes reviews of research related to important topics of interest to practitioners, practice wisdom from the field, an update on evaluation issues, and summaries of new teaching and intervention resources. Volume 2, Issue 4, Winter 1996, focuses on caregiving for the elderly.

The King's Fund
⟨www.kingsfund.org.uk/⟩

The King's Fund is an independent health care charity working for better health in London and across the United Kingdom. It gives grants and carries out research and development work to bring about better health policies and services. The King's Fund spearheaded the development of the recent *Quality Standards for Local Carer Support Services* approved by the British government in February 2000. More details on the new project "Quality Support to Carers" can be found at The Health and Social Care Carer Support page at ⟨www.kingsfund.org. uk/eHealthSocialCare/html/carers.htm⟩. They have a useful tool, the *Carers Compass for Primary Care*, which can be downloaded in PDF format at ⟨www.kings-fund.org.uk/eHealthSocialCare/assets/applets/penny_compass1.pdf⟩. The *Carers Compass* is a booklet/checklist designed to aid primary care teams in meeting eight key needs of carers and thus improve the quality of their care. (Reminder: Carer is the British equivalent of family caregiver.) This site has extensive annotated links to a wide variety of European health and social care organizations, as well as to topic-specific search engines—a treasure trove.

National Aging Information Center: A Service of the Administration on Aging
⟨www.aoa.dhhs.gov/NAIC/Notes/caregiverresource.html⟩

A warehouse of information, this site has links to websites and articles related to aging and family caregiving.

National Family Caregivers Association (NFCA)
⟨www.nfcacares.org/⟩

NFCA is a grassroots membership organization created to educate, support, empower, and speak up for the millions of Americans who care for chronically ill, aged, or disabled loved ones. Through its services in the areas of information and education, support and validation, public awareness and advocacy, NFCA strives to minimize the disparity between a caregiver's quality of life and that of mainstream Americans. NFCA offers a number of publications, including *Take Care! Self Care for the Family Caregiver*, a quarterly newsletter providing can-do advice, resources and Q & A. This publication and other resource materials from the NFCA, including *A National Report on the Status of Caregiving in America* (2000), can be purchased at ⟨www.comcat.com/~nfca/securepubs.html⟩.

National Parent Information Network
⟨npin.org/library/pre1998/n00225/n00225.html⟩

Family Caregiving, by Nancy Beekman. Full-text article online about caregivers, addressing caregiver burden, effective coping strategies, and ongoing challenges.

Well Spouse Foundation
⟨www.wellspouse.org/⟩

The Well Spouse Foundation is a national, not-for-profit membership organization that gives support to husbands, wives, and partners of the chronically ill and/or disabled. Look at the bimonthly newsletter, *Mainstay*, found at ⟨www.well-spouse.org/mainstay.html⟩.

For more dementia-specific sites, please refer to the online journal *Innovations in End-of-Life Care* at ⟨www.edc.org/lastacts⟩. The archived issue Only Connect: Promoting Meaning in the Lives of Patients with Advanced Dementia, Vol. 1, No. 4, 1999, contains many more resources.

Part Four: On Grief and Bereavement

A. ORIGINAL TOOLS FROM CONTRIBUTORS

1. Breakout Session Topics Handout.
Copyright © 2001 UCSF Children's Hospital. Reprinted with permission.

Breakout Session Topics Handout

June 10 and 11, 2000

A	B	C
Saturday, June 10 Breakout 1 *1:15–2:45 p.m.*	**Saturday, June 10** Breakout 2 *4:15–5:45 p.m.*	**Sunday, June 11** Breakout 3 *9:45–11:15 a.m.*
1. A Father's Grief *Fireside Room*	1. Grief and Marriage *Willow Lodge*	1. Young Adult Siblings *Willow Lodge*
2. Beyond the First Year *Buckeye Room*	2. Dreams and Unusual Happenings *Buckeye Lodge*	2. Grief and Marriage *Fireside Room*
3. Death of an Only Child *Buckeye Lodge*	3. Beyond the First Year *Buckeye Room*	3. Anger and Guilt *Pine Lodge*
4. Anger and Guilt *Cypress Lodge*	4. Dealing with Friends & Family *Fireside Room*	4. Spirituality *Buckeye Room*
5. Supporting Siblings *Pine Lodge*	5. Issues Re: Having More Children *Eucalyptus Lodge*	5. Taking Stock *Cypress Lodge*
6. Young Adult Siblings *Willow Lodge*	6. Anniversaries & Special Occasions *Pine Lodge*	6. Spanish Speaking Family Support Group *Buckeye Lodge*
7. First Year of Grief *Eucalyptus Room*	7. Experiencing the Moment of Death *Cypress Lodge*	
8. Spanish Speaking Family Support Group *Teacher's Lodge*	8. Spanish Speaking Family Support Group *Teacher's Lodge*	

2. Children's Program Bereavement Retreat Schedule

Copyright © 2001 UCSF Children's Hospital. Reprinted with permission.

Working Document: Activities for different age groups of children for the three time slots on Saturday and one on Sunday morning.

Children's Program Bereavement Retreat Schedule

SATURDAY JUNE 10, 2000

10:30–11:50 a.m. Children, 3–12 years old

Ice breaker: (large group) Everyone who likes pizza . . .
Gathering into group: Everyone who has had a brother/sister die . . .
Light candle
Introduction to project: Memory box for sibling or other person/loss
Split the larger group into three groups by age and identify leader and helpers for each group:
3-5 years old: List names of staff who will run this group.
6-8 years old: List names of staff who will run this group.
9-12 years old: List names of staff who will run this group.
Anagram: Use each letter in name of sibling or self as first letter of a word that describes the sibling or the participant (may need to adapt with younger kids).
Project: Memory Boxes, Memory Wheel (collage), Memory Book
Theme: Remembering, working through/processing, feelings.
[The children could cut out/color pre-made feeling faces representing different emotions.] Focus on sibling who died and relationship with surviving sibling.
Closure: Share boxes/collages/memory book page(s) in circle (three separate groups). Share feelings chosen, and come together around candle for wish circle. (May want to re-evaluate coming back together based on numbers/ages).
Group facilitators: List names of staff who will run this activity.

10:30–11:50 a.m. Teens, 13–17 years old
Ropes Course

Early afternoon: Preschoolers, 3–5 years old
1:00–3:00 p.m.   *Ice breaker*: Throw ball to friend, say name, favorite food, color (5 min.)
Intro: Video (15 min.)
Project: Three play/art stations (25–30 min each)
1. Hand tracing/saying goodbye coloring page
2. Play dough/family figure play area
3. Book area/charades in acting out feelings
Prompts/suggestions for guiding the groups:

> Why are we all here this weekend? Who in your family died? Some people may have been little babies or not even been born yet when brother/sister got so sick that he or she died. People may have come together at a funeral to say goodbye to your brother or sister. There may have been music, singing, and prayers. Do you remember the funeral? Did you go to the funeral? What was that like for you (if did or did not go)? It is hard to say "Goodbye" to your brother or sister when they die because they will not come back to live with your family . . . you can't play with them anymore. But we have pictures and memories. . . . What do you remember about your brother or sister? When we think about our brother or sister, we have many different kinds of memories and feelings— sad, mad, funny, happy. . . .

Issues of saying goodbye, family constellation/changes, and feelings can be addressed more specifically in each smaller group.
Theme: Saying goodbye, family life changes, memories (remembering) and feelings
Closing: Reading of *Swan Sky* (15 min.)

Children, 6–12 years old
Project: Make masks
Teens, 13–17 years old
Swimming/sports activity

Late afternoon: Preschoolers, 3–5 years old
3:15–5:15 p.m.   Creek walk, story time
Children, 6–12 years old
Sports activity/swimming/make masks for Sunday morning art project

Teens, 13–17 years old

Ice breaker: Paired interviews (Teens pick numbers out of hat. Those who pick matched pairs are partners for this activity. Each person interviews the partner for 3 minutes and then at the end, larger group re-forms, and each person introduces his or her partner to the group. Timekeeper needs to be clear about time to switch so that both partners get equal time.)

Introduction: Light a candle and explain the theme of this activity: mandala/shields of strength/dream catchers

Project: Mandalas and/or dream catchers

Theme: Remembering good and bad times, letting go of painful memories and holding on to good memories, strategies that help you to cope/have courage or strength

Closure: Candle, sharing of project

Group facilitators: List names of staff who will run this activity.

SUNDAY JUNE 11, 2000

9:45–12:30 p.m. Preschoolers, 3–5 years old

9:45–10:00 a.m.   Debrief from memorial service
10:00–11:00 a.m. Decorate picture mats
11:00–11:30 a.m. Songs and dance
11:30–12:30 p.m. Make book: All about Me

Introduction: Sharing of family members

Projects: Make family pictures in decorative mat; Book: All about Me

Book to read aloud: Badger's Parting Gifts (This book emphasizes what is special about each person in family. Stress that they are special.)

Extra activity: Music/songs/dance by Bread and Roses (between art projects from 11:00 to 11:30 a.m.)

Group facilitators: List names of staff who will run this activity.

9:45–12:30 p.m. Children, 6–8 years old

9:45–10:15 a.m.   Debrief from memorial service
10:15–10:45 a.m. Story teller
10:45–12:30 p.m. Masks

Introduction: Feelings: inside feelings/outside feelings

Project: Decorate masks (children made paper maché masks on Saturday with counselors.)

Theme: Feelings are normal, no right or wrong, okay to share feelings and okay not to share. You are in control over how much you choose to share. Everyone reacts differently. We are all unique and special.

Closure: Share mask and something special about "you" (may want to fine-tune this as small group)

Extra activity: Story teller

Group facilitators: List names of staff who will run this activity.

9:45–12:30 p.m. Children, 9–12 years old

9:45–10:15 a.m. Debrief from memorial service
10:15–11:45 a.m. Rock Ceremony
11:45–12:30 p.m. Mime

Introduction: Change and growth; how experiences can change us, good and bad influences, work hard on finding good or positive. Through hard times, can grow stronger, more empathic, more sensitive and aware of making the most of our own lives. Explain analogy of rough rock and polished stone.

Project: Pick rough rock, choose polished stone, make medicine pouch.

Closure: Share meaning behind stone chosen, light candle.

Theme: Same as above. We can be in control of our feelings, let go of sad, scary ones, hold on to good, happy ones, grow stronger and more beautiful through this hard experience.

Extra activity: Mime

Group leader facilitators: List names of staff who will run this activity.

9:45–12:30 p.m. Teens, 13–17 years old

9:45–10:15 a.m. Debrief from memorial service
10:15–11:45 a.m. Rock Ceremony (make pouches?)
11:45–12:30 p.m. Kickball or other sport activity

Introduction: Change and growth; metamorphosis, how experiences can change us; good and bad influences, work hard on finding good or positive. Through hard times, we can grow stronger, more empathic, more sensitive and aware of making the most of our own lives.

Project: Find rough rock, choose polished stone, Rock Ceremony (Pass rock in circle with silent wishes, music in background.)

Sharing Time/Closure: (Pick two or three questions/ issues to share; e.g., how experience has changed us, in a positive way? In general, what helps when you are sad or down? (The point here is to identify what their existing coping strategies are and build on them.)

Theme: As above, validate importance of remembering sibling, but also acknowledge that we must go on with life, taking a tragedy and with a lot of "tumbling," hard work, love, and support, we can grow from the experience . . . feel whole, beautiful, and strong.

Extra activity: Make pouches: Need felt and embroidery thread.

Group facilitators: List names of staff who will run this activity.

3. **Family Bereavement Retreat Breakout Session Topics by Location**
Copyright © 2001 UCSF Children's Hospital. Reprinted with permission.

Family Bereavement Retreat Breakout Session Topics by Location

SATURDAY, JUNE 10, 2000

Adults		Children/Teens/Young Adults	
9:30–10:15 a.m.	Registration in Buckeye Room	10:00–10:15 a.m.	Preschoolers/ Children/Teens: Meet counselors outside of Buckeye Room
10:30–11:50	Keynote Address: "Befriending Grief" (Buckeye Room)	10:30–11:50	Preschooler: Art Project/Support Group Children: Art Project/Support Group Teens: Ropes Course
		10:30-11:50	Young Adults: Keynote Address
12:00–12:45 p.m.	LUNCH	12:00–12:45 p.m.	LUNCH
1:15–2:45	Breakout Session #1 (Locations posted outside of Buckeye Room)	1:00–3:00	Preschoolers: Art Project/Support Group
			Children: Ropes Course Teens: Swimming/ Sports Activity
		1:15–2:45	Young Adults: Support Group
2:50–3:00	SNACK in the Buckeye Room	3:00–3:15	Children's SNACK in Maple Room
2:50–4:05	Writing through Grief Workshop (SNACK provided)		
3:05–4:05	Nature Walk	2:50–4:05	Young Adults: Writing Workshop
		3:15–5:45	Preschoolers: Creek Walk/Story Time Children: Sports Activity/Swimming Teens: Art Project/ Support Group
4:15–5:45	Breakout Session #2	4:15–5:45	Young Adults: Nature Walk

6:00–6:45	DINNER
6:45–7:30	FREE TIME
7:30–9:30	Family Entertainment:
	Square Dance on patio outside of dining hall (all welcome)
	Children's movie and activities inside of dining hall

SUNDAY, JUNE 11, 2000

Adults		Children/Teens/Young Adults	
8:00–8:45 a.m.	BREAKFAST	8:00–8:45 a.m.	BREAKFAST
9:00–9:30	A Special Time for Remembering: Gather at Buckeye Room (Parents bring children to Buckeye Room after ceremony to meet counselors)	9:45–12:30 p.m.	Preschooler: Art/Support Group/Sports Children: Art/Support Sports Teens: Art/Support Group/Sports Young Adults:
9:45–11:15	Breakout Session #3	9:45–11:15	Support Group Young Adults:
11:30–12:30 p.m.	Closing Address: "The Mourning Process: Healing after Loss" (Buckeye Room)	11:30–12:30	Closing Address
12:30–1:15	Lunch and Evaluations		
1:30	Goodbye and Departure		

B. WEBSITES RELATED TO CONTRIBUTORS

AARP Grief and Loss Programs
⟨www.aarp.org/griefandloss/home.html⟩

AARP (American Association of Retired Persons), a nonprofit advocacy organization, offers an array of resources for bereaved persons, including the AARP Widowed Persons Service, a community-based program in which trained widowed volunteers reach out to the newly widowed. Established in 1973, this program is based on the "Widow to Widow" research of Dr. Phyllis Silverman.

American Pain Foundation
⟨www.painfoundation.org⟩

This nonprofit information resource and patient advocacy organization aims to improve the quality of life of persons with pain and raise public awareness and understanding of pain. The site includes a pain care bill of rights, pain action guide, legislative updates, and patient information that can be searched by disease type, as well as other resources and links.

Mount Ida College, National Center for Death Education
⟨www.mountida.edu⟩

Find information about Mt. Ida's National Center for Death Education by clicking on "Offices and Services" and then scroll down. Dr. Carol Wogrin serves as executive director and Dr. Phyllis Silverman is on the advisory board. The National Center for Death Education offers workshops and a summer seminar on various dimensions of death and dying for health care professionals.

Phyllis R. Silverman
⟨www.phyllisrsilverman.com/⟩

Dr. Silverman's personal website with information about her published work.

Project on Death in America
⟨www.soros.org/death/⟩

Sponsored by the Soros Foundation, the mission of the Project on Death in America is to understand and transform the culture and experience of dying and bereavement through initiatives in research, scholarship, the humanities, and the arts and to foster innovations in the provision of care, public education, professional education, and public policy.

Supportive Care of the Dying: A Coalition for Compassionate Care
⟨www.careofdying.org/⟩

The three priorities of the coalition are research, developing models of comprehensive, community-based, supportive care for dying people, and creating a professional development program. The site has a variety of tools and resources, as well as back issues of *Supportive Voice*, the newsletter of the coalition.

C. OTHER RELEVANT WEBSITES

The resources included in "On Grief and Bereavement" are primarily focused toward the grieving individual. Families and communities who are coping with grief and loss, especially traumatic loss, will find additional resources in the November–December 2001 issue of *Innovations* entitled *Coping with Loss*. This archived issue can be found at ⟨www.edc.org/lastacts/⟩.

The Special Feature on page 237 entitled Online Bereavement Support contains an annotated list of grief and bereavement websites. The following list contains additional relevant sites.

Arizona State University, Prevention Resource Center
⟨www.azprevention.org⟩

The Prevention Research Center (PRC) was established in 1984 to develop, evaluate, and disseminate prevention programs for children and families in high-stress situations. It is one of four research centers funded by the Prevention Branch of the National Institute of Mental Health. Research at the Center focuses on children and families experiencing four different stressors: parental divorce, poverty, bereavement, and parental job loss. *Coping with Loss*, the November–December 2001 online issue of *Innovations in End-of-Life Care* features the Family Bereavement Program, of the PRC, directed by Dr. Irwin Sandler. To read more about this program, go to ⟨www.edc.org/lastacts⟩ to access archived issue Vol. 3, No. 6., 2001.

Association for Death Education and Counseling
⟨www.adec.org⟩

A multidisciplinary professional organization dedicated to promoting excellence in death education, bereavement counseling, and care of the dying. The Association for Death Education and Counseling envisions a world in which death, dying, grief, and bereavement are recognized as significant aspects of the human experience. Current information in the field of thanatology and counseling, as well as links to special interest topics on grief and bereavement, can be found here.

Before Their Time
⟨www.beforetheirtime.org/⟩

Before Their Time is a collection of memorial songs that aims to provide comfort to people after the death of someone close and help them to heal. Besides offering musical comfort that may make grieving less painful and lonely, this album project is designed to raise money and visibility for two organizations that provide services to individuals and families going through end-of-life experiences. All net revenue from album sales will go to Hospice VNH, which provides both assistance for the terminally ill and bereavement support to survivors in Vermont and New Hampshire, and the New Hampshire Youth Suicide Prevention Association, a nonprofit organization that has provided educational and intervention programs since 1994.

Bereavement Magazine: A Journal of Hope and Healing
⟨www.bereavementmag.com⟩

Designed to be "a support group in print," Bereavement Magazine includes articles, stories, and poetry. Readers have full access to archived issues at this site, as well as access to some material available only on the Web.

Louis D. Brown Peace Institute
⟨www.institute4peace.org⟩

Named for the young victim of a Boston-area gang shooting, the Institute for Peace was founded in 1994 by the parents of Louis D. Brown, in order to continue the peacemaking legacy of their son. The institute offers a peace curriculum, training workshops, and survivor outreach.

Cancer.gov
⟨www.cancer.gov⟩

Cancer.gov's mission is to provide recent and accurate cancer information from the National Cancer Institute (NCI), the federal government's principal agency for cancer research, to the public. Features a PDQ (Physician Data Query) on grief, loss, and bereavement for patients and another for health professionals. Search on the terms "grief and bereavement."

Centering Corporation
⟨www.centering.org⟩

This site aims to provide access to grief resources available on the Web. They also work to develop needed books and caring workshops on grief for adults and children.

The Centre for Grief Education
⟨www.grief.org.au⟩

An independent, nonprofit organization started in 1996 and based in Melbourne, Australia, the Centre for Grief Education offers links to education programs, individual counseling, a journal called "Grief Matters," a bereavement support directory, and grief support information.

Toolkit of Instruments to Measure End-of-Life Care (TIME)
⟨www.chcr.brown.edu/pcoc/toolkit.htm⟩

Dr. Joan Teno has built a "toolkit" that provides a comprehensive list of tools and references, including measurement instruments related to palliative care. This site contains annotated bibliographies of tools for specific domains, including quality of life, pain and other symptoms, emotional and cognitive symptoms, functional status, survival time and aggressiveness of care, advance care planning, continuity of care, spirituality, grief and bereavement, and patient-centered reports and rankings (aka statisfaction) for the quality of care and caregiver well-being. Take special note of the Tools to Assess Grief ⟨www.gwu.edu/~cicd/toolkit/grief.htm⟩, including the "After-Death Bereaved Family Member Interview" and the Grief and Bereavement Literature Review.

Compassion Books
⟨www.compassionbooks.com⟩

Compassion Books offers many excellent books, audiotapes, and videos on the topics of grief, death, and dying. The resources have been collected from hundreds of publishers, both small and large, and have been carefully reviewed by knowledgeable professionals and others who have experience with grief, loss, and death.

The Compassionate Friends
⟨www.compassionatefriends.org/⟩

The Compassionate Friends is a national nonprofit, self-help support organization that offers friendship and understanding to bereaved parents, grandparents, and siblings. The mission of The Compassionate Friends is to assist families toward the positive resolution of grief following the death of a child of any age and to provide information to help others to be supportive.

The Dougy Center: The National Center for Grieving Children and Families
⟨www.dougy.org⟩

This center, based in Portland, Oregon, offers support services to children, teens, and adult caregivers grieving a death. The site has information about training, books, videos, and training manuals for those interested in constructing grief programs in their own communities.

Dr. John Grohol's Mental Health Page
⟨www.grohol.com⟩

A dedicated and Web-savvy mental health professional, Dr. Grohol has created a site with numerous links to resources and online support groups. Visitors may search for information on grief and bereavement.

Mothers Against Drunk Driving
⟨www.madd.org⟩

With more than 600 chapters across the United States, MADD's focus is to look for effective solutions to the drunk driving and underage drinking problems, while supporting those who have already experienced the pain of these senseless crimes.

OncoLink
⟨www.oncolink.com⟩

Full of links and information on cancer, ranging from diagnosis, treatment, clinical trials, to support, OncoLink contains many articles on death, grief, and bereavement. Find information on bereavement counseling here, as well as links to book reviews and additional resources about the grief process.

Suicide Information and Education Centre
⟨www.suicideinfo.ca⟩

The Suicide Information and Education Centre (SIEC) is a special library and resource center providing information on suicide and suicidal behavior. Click on the library and search with keywords to access the full range of this site's information and resources. Access a list of recommended reading on grief and loss in the aftermath of suicide at ⟨www.suicideinfo.ca/resources/booklists.pdf⟩.

Part Five: Promoting Better Pain Management in Long-Term Care Facilities

A. ORIGINAL TOOLS FROM CONTRIBUTORS

1. Tools from the Medical College of Wisconsin (MCW) Palliative Care Program

a. Facility Needs Assessment

Copyright © 2000 by the US Cancer Pain Relief Committee. Reprinted by permission of Elsevier Science. From Weissman DE, Griffie J, Muchka S, Matson S. Building an institutional commitment to pain management in long-term care facilities. *Journal of Pain and Symptom Management.* 2000;20(1):35–43.

Facility Needs Assessment

Date: _____

Facility Name: _____

Address: _____

Telephone: ( ) _____   FAX: ( ) _____

Director of Nursing: _____

Medical Director: _____

1. Number of beds in facility: _____

2. Specialty units: (check all that apply)

Alzheimer's   _____   Medicare   _____

Subacute   _____   Hospice   _____

Rehab   _____   Other (please state) _____

3. Does your facility contract with a hospice agency or agencies?
Yes _____   No _____

If yes, please list agencies: _____

4. Are Certified Medication Assistants utilized?
Yes _____   No _____

5. Is there a pharmacist on site?
Yes _____   No _____

6. Is infusion therapy provided? (IVs, Subcu, PCA, etc.)
Yes _____   No _____

If yes, how is the service provided?
Facility staff   _____   Contract agency   _____

---

7. List policies and procedures for pain management practices currently in place.

_____

_____

_____

_____

8. Are standardized pain assessment tools in place at this time?

For the cognitively intact resident?   Yes _____   No _____

For the cognitively impaired resident?   Yes _____   No _____

9. What is your current facility standard for when pain assessment is done?

(check all appropriate answers)

Admission   _____   Change of condition   _____

Monthly   _____   Change of medication   _____

Quarterly   _____   Annually   _____

Other (please explain)_____

No standard at this time   _____

b. Guidelines for Analgesic Drug Orders

MCW researchers developed these guidelines to help agencies formulate their own policies and procedures about the use of analgesics.

Guidelines for Analgesic Drug Orders

Purpose: The following criteria will serve as a guide for evaluating analgesic orders. The purpose is to assure appropriate use of analgesics based upon individual patient assessment. These guidelines are adapted from the AHCPR Standards for Acute and Cancer Pain Management.[1,2]

Critical Points

1. The character of the pain has been documented on assessment so that the health care provider writing the medical orders can determine the type of pain that the patient is experiencing. For example, burning, shooting pain has been characterized as neuropathic.
2. Drugs used for pain management are based upon severity of pain.
3. If an opioid is required for severe pain, morphine is the drug of choice. For acute pain, the route of choice is IV; for chronic pain, the route is po. If a patient is unable to take po medications, IV, subcutaneous, buccal, sublingual, rectal, and transdermal routes are considered before IM.
4. Patients who report constant pain should receive long-acting medication, with a short-acting medication ordered prn for breakthrough pain.
5. Long-acting oral analgesic agents are not used for the management of acute postoperative pain (first 48–72 hours).
6. Patients who report intermittent pain have medications ordered on a prn basis.
7. Only one combination analgesic (opioid and nonopioid, e.g., Vicodin, Tylenol #3) is ordered for prn breakthrough pain.
8. Only one opioid is ordered for continuous moderate to severe pain (e.g., continuous opioid infusion or MS Contin or Oramorph SR or Kadian or OxyContin, or Duragesic.)
9. Short-acting po opioids are ordered at intervals no longer than four hours.
10. Consider using adjuvant analgesics for nonopioid responsive neuropathic pain.
11. An appropriate plan for a bowel regimen is ordered.
12. A plan is in place for a pharmacologic and/or nonpharmacologic intervention for patients prior to activities that are reported to cause or increase pain.
13. A pain management flow sheet is initiated on all patients rating pain as moderate, that is, $\geq 5/10$, $\geq 3/5$, or $\geq 2/3$ on admission.

14. Orders for nonpharmacologic interventions are present and are clearly stated as part of the nursing and medical plan of care.
15. Meperidine (Demerol) is used only for short-term procedural pain. Doses of greater than 600 mg per 24 hours should be avoided.
16. Propoxyphene (Darvocet N, Darvon) is avoided due to weak analgesic effect and potential toxicity.[3]

REFERENCES

1. Acute Pain Management Guideline Panel. *Acute Pain Management: Operative or Medical Procedures and Trauma.* Clinical Practice Guideline. AHCPR Pub. No. 92-0032. Rockville, MD: Agency for Health Care Policy and Research, Public Health Service, U.S. Department of Health and Human Services, February 1992.
2. Jacox A, Carr DB, Payne R, et al. *Management of Cancer Pain Clinical Practice Guideline No. 9.* AHCPR Publication No. 94-0592. Rockville, MD: Agency for Health Care Policy and Research, U.S. Department of Health and Human Services, Public Health Service, March 1994.
3. Inturrisi, C, Colburn, W, Verebey, K, Dayton, H., Woods, G., O'Brien, C. Propoxyphene and norpropoxyphene kinetics after single and repeated doses of propoxyphene. *Clinical Pharmacology and Therapeutics.* February 1982:157–167.

c. Three-Person Pain Assessment Role-Playing Exercise

Copyright ©2000 MCW Research Foundation. Permission granted to modify or adopt provided written credit is given to the Medical College of Wisconsin. Reprinted with permission from Griffie J, Weissman DE. *Nursing Staff Education Resource Manual: A Six Session Inservice Education Program in Pain Management for Long-Term Care Facilities.* Milwaukee: Medical College of Wisconsin, 2000.

Three-Person Pain Assessment Role-Playing Exercise

NURSE INTERVIEWER SCENARIO

You are a nurse seeing Mrs. K., a 75-year-old female with degenerative arthritis. You met her once, shortly after she was first seen by your agency. You have been away for the past 10 days and return now to find that pain is reported to be an increasing problem. You are going to see her/care for her. All the information you have is that staff is increasingly concerned because she has been using/requesting more analgesics and appears to be a bit withdrawn. Her analgesic orders are for a hydrocodone/acetaminophen product, Tylenol #3, and Extra-Strength Tylenol. Mrs. K. is awaiting your visit.

PATIENT SCENARIO

History

You are Mrs. K., a 75-year-old woman with chronic arthritis. Two weeks ago, you were admitted to Happy Valley Care Center/Happy Valley Home Care following a fall and broken arm. Although the arm is healing well, you will likely need long-term institutional care as you are unable to care for yourself due to the arthritis and having no home support.

Your pain has become worse over the past month and it is limiting your mobility. You note an aching pain in both hips, the right hip worse than left, as well as your lower back and right shoulder. The pain had been intermittent for years, but for the past month it has been almost continuous. The right hip pain is the biggest problem. It is becoming more intense with movement, especially at night. The pain wakes you up at night and you have trouble falling back to sleep. The pain is much worse whenever you get out of bed. Your current pain score using a 0–10 scale is 5/10 and will go to an 8/10 at night and with movement. The pain never goes below 3/10. Your goal for pain relief is to be able to sleep at night without pain.

Up until six months ago you were able to get by with prn NSAIDs. Six months ago your doctor told you to stop the NSAID because there was something wrong with your kidneys. You are not sure what the problem is. Since then, you have been taking Tylenol #3 and a hydrocodone/acetaminophen product. Current medications orders:

- Tylenol Extra Strength, 1 tab po q 6 hours prn, general discomfort.
- Tylenol #3, 1 tab po q 6 hours, prn pain.
- Hydrocodone/acetaminophen, 1 tab po q 6 hours, prn for severe pain.

You have been asking for pain medication more frequently in the past week, although you really hate to take drugs. In fact, you think that some of the medication made you fall in the first place. Depending on the nurse that is working with you, you either receive 1 Tylenol #3 or 1 hydrocodone/acetaminophen every 6 hours. Tylenol #3 gives you no relief. The hydrocodone/acetaminophen starts working in about 30 minutes, reducing the pain from 8/10 to 3–4/10, but relief only lasts about three hours. A heating pad to your back has helped the back pain, but not the hip pain.

Social History

Prior to admission to the nursing home, you had been living alone. You are a widow with two children who live within 45 minutes of Happy Valley. You have noticed a decreased appetite over the past two weeks and have been less interested in social activities, preferring to stay in your bedroom. You are afraid that increasing pain will mean that you need surgery. Several years ago, your best friend had hip surgery and died a few days after the operation. You last saw your physician about two weeks ago, but did not tell him/her that the pain was getting worse because you feared he/she would insist on surgery.

Appearance, Affect, and Responses to Interviewer

During the interview, you should be seated and appear to be uncomfortable, often shifting position in your chair. Your affect should be depressed, with little expression, responding in short answers and frequent sighs. Your affect should indicate a "what does it matter" attitude. If asked, reply "Of course I'm depressed, I'm in pain. I probably will need surgery. I might as well be dead." Only if prompted about your concerns should you reveal that you are afraid of surgery because of what happened to your friend. Only if prompted should you reveal that you are afraid to tell your physician about the worsening pain because of your fear of surgery.

OBSERVER SCENARIO

Your job is to watch the interview process. Check off the following components of the assessment as they are completed. Once the pain assessment is completed, discuss the process and your observations with your team. Was the interviewer successful in obtaining a full assessment?

Location/s	yes _____	no _____
Description/quality	yes _____	no _____
Pain rating/intensity	yes _____	no _____
Patient goals for relief	yes _____	no _____
Pattern/timing	yes _____	no _____
Analgesic history	yes _____	no _____
Strategies that help	yes _____	no _____
Exacerbating activities	yes _____	no _____
Emotional state	yes _____	no _____
Support systems	yes _____	no _____
Effect on ADLs (including sleep)	yes _____	no _____

d. Pain Algorithms

Copyright © 2000 by MCW Research Foundation. Reprinted with permission. Permission granted to modify or adopt provided written credit is given to the Medical College of Wisconsin.

Nursing leaders in Wisconsin Long Term Care Coalition to Improve Pain Management believed there was a need for an educational tool that could guide nurses through the analgesic management of pain. Based on a complete pain assessment, algorithms were designed to guide nurses through the pharmacological and nonpharmacological management of pain. Pain is categorized as Mild (1-3), Moderate (4-6), or Severe (7-10). Using the algorithms, the nurse can suggest appropriate interventions for management of the resident's pain.

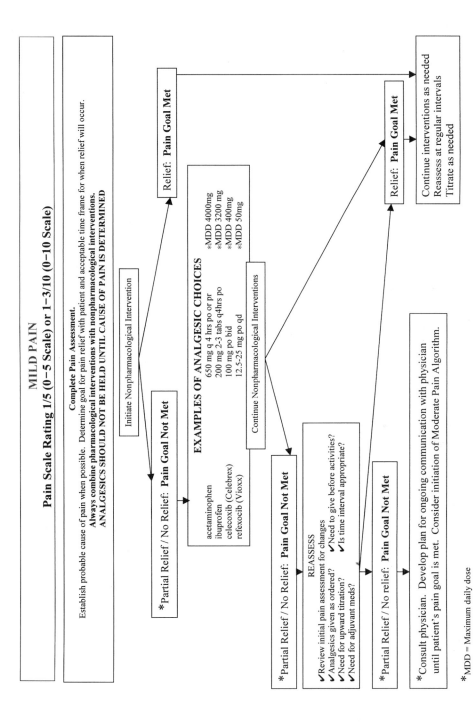

MILD PAIN
Pain Scale Rating 1/5 (0–5 Scale) or 1–3/10 (0–10 Scale)

Complete Pain Assessment.

Establish probable cause of pain when possible. Determine goal for pain relief with patient and acceptable time frame for when relief will occur.
Always combine pharmacological interventions with nonpharmacological interventions.
ANALGESICS SHOULD NOT BE HELD UNTIL CAUSE OF PAIN IS DETERMINED

Initiate Nonpharmacological Intervention

Relief: **Pain Goal Met**

*Partial Relief / No Relief: **Pain Goal Not Met**

EXAMPLES OF ANALGESIC CHOICES

acetaminophen	650 mg q 4 hrs po or pr	*MDD 4000mg
ibuprofen	200 mg 2-3 tabs q4hrs po	*MDD 3200 mg
celecoxib (Celebrex)	100 mg po bid	*MDD 400mg
refexocib (Vioxx)	12.5-25 mg po qd	*MDD 50mg

Continue Nonpharmacological Interventions

Relief: **Pain Goal Met**

Continue interventions as needed
Reassess at regular intervals
Titrate as needed

*Partial Relief / No Relief: **Pain Goal Not Met**

REASSESS
✔Review initial pain assessment for changes
✔Analgesics given as ordered? ✔Need to give before activities?
✔Need for upward titration? ✔Is time interval appropriate?
✔Need for adjuvant meds?

*Partial Relief / No relief: **Pain Goal Not Met**

*Consult physician. Develop plan for ongoing communication with physician
until patient's pain goal is met. Consider initiation of Moderate Pain Algorithm.

*MDD = Maximum daily dose

©2000 MCW Research Foundation
Permission granted to modify or adopt provided written credit is given to the Medical College of Wisconsin.

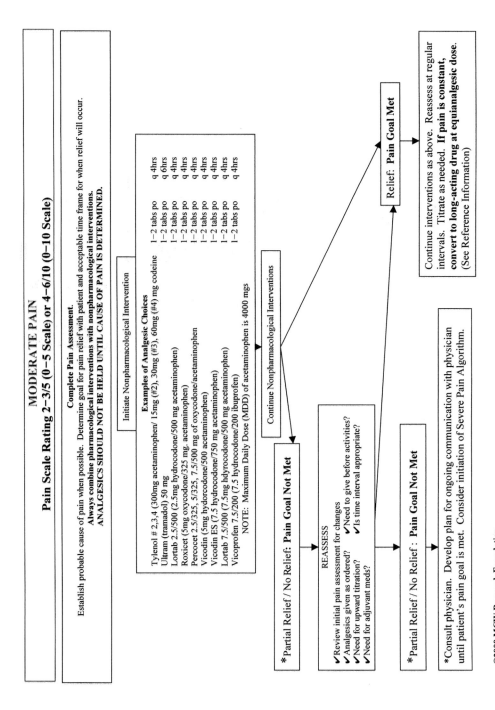

MODERATE PAIN
Pain Scale Rating 2–3/5 (0–5 Scale) or 4–6/10 (0–10 Scale)

Complete Pain Assessment.

Establish probable cause of pain when possible. Determine goal for pain relief with patient and acceptable time frame for when relief will occur. Always combine pharmacological interventions with nonpharmacological interventions. **ANALGESICS SHOULD NOT BE HELD UNTIL CAUSE OF PAIN IS DETERMINED.**

Initiate Nonpharmacological Intervention

Examples of Analgesic Choices

Tylenol # 2,3,4 (300mg acetaminophen/ 15mg (#2), 30mg (#3), 60mg (#4) mg codeine	1–2 tabs po	q 4hrs
Ultram (tramadol) 50 mg	1–2 tabs po	q 6hrs
Lortab 2.5/500 (2.5mg hydrocodone/500 mg acetaminophen)	1–2 tabs po	q 4hrs
Roxicet (5mg oxycodone/325 mg. acetaminophen)	1–2 tabs po	q 4hrs
Percocet 2.5/325, 5/325, 7.5/500 mg of oxycodone/acetaminophen	1–2 tabs po	q 4hrs
Vicodin (5mg hydorcodone/500 acetaminophen)	1–2 tabs po	q 4hrs
Vicodin ES (7.5 hydrocodone/750 mg acetaminophen)	1–2 tabs po	q 4hrs
Lortab 7.5/500 (7.5mg hdyrocodone/500 mg acetaminophen)	1–2 tabs po	q 4hrs
Vicoprofen 7.5/200 (7.5 hydrocodone/200 ibuprofen)	1–2 tabs po	q 4hrs

NOTE: Maximum Daily Dose (MDD) of acetaminophen is 4000 mgs

Continue Nonpharmacological Interventions

Relief: **Pain Goal Met**

Continue interventions as above. Reassess at regular intervals. Titrate as needed. **If pain is constant, convert to long-acting drug at equianalgesic dose.** (See Reference Information)

*Partial Relief / No Relief: **Pain Goal Not Met**

REASSESS

✔Review initial pain assessment for changes
✔Analgesics given as ordered?   ✔Need to give before activities?
✔Need for upward titration?   ✔Is time interval appropriate?
✔Need for adjuvant meds?

*Partial Relief / No Relief : **Pain Goal Not Met**

*Consult physician. Develop plan for ongoing communication with physician until patient's pain goal is met. Consider initiation of Severe Pain Algorithm.

©2000 MCW Research Foundation
Permission granted to modify or adopt provided written credit is given to the Medical College of Wisconsin.

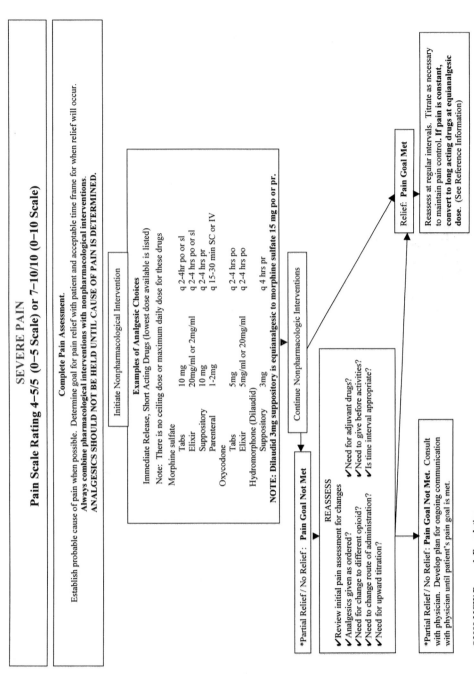

SEVERE PAIN

Pain Scale Rating 4–5/5 (0–5 Scale) or 7–10/10 (0–10 Scale)

Complete Pain Assessment.

Establish probable cause of pain when possible. Determine goal for pain relief with patient and acceptable time frame for when relief will occur. **Always combine pharmacological interventions with nonpharmacological interventions. ANALGESICS SHOULD NOT BE HELD UNTIL CAUSE OF PAIN IS DETERMINED.**

Initiate Nonpharmacological Intervention

Examples of Analgesic Choices

Immediate Release, Short Acting Drugs (lowest dose available is listed)
Note: There is no ceiling dose or maximum daily dose for these drugs

Morphine sulfate
Tabs	10 mg	q 2–4hr po or sl
Elixir	20mg/ml or 2mg/ml	q 2–4 hrs po or sl
Suppository	10 mg	q 2–4 hrs pr
Parenteral	1–2mg	q 15–30 min SC or IV

Oxycodone
Tabs	5mg	q 2–4 hrs po
Elixir	5mg/ml or 20mg/ml	q 2–4 hrs po

Hydromorphone (Dilaudid)
Suppository	3mg	q 4 hrs pr

NOTE: Dilaudid 3mg suppository is equianalgesic to morphine sulfate 15 mg po or pr.

Continue Nonpharmacologic Interventions

*Partial Relief / No Relief : **Pain Goal Not Met**

REASSESS

✔Review initial pain assessment for changes
✔Analgesics given as ordered?   ✔Need for adjuvant drugs?
✔Need for change to different opioid?   ✔Need to give before activities?
✔Need to change route of administration? ✔Is time interval appropriate?
✔Need for upward titration?

*Partial Relief / No Relief : **Pain Goal Not Met.** Consult with physician. Develop plan for ongoing communication with physician until patient's pain goal is met.

Relief: **Pain Goal Met**

Reassess at regular intervals. Titrate as necessary to maintain pain control. **If pain is constant, convert to long acting drugs at equianalgesic dose.** (See Reference Information)

©**2000 MCW Research Foundation**
Permission granted to modify or adopt provided written credit is given to the Medical College of Wisconsin.

2. Subacute and Extended Care: Pain Management Guidelines

Copyright © 2000 by Franciscan Woods, Covenant Healthcare. Reprinted with permission.

---

1. Initiate
   - Admission—scheduled analgesics
   - Admission—pain acknowledged or observed
   - Any new report of pain or change in pain status

2. Use
   - For up to three days with initiation of scheduled analgesics (continue use if patient's goal not met)
   - All prn pain management medications
   - While pain is a Medicare/insurance qualifier

3. Evaluate
   - Evaluate data according to pain management principles

B. WEBSITES RELATED TO CONTRIBUTORS

End-of-Life Physician Education Resource Center (EPERC)
⟨www.eperc.mcw.edu/⟩

The purpose of EPERC is to assist physician educators and others in locating high-quality, peer-reviewed training materials. This website supports the identification and dissemination of information on end-of-life training materials, publications, conferences, and other opportunities. EPERC is supported by The Robert Wood Johnson Foundation and located at the Medical College of Wisconsin.

Mayday PainLink
⟨www.edc.org/PainLink/⟩

An extensive list of annotated links to pain-related websites can be found at ⟨www.edc.org/PainLink/plweb.html⟩. Mayday *PainLink* is a virtual community of institutions and practitioners committed to improving their pain management practices developed by staff at the Center for Applied Ethics and Professional Practice at EDC in Newton, Massachusetts, and initially funded by the Mayday Fund. The site has both public and members-only sections.

Palliative Medicine Program at the Medical College of Wisconsin
⟨www.mcw.edu/pallmed⟩

This site offers a variety of educational services and information for health care professionals about pain management and end-of-life care.

Wisconsin Cancer Pain Initiative: A World Health Organization Demonstration Project
⟨www.wisc.edu/wcpi/wcpihome.htm⟩

The "Making pain management a priority in all health care settings" page includes a short description of the Medical College of Wisconsin Long-Term Care Pain Management program featured in Part Five of *Innovations*. The WCPI is a member of the American Alliance of Cancer Pain Initiatives. Viewers can click on a map to look up their state's initiative.

C. OTHER RELEVANT WEBSITES

American Association of Homes and Services for Aging (AAHSA)
⟨www.aahsa.org/⟩

The American Association of Homes and Services for the Aging (AAHSA) represents nonprofit organizations dedicated to providing high-quality health care, housing, and services to the nation's elderly. The website includes information on the organization, its resources, and programs.

American College of Health Care Administrators (ACHCA)
⟨www.achca.org⟩

ACHCA is a professional society dedicated to advancing the standards of long-term care, from skilled nursing to assisted living to subacute care.

American Medical Directors Association (AMDA)
⟨www.amda.com/⟩

This is a national professional organization committed to the continuous improvement of the quality of patient care by providing education, advocacy, information, and professional development for medical directors and other physicians who practice in long-term care. Viewers can enter "pain management" into the search feature to create a list of documents that can be downloaded, including "CNA Retention—What the Medical Director Can Do to Help."

American Pain Society
⟨www.ampainsoc.org/⟩

The mission of the American Pain Society is to serve people in pain by advancing research, education, treatment, and professional practice. APS is a nonprofit membership society and welcomes broad participation from all disciplines. Resources include the most recent information on public policy updates, reference tools, and advances in pain management.

Cancer Pain Release
⟨www.whocancerpain.wisc.edu⟩

This publication of the World Health Organization Collaborating Center for Policy & Communications in Cancer Care now posts back issues online. The issue entitled "Resources for Patient Education About Pain Relief in Cancer," Vol. 13, Nos. 3–4, 2000, offers an invaluable listing of books, videos, websites, CD-ROMS, and audiotapes in English, French, and Spanish.

Center for Community Change
⟨www.communitychange.org⟩

An organization committed to helping poor people improve their communities and change policies and institutions that affect their lives by developing their own strong organizations. This site has specific pages with resources devoted to "Changing Policies" and "Building Organizations" that may be of particular interest to pain management change agents.

Community–State Partnerships to Improve End-of-Life Care
⟨www.midbio.org/npopolicybrief.htm⟩

This page lists policy briefs, which can be downloaded. Issues 5, 6, 7, and 8 focus on improving long-term care. Issue 5: "Promising Educational Initiatives for Staff, Regulators, and Families" is of particular interest. Community–State Partnerships is housed at the Midwest Bioethics Center in Kansas City, Missouri. Myra Christopher, president and CEO of Midwest Bioethics Center, is national director of the Community–State Partnerships program. A grant program funded by The Robert Wood Johnson Foundation, Community–State Partnerships to Improve End-of-Life Care has awarded $11.25 million to 23 broad-based, multidisciplinary coalitions working to promote policy change and support for high-quality, comprehensive end-of-life care.

Cynergy Group, Opioid Conversion Calculator
⟨www.cynergygroup.org⟩

The Opioid Conversion Calculator is a tool for determining equi-analgesic doses of opioid drugs. Viewers can input the patient's current regimen and specify a drug to convert to, and the calculator gives you an equivalent dose of the new drug. A wide variety of drugs and routes can be specified. The Calculator is a synthesis of widely accepted equivalencies, recent information reported in the literature, clinical experience, and collaboratively acquired expert opinions. The site has also tried to include distilled "best practice" recommendations where possible. Go to the following page for disclaimer and proceed to the opioid converter: ⟨www.cynergygroup.org/cgi-bin/calc/disclaimer.asp⟩.

The John A. Hartford Foundation Institute for Geriatric Nursing
⟨www.hartfordign.org⟩

This site has a Publications page, which includes a newsletter called *Try This*. Each issue focuses on a particular topic (geriatric depression, pain assessment, cognitive impairment) and reviews a sample tool for assessing this domain. The tools are posted and can be downloaded. See for example, "Assessing Pain in Older Adults," which includes the visual analog scale and a faces scale for measuring pain intensity.

Joint Commission on Accreditation of Healthcare Organizations (JCAHO) Pain Standards for 2002
⟨www.jcaho.org/htba/index.htm⟩

This page of the JCAHO website features various topics of interest, including general information, clarifications, revisions, frequently asked questions, field reviews, manual supplements, and more.

National Association of Directors of Nursing Administration in Long Term Care (NADONA)
⟨www.nadona.org⟩

Of particular interest are archived articles from *The Director* found at ⟨www.nadona.org/director.html⟩. These include a three-part series on the evolving role of CNAs, as well as a short piece on pain entitled "Pain On Hold!"

Wong–Baker FACES Pain Rating Scale
⟨www.us.elsevierhealth.com/WOW/faces.html⟩

Explanation of the development of this popular pain rating scale as well as a version that can be downloaded and necessary permission forms to complete if users wish to use the scale.

Part Six: Quality of Life

A. ORIGINAL TOOLS FROM CONTRIBUTORS

Edmonton Palliative Care Program
⟨www.palliative.org/⟩

The Clinical Assessment page at ⟨www.palliative.org/pc_assess.html⟩ lists the Edmonton Program's most useful tools with hotlinks to each. Readers can access the Edmonton Symptom Assessment System (ESAS), both the numerical and visual analog versions, and a graph for tracking changes in scores over time and the Edmonton Comfort Assessment Form (ECAF), a tool for caregivers to complete when patients are unable to complete the ESAS themselves, and other tools. (The ECAF was previously known as the Edmonton Discomfort Assessment Form.) The Edmonton Palliative Care Program site is organized for both professional and nonprofessional audiences, offered by the Division of Palliative Medicine, Department of Oncology, University of Alberta, Edmonton, Canada, and the Edmonton Regional Palliative Care Program. Content includes clinical information, patient assessment tools, cancer material, and links to related resources.

B. WEBSITES RELATED TO CONTRIBUTORS

European Association for Palliative Care (EAPC)
⟨www.eapcnet.org⟩

Founded with 40 individual members in 1988, the EAPC is now a federation of national and regional societies of palliative care representing more than 25,000 individuals across Europe and other parts of the world. This website includes information about the EAPC and its activities, with details about publications and congresses, and a directory of participating organizations with contact names and addresses. Many resources are available in French and English. Professor Vittorio Ventafridda is one of the founders of this organization. A number of *Innovations* editorial board members play leadership roles in this organization, including Stein Kaasa, MD, PhD, who currently serves as president of the EAPC.

International Association for Hospice & Palliative Care (IAHPC)
⟨www.hospicecare.com⟩

IAHPC is a nonprofit international organization dedicated to the development and improvement of palliative care worldwide by encouraging countries to come up with their own models of palliative care provision rather than expecting them to copy models more appropriate to affluent countries. IAHPC is currently chaired by Dr. Eduardo Bruera, founder of the Edmonton Program. The October 2000 issue of the IAHPC newsletter includes "The Palliative Medicine Argentine Program–FEMEBA" by Dr. Roberto Wenk, Dr. Mariela Bertolino, and Dr. Jorge Ochoa at ⟨www.hospicecare.com/Newsletters/october2000/page4.html⟩.

C. OTHER RELEVANT WEBSITES

Dying Well
⟨**www.dyingwell.org**⟩

Dr. Ira Byock, past president of the American Academy of Hospice and Palliative Medicine, provides written resources for patients and families facing life-limiting illness and their professional caregivers. You may find the *Missoula–Vitas Quality of Life Index*, a measurement tool for assessing quality of life during the final stages of terminal illness at ⟨www.dyingwell.com/MVQOLI.htm⟩.

Toolkit of Instruments to Measure End-of-Life Care (TIME)
⟨**www.chcr.brown.edu/pcoc/toolkit.htm**⟩

Dr. Joan Teno has built a "toolkit" that provides a comprehensive list of tools and references, including measurement instruments related to palliative care. This site contains annotated bibliographies of tools, including a substantial section on quality of life instruments at ⟨www.chcr.brown.edu/pcoc/Quality.htm⟩.

Appendix C: End-of-Life Care Websites

We have divided these wide-ranging sites into five groups: general sites of interest, journals, professional associations, professional education, and a list of targeted grant-giving organizations.

A. SITES OF GENERAL INTEREST

Administration on Aging
⟨www.aoa.gov/⟩

This US government agency website has many useful resources for older Americans and family caregivers.

Aging with Dignity
⟨www.agingwithdignity.org⟩

Aging with Dignity is a nonprofit organization with the goal of improving care for those near the end of life. *Five Wishes*, an easy-to-use advance directive, is available at this site.

American Alliance of Cancer Pain Initiatives (AACPI)
⟨www.aacpi.org/⟩

As voluntary grassroots organizations, Cancer Pain Initiatives are composed of nurses, physicians, pharmacists, representatives of clinical care facilities, higher education, and government. These state-based initiatives and their participants provide education, training, information, and organizational support to health care providers, cancer patients, and their families.

American Association of Retired Persons (AARP)
⟨www.aarp.org⟩

AARP is a nonprofit, nonpartisan membership organization focused on improving the quality of life for all people as they get older. The Health and Wellness page provides a wide range of links to information on issues such as caregiving, Medicare, and coping with loss.

American Pain Foundation
⟨www.painfoundation.org⟩

This nonprofit information resource and patient advocacy organization aims to improve the quality of life of persons with pain and to raise public awareness and understanding of pain. The site includes a pain care bill of rights, pain action guide, legislative updates, and patient information that can be searched by disease type, as well as other resources and links. The foundation is based in Baltimore, Maryland.

Americans for Better Care of the Dying (ABCD)
⟨www.abcd-caring.org⟩

ABCD is a nonprofit public advocacy organization, which publishes *ABCD Exchange*, a bimonthly newsletter online at ⟨www.abcd-caring.org/newsletter.htm⟩ and in print.

Association internationale Ensemble contre la douleur
⟨www.sans-douleur.ch/⟩

Ensemble contre la douleur is a francophone nonprofit organization founded in 1997 in Geneva, Switzerland, by leaders in pain management. The site hosts information primarily in French, including information on its two campaigns: *Vers un hôpital sans douleur* (Toward a Pain-Free Hospital) and *Vivre avec le cancer sans douleur* (Living with Cancer without Pain). The site hosts a bibliography with both French and English entries, as well as a resource page providing links to French and English pain-related websites and a listserv for French speakers.

Australasian Palliative Link International (APLI)
⟨petermac.unimelb.edu.au/apli/index.html⟩

APLI is a group of palliative care personnel and supporters interested in the development of palliative care globally. The site includes past newsletters, links, and names and addresses of palliative care contacts in Australia. The site is hosted by the Peter MacCallum Cancer Institute site in East Melbourne, Australia.

Beth Israel Medical Center's *Stop Pain*! Website
⟨www.StopPain.org⟩

This is an extensive site, addressing many topics in depth. Find resources for educators, physicians, nurses, patients, and caregivers. It includes many tools for supporting patients and their families.

Cancer.gov
⟨www.cancer.gov/⟩

Cancer.gov is a gateway to recent and accurate cancer information and resources from the National Cancer Institute, the federal government's principal agency for cancer research. The section on support and resources at ⟨www.cancer.gov/cancer_information/support/⟩ contains information on hospice and transitional care planning for both patients and health professionals. The site also includes a thorough list of links to other cancer-related websites.

Cancer Pain Release
⟨www.whocancerpain.wisc.edu⟩

Cancer Pain Release is the publication of the World Health Organization global communications program to improve cancer pain control and palliative and supportive care.

Carers: Government Information for Carers
⟨www.carers.gov.uk⟩

A British governmental site with a great deal of information for family caregivers, called *carers* in the United Kingdom.

Center for Applied Ethics and Professional Practice, Education Development Center, Inc.
⟨www.edc.org/CAE⟩

The center designs, implements, and evaluates solutions to health and community problems, accomplishing change in ways that respect the often-conflicting values of a pluralistic society. A major current focus is on ensuring the wise and effective use of biomedical technologies and scientific knowledge to improve the quality of life and the health of the public. *Innovations in End-of-Life Care* is one of several current projects designed to improve terminal and palliative care.

Center for Bioethics, University of Minnesota
⟨www.bioethics.umn.edu⟩

The mission of the University of Minnesota's Center for Bioethics is to advance and disseminate knowledge concerning ethical issues in health care and the life sciences. The center conducts original interdisciplinary research, offers educational programs and courses, fosters public discussion and debate through community service activities, and assists in the formulation of public policy.

Center to Advance Palliative Care (CAPC)
⟨www.capcmssn.org⟩

Established by The Robert Wood Johnson Foundation to promote wider access to excellent palliative care in hospitals and health systems in the United States, CAPC aims to provide assistance in the planning, development, and implementation of hospital and health system based palliative care programs. The site includes a variety of resources and materials.

Center to Improve Care of the Dying (CICD)
⟨www.medicaring.org⟩

The Center to Improve Care of the Dying is an interdisciplinary team of committed individuals engaged in research, public advocacy, and education activities to improve the care of the dying and their families.

Centers for Medicare & Medicaid Services (CMS)
⟨www.hcfa.gov⟩

Formerly the Health Care Financing Administration, this U.S. government agency provides health insurance for 74 million Americans through Medicare, Medicaid, and other government programs.

Dying Well
⟨www.dyingwell.org⟩

Dr. Ira Byock, past president of the American Academy of Hospice and Palliative Medicine, provides written resources for patients and families facing life-limiting illness and their professional caregivers.

Edmonton Palliative Care Program
⟨www.palliative.org/⟩

An extensive palliative care site for both professional and nonprofessional audiences offered jointly by the Division of Palliative Medicine and Department of Oncology at the University of Alberta in Edmonton, Canada, and the Edmonton Regional Palliative Care Program. The purpose of the site is to acquaint the visitor with the basic philosophy of palliative care and its workings in large or small centers. Content includes clinical information, patient assessment tools, cancer material, and links to related resources.

Growth House, Inc.
⟨www.growthhouse.org/⟩

A search engine that offers access to a comprehensive collection of reviewed resources for end-of-life care. The Inter-Institutional Collaborating Network on End-of-Life Care (IICN) links health care organizations through a shared network.

The Hastings Center
⟨www.thehastingscenter.org⟩

The Hastings Center is an independent, nonpartisan, interdisciplinary research institute that studies ethical and social issues in medicine, the life sciences, and the professions. The center publishes *The Hastings Center Report*, a bimonthly journal featuring articles on a variety of issues in bioethics.

Health on the Net Foundation
⟨www.hon.ch/home.html⟩

Health on the Net Foundation (HON) is a nonprofit organization, headquartered in Geneva, Switzerland. The purpose of the foundation is to advance the development and application of new information technologies, notably in the fields of health and medicine. The Health on the Net Code of Conduct (HONcode) has been created in response to concerns expressed to the Health on the Net Foundation regarding the varying quality of medical and health information currently available on the Web.

HELP: Helpful Essential Links to Palliative Care
⟨www.dundee.ac.uk/MedEd/help/welcome.htm⟩

This site is hosted by the Centre for Medical Education at the University of Dundee in collaboration with the U.K. charity Macmillan Cancer Relief. Intended for an audience of medical professionals, this site has an emphasis on management of advanced cancer. Content includes pain management, management of distressing symptoms, communication issues, and emotional support for persons facing death and their loved ones.

Hospice Cares Online Community
⟨www.hospice-cares.com/oc_home.html⟩

The purpose of this site is to promote the hospice philosophy by providing an interactive gathering place for the online hospice community and a comprehensive index of the hospice related information available over the Internet and by adding to that body of information with original articles. The site includes an extensive list of links, articles, and a chat forum.

Hospice Foundation of America (HFA)
⟨www.hospicefoundation.org/⟩

Hospice Foundation of America is the nation's largest charity whose sole mission is to promote the hospice concept of care and is supported primarily by individual donations. Information about annual teleconferences available from the home page. For 2002, the initiative was "Living with Grief: Loss in Later Life." These teleconferences are available for purchase on video, dating back to 1996.

Initiative to Improve Palliative Care for African-Americans (IIPCA)
⟨www.iipca.org⟩

Founded by Dr. Richard Payne, Dr. LaVera Crawley serves as executive director and Terrie Reid Payne serves as deputy director. IIPCA promotes a research, education and policy agenda to improve care for African American patients facing serious illness. The website and organization are supported by the Open Society Institute and the Project on Death in America. See the Activities page for a list of recent publications and presentations.

Institute for Healthcare Improvement (IHI)
⟨www.ihi.org/⟩

IHI is a Boston-based, independent, nonprofit organization working since 1991 to accelerate improvement in health care systems in the United States, Canada, and Europe by fostering collaboration, rather than competition, among health care organizations.

Joint Commission on Accreditation of Healthcare Organizations (JCAHO)
⟨www.jcaho.org⟩

The Joint Commission evaluates and accredits nearly 18,000 health care organizations and programs in the United States. An independent, nonprofit organization, JCAHO is the nation's predominant standards-setting and accrediting body in health care.

Last Acts Fact Sheets
⟨www.lastacts.org/scripts/la_res01.exe?FNA=FactSheets__Ala_res_NewHome_html⟩

Last Acts has compiled a series of "fact sheets" and "tip sheets" that present basic information on a variety of aspects of end-of-life care. These fact sheets cover topics such as starting the conversation about end-of-life care, challenges for working caregivers, advance planning, legal issues, nutrition, and others in a clear and candid way that family members may find helpful. Readers are encouraged to print and reproduce any of these sheets. Adobe Acrobat Reader is required to view these documents. Download Acrobat for free at ⟨www.adobe.com⟩.

Mayday Pain Project
⟨www.painandhealth.org⟩

The major goal of the Mayday Pain Project is to increase awareness and provide objective information concerning the treatment of pain. This site is set up to be an index for visitors and contains carefully chosen links and resources.

Midwest Bioethics Center (MBC)
⟨www.midbio.org⟩

MBC is a community-based ethics center dedicated to the mission of integrating ethical considerations into health care decision making throughout communities. The center offers workshops and educational programs for professionals and lay people alike, assists health care providers throughout the United States in grappling with ethical issues in clinical work, and assists administrators in integrating ethics into the organizational structure. MBC houses the Community–State Partnerships to Improve End-of-Life Care grant program funded by The Robert Wood Johnson Foundation.

National Alliance for Caregiving (NAC)
⟨www.caregiving.org/⟩

The National Alliance for Caregiving is a nonprofit joint venture created in 1996 to support family caregivers of the elderly and the professionals who serve them. NAC strives to increase public awareness of issues facing family caregivers.

National Council for Hospice and Specialist Palliative Care Service
⟨www.hospice-spc-council.org.uk/index.htm⟩

The council is the representative and coordinating body for all those working in hospice and specialist palliative care in England, Wales, and Northern Ireland. The website provides a number of publications on hospice care intended both for the general public and for professional care providers, including a directory of all hospice services in the United Kingdom. An excellent source of links and palliative care resources worldwide, this site includes the "ABC of Palliative Care," a compilation of key articles published in the *British Medical Journal* between September 1997 and February 1998 at 〈www.hospice-spc-council.org.uk/informat.ion/abcofpc.htm〉.

National Family Caregivers Association (NFCA)
〈**www.nfcacares.org/**〉

NFCA is a grass-roots organization created to educate, support, empower and speak up for the millions of Americans who care for chronically ill, aged, or disabled loved ones. Through its services in the areas of information and education, support and validation, public awareness and advocacy, NFCA strives to minimize the disparity between a caregiver's quality of life and that of mainstream Americans.

OncoLink
〈**www.oncolink.com/**〉

A comprehensive guide to cancer information provided by the University of Pennsylvania Cancer Center. Designed for both professionals and patients, the site includes information on specific types of cancer, medical specialties, global resources, psychological support and personal experiences, clinical trials, conferences and meetings, and prevention and detection.

On Our Own Terms: Moyers on Dying
〈**www.pbs.org/wnet/onourownterms/**〉

In a four-part, six-hour television series, Bill Moyers crosses the country from hospitals to hospices to homes to capture stories and candid conversations from multiple perspectives on this topic. The website features end-of-life care resources and community action plans, as well as providing readers with the tools to engage in an ongoing dialogue about facing the end of life. Viewers can order videotapes of the series.

PainLink
〈**www.edc.org/PainLink/**〉

PainLink is a virtual community of institutions and practitioners committed to improving their pain management practices developed by staff at the Center for Applied Ethics and Professional Practice at EDC in Newton, Massachusetts and was initially funded by the Mayday Fund. The site has both public and members-only sections.

An extensive annotated list of pain-related websites and resources is available to the public.

Palliative-medicine mailbase
⟨www.mailbase.ac.uk/lists/palliative-medicine/⟩

A listserv for clinicians and others involved and interested in palliative care. Based in the United Kingdom, it regularly includes voices from South Africa, New Zealand, Australia, and the continent. The list allows for discussion on all aspects of palliative medicine and care. Its aim is to facilitate communication between practitioners involved in research or educational initiatives and also allow the exchange of information or advice related to clinical matters.

Partnership for Caring: America's Voices for the Dying
⟨www.partnershipforcaring.org⟩

Formerly "Choice in Dying," this is a national nonprofit organization devoted to raising consumer expectations and demand for excellent end-of-life care. The site offers resources for talking about end-of-life choices and provides state-specific advance directive documents.

Princess Royal Trust for Carers
⟨www.carers.org/⟩

This organization sponsors Carer Centres throughout the United Kingdom for the six million adult carers there. (Carer is the British term for an unpaid family caregiver.) They estimate that there are also 50,000 young carers, or people under the age of eighteen, who are providing care for parents or siblings. The site offers an online carer discussion group and chat room, as well as an extensive list of links to sites based in the United Kingdom on a wide variety of related topics.

Ready or Not: A Study Guide for Medical School Faculty
⟨www.edc.org/Innovations/ReadyorNot⟩

This sixteen-page study guide by Anna L. Romer, EdD, and Mildred Z. Solomon, EdD, is designed for medical school faculty to use in conjunction with the video *Ready or Not*. The video is an intimate behind-the-scenes portrait of a small number of first-year medical students enrolled in the course "Living with Life-Threatening Illness" at Harvard Medical School. The course, developed by Susan Block, MD, and J. Andrew Billings, MD, pairs first-year medical students with terminally ill patients. In this study guide, medical faculty will find ways to use the video to enhance students' comfort and skill caring for dying patients and, more generally, to enhance their ability to forge meaningful relationships with patients, regardless of health status.

Supportive Care of the Dying: A Coalition for Compassionate Care
⟨www.careofdying.org/⟩

The three priorities of the coalition are research, developing models of comprehensive, community-based, supportive care for dying people, and creating a professional development program. The site has a variety of tools and resources and back issues of *Supportive Voice*, the newsletter of the coalition.

TALARIA: The Hypermedia Assistant for Cancer Pain Management
⟨www.talaria.org⟩

This site has a hypermedia presentation of the *Clinical Practice Guideline on the Management of Cancer Pain*, a publication of the Agency for Healthcare Research and Quality (formerly AHCPR). The site also has other resources for technical information on pain, including the complete text of *Current and Emerging Issues in Cancer Pain: Research and Practice*, edited by C.R. Chapman and K. Foley and published by Lippincott-Raven in 1993.

Toolkit of Instruments to Measure End-of-Life Care (TIME)
⟨www.chcr.brown.edu/pcoc/toolkit.htm⟩

Dr. Joan Teno has built a "toolkit" that provides a comprehensive list of tools and references, including measurement instruments related to palliative care. This site contains annotated bibliographies of tools for specific domains, including quality of life, pain and other symptoms, emotional and cognitive symptoms, functional status, survival time and aggressiveness of care, advance care planning, continuity of care, spirituality, grief and bereavement, and patient-centered reports and rankings (aka statisfaction) for the quality of care and caregiver well-being.

Wisconsin Cancer Pain Initiative:
A World Health Organization Demonstration Project
⟨www.wisc.edu/wcpi/wcpihome.htm⟩

The Wisconsin Cancer Pain Initiative is dedicated to overcoming the barriers that prevent the relief of cancer pain. It is a voluntary, grass-roots organization of health care professionals and representatives of higher education and government. It has five major areas of service: public education, patient education, professional education, regulatory updates, and making pain management a priority in all health care settings.

B. JOURNALS

American Journal of Hospice and Palliative Care
⟨www.hospicejournal.com/pn01000.html⟩

British Medical Journal (BMJ)
⟨www.bmj.com⟩

N.B. Access is free. For BMJ's collected resources on palliative care see
⟨www.bmj.com/cgi/collection/palliative_medicine⟩.

European Journal of Palliative Care (EJPC)
⟨www.ejpc.co.uk⟩

Innovations in End-of-Life Care, online
⟨www.edc.org/lastacts/⟩

International Journal of Palliative Nursing
⟨www.internationaljournalofpalliativenursing.com⟩

Journal of Pain and Symptom Management
⟨www.elsevier.nl/locate/jpainsymman⟩

Journal of Palliative Care
⟨www.ircm.qc.ca/bioethique/english/publications/
journal_of_palliative_care⟩

**Journal of Palliative Medicine in collaboration with Innovations in
End-of-Life Care**
⟨www.liebertpub.com/jpm⟩

Journal of the American Geriatrics Society (JAGS)
⟨www.blackwellscience.com/journals/geriatrics/index.html⟩

Palliative Medicine
⟨www.arnoldpublishers.com/journals/pages/pal-med02692163.htm⟩

Progress in Palliative Care
⟨www.leeds.ac.uk/lmi/ppc/intro.html⟩

C. PROFESSIONAL ASSOCIATIONS

American Academy of Hospice and Palliative Medicine (AAHPM)
⟨www.aahpm.org/⟩

The AAHPM is an organization of physicians and other medical professionals dedicated to excellence in palliative medicine and the prevention and relief of suffering among patients and families by providing education and clinical practice standards, fostering research, and facilitating personal and professional development of its members.

American Academy on Physician and Patient (AAPP)
⟨www.physicianpatient.org/⟩

AAPP is a professional society dedicated to research, education, and professional standards in doctor–patient communication. Its goal is no less than to change the practice of medicine by helping doctors to relate more effectively to each patient. The site includes announcements about upcoming training courses and publications.

American Association of Critical-Care Nurses
⟨www.aacn.org⟩

The American Association of Critical-Care Nurses (AACN) is the world's largest specialty nursing organization with more than 68,000 members. Information about the AACN is available at this website or by calling 800-899-AACN.

American College of Health Care Administrators (ACHCA)
⟨www.hospitalconnect.com⟩

A professional society dedicated to advancing the standards of long-term care, from skilled nursing to assisted living to subacute care.

American Hospital Association (AHA)
⟨www.hospitalconnect.com⟩

The American Hospital Association is a national organization, with close to 5,000 institutional, 600 associate, and 37,000 personal members, that represents and serves all types of hospitals, health care networks, and their patients and communities. Each year AHA hosts the Circle of Life Award to recognize and reward excellence in end-of-life care. Application information is available online.

American Medical Directors Association
⟨www.amda.com/⟩

This is a national professional organization committed to the continuous improvement of the quality of patient care by providing education, advocacy, information, and professional development for medical directors and other physicians who practice in long-term care.

American Pain Society
⟨www.ampainsoc.org/⟩

The mission of the American Pain Society is to serve people in pain by advancing research, education, treatment, and professional practice. APS is a nonprofit membership society and welcomes broad participation from all disciplines. Resources include the most recent information on public policy updates, reference tools, and advances in pain management.

American Society of Bioethics & Humanities (ASBH)
⟨www.asbh.org/⟩

The purpose of the ASBH is to promote the exchange of ideas and foster multi-disciplinary, interdisciplinary, and interprofessional scholarship, research, teaching, policy development, professional development, and collegiality among people engaged in all the endeavors related to clinical and academic bioethics and the health-related humanities.

American Society of Law, Medicine & Ethics (ASLME)
⟨www.aslme.org/⟩

The mission of ASLME is to provide high-quality scholarship, debate, and critical thought to the community of professionals at the intersection of law, health care, policy, and ethics.

American Society on Aging (ASA)
⟨www.asaging.org/⟩

Offers educational programs, conferences, and publications. Recently sponsored a joint conference with the National Council on Aging, which included a pre-conference special program "Meeting the Needs of Family Caregivers."

Association for Death Education and Counseling (ADEC)
⟨www.adec.org⟩

Founded in 1976, the Association for Death Education and Counseling (ADEC) is a multidisciplinary organization dedicated to improving the quality of death education, counseling, and caregiving; to promoting research; and to providing support, stimulation, and encouragement to its members and those studying and working in death-related fields.

European Association for Palliative Care (EAPC)
⟨www.eapcnet.org/⟩

The EAPC was founded with 40 individual members in 1988. It is now a federation of national and regional societies of palliative care, representing more than 25,000 individuals across Europe and other parts of the world. The website serves as an information source about the EAPC and its activities, including descriptions of publications and congresses. The site also offers a directory of participating organizations around the world, including contact names and addresses. Many resources are available in French and English. A number of *Innovations* editorial board members play leadership roles in this organization, including Dr. Stein Kaasa, MD, PhD, who is the president.

Hospice & Palliative Nurses Association (HPNA)
⟨www.hpna.org/index.htm⟩

The purpose of this professional association is to exchange information, experiences, and ideas; to promote understanding of the specialties of hospice and palliative nursing; and to study and promote hospice and palliative nursing research.

International Association for Hospice & Palliative Care (IAHPC) ⟨www.hospicecare.com⟩

IAHPC is a nonprofit international organization dedicated to the development and improvement of palliative care worldwide by encouraging countries to develop their own model of palliative care provision rather than expecting them to copy models more appropriate to affluent countries. IAHPC is currently chaired by Dr. Eduardo Bruera. Readers can join the IAHPC at this website, as well as access its many resources. These include "World Palliative Care Reports," which are short summaries of state of the art palliative care in specific countries, a monthly newsletter, an extensive ethics page, updates on IAHPC activities, and links to key palliative care journals and organizations.

International Association for the Study of Pain (IASP) ⟨www.iasp-pain.org/⟩

The International Association for the Study of Pain is an international, multidisciplinary, nonprofit professional association dedicated to furthering research on pain and improving the care of patients with pain. *Pain: Clinical Updates*, the IASP newsletter, is available on the Web at <www.iasp-pain.org/PCUOpen.html>. The IASP homepage also offers extensive links to other pain resources at ⟨www.iasp-pain.org/ressopen.html⟩.

National Funeral Directors Association: NFDA Online ⟨www.nfda.org/⟩

Information for funeral directors as well as a search feature to find a funeral home or online obituary. Includes consumer protection guidelines and other consumer resources.

National Hospice and Palliative Care Organization (NHPCO) ⟨www.nhpco.org/⟩

Formerly the NHO, this is the largest nonprofit membership organization representing hospice and palliative care programs and professionals in the United States.

Sociedad Española de Cuidados Paliativos (SECPAL) ⟨www.secpal.com/⟩

This is the website for the Spanish Association of Palliative Care; all content is in Spanish. Extensive information on the association as well a clinical guide to palliative care entitled *Guias y Manuales: Cuidados Paliativos—Recomendaciones de la Sociedad Española de Cuidados Paliativos* are available at ⟨www.secpal.com/guia_gral.html⟩ and access to the journal *Medicina Paliativa* is at ⟨www.secpal.com/revi_gral.html⟩.

D. PROFESSIONAL EDUCATION

Education for Physicians on End-of-Life Care (EPEC) ⟨www.epec.net⟩

This project specializes in physician education and training through its core curriculum on essential clinical competencies required to provide quality end-of-life care.

End-of-Life Nursing Education Consortium (ELNEC) ⟨www.aacn.nche.edu/elnec⟩

A comprehensive, national education project to improve end-of-life care by nurses, ELNEC is a partnership of the American Association of Colleges of Nursing (AACN) and the Los Angeles-based City of Hope Cancer Center, supported by The Robert Wood Johnson Foundation. *Peaceful Death: Recommended Competencies and Curricular Guidelines for End-of-Life Nursing Care* and other publications and resources can be found here.

End of Life Physician Education Resource Center (EPERC) ⟨www.eperc.mcw.edu/⟩

The purpose of EPERC is to assist physician educators and others in locating high-quality, peer-reviewed training materials. This website supports the identification and dissemination of information on end-of-life training materials, publications, conferences, and other opportunities. EPERC is supported by The Robert Wood Johnson Foundation and is located at the Medical College of Wisconsin.

John A. Hartford Foundation
Institute of Geriatric Nursing
⟨www.hartfordign.org⟩

The institute was founded in 1996 and is housed at New York University, at the Steinhardt School of Education, Division of Nursing. This site includes training information and publications to enhance geriatric nursing knowledge and skill. See the "What's New" page for the Try This series, edited by Meredith Wallace, RN, MSN, PhD (cand). This series offers short descriptions of best practices in nursing care to older adults and specific assessment tools that can be downloaded. Past topics include among others: cognitive assessment, geriatric depression scale, sexuality.

Palliative Medicine Program at the Medical College of Wisconsin ⟨www.mcw.edu/pallmed⟩

This site offers a variety of educational services and information for health care professionals about pain management and end-of-life care.

VA Faculty Leaders Project for Improved Care at the End of Life ⟨www.va.gov/oaa/flp/⟩

The VA Faculty Leaders Project is a two-year initiative of the Office of Academic Affiliations, Department of Veterans Affairs (VA). Its goal is to develop benchmark curricula for end-of-life care, and palliative care as well as strategies for their implementation, for training resident physicians. This project is supported by The Robert Wood Johnson Foundation.

E. TARGETED GRANT-GIVING ORGANIZATIONS

The King's Fund ⟨www.kingsfund.org.uk/⟩

The King's Fund is an independent health care charity working for better health in London and across the United Kingdom. It gives grants and carries out research and development work to bring about better health policies and services.

Last Acts ⟨www.lastacts.org⟩

A national coalition to improve care and caring near the end of life. The goal of the campaign is to bring death-related issues out in the open and to help individuals and organizations to pursue better ways to care for the dying. This site has many resources and links to grantees.

National Institutes of Health (NIH) ⟨www.nih.gov⟩

One of eight health agencies of the U.S. Public Health Services, the NIH is a major funder of scientific research in the United States.

Project on Death in America (PDIA) ⟨www.soros.org/death⟩

PDIA's mission is to understand and transform the culture and experience of dying and bereavement through initiatives in research, scholarship, the humanities, and the arts and to foster innovations in the provision of care, public education, professional education, and public policy. The PDIA site provides a comprehensive overview of the Project on Death in America Faculty Scholars program, grants program, and funding initiatives.

Promoting Excellence in End-of-Life Care
⟨**www.promotingexcellence.org/**⟩

A national program office of The Robert Wood Johnson Foundation with direction and technical assistance provided by the Practical Ethics Center at the University of Montana. Promoting Excellence is currently funding 22 projects to improve palliative care in different parts of the United States.

United Hospital Fund (UHF)
⟨**www.uhfnyc.org/**⟩

The United Hospital Fund's mission is to shape positive change in health care for the people of New York. Its Palliative Care Initiative has gathered extensive data about hospital deaths and is now developing, implementing, and testing a variety of approaches to improve care for dying patients in five hospitals. Site includes the executive summary of *The Challenge of Caring for Patients near the End of Life: Findings from the Hospital Palliative Care Initiative*.

Contributors and Core Team

Mary Arata, BSN, RN, OCN, has worked with oncology and hospice patients for twenty years in both acute care and long-term care settings. She regularly lectures on pain management to senior groups, played a key role in the development of a subacute oncology unit at Franciscan Woods, part of Covenant Healthcare in Brookfield, Wisconsin, and provides ongoing education to the staff there. Currently, Ms. Arata is a member of the Covenant Pain Resource Team. In addition, she serves on a community advisory board for the development of palliative care programs in long-term care settings.

Ellen Bartoldus, MSW, CSW, earned her master's in social work from Fordham University and a certificate from Columbia University and the Albert Einstein College of Medicine in Bioethics and the Medical Humanities. She is currently the administrator of Lutheran Home for the Aging, part of Wartburg Lutheran Services (WLS), which operates four nursing homes, four adult day health care programs, a long-term home health care program, and a mobile meals program. Ms. Bartoldus also holds the position of ethics officer with WLS and chairs its interfacility ethics committee. She has been co-principal investigator for the Brooklyn Hospital/Wartburg Caregivers Project since its inception in 1998 and has been responsible for providing social work supervision and workshop design and implementation to the project.

Mariela Bertolino, MD, earned her medical degree from the Universidad Nacional de La Plata, Argentina, in 1987. She completed a residency in Internal Medicine at Sanatorio Güemes y Hospital E. Fernandez in Buenos Aires, Argentina, and then went on to receive further training at the Edmonton General Hospital, Palliative Care Unit in Alberta, Canada, and the Centre de Soins Palliatifs at the Hôtel Dieu in Paris. Since 1996, Dr. Bertolino has served as the medical director of the Palliative Care Unit at the Hospital Tornú–FEMEBA Foundation, where she has also coordinated the Curso de Postgrado de Actualización en Cuidados Paliativos.

Douglas Bishop has been a teacher to students ranging in age from 1 to 90 and currently teaches English as a Second Language at a middle school in Lowell, Massachusetts. As a poet, he has performed in places as far away as Israel and Guatemala, but he now appears primarily in the Boston area.

Marilyn Bookbinder, PhD, RN, is the director of nursing, Department of Pain Medicine and Palliative Care, Beth Israel Medical Center, and adjunct assistant professor at New York University School of Nursing. She is the former director of nursing research at Memorial Sloan–Kettering Cancer Center and currently principal investigator for "Benchmarking for the Care of the Imminently Dying Inpatient: A CQI Project to Improve End-of-Life Care." She serves on the faculty for the National Oncology Nursing Society's Research Utilization Short Course and Evaluator for the Project Team on End-of-Life Care. In addition, she serves on the faculty for a United Hospital Fund of New York and Center to Improve Care of the Dying/Institute for Healthcare Improvement quality improvement initiative in palliative care. She has authored and lectured extensively on building best practices using quality improvement models.

Nereida Borrero, RN, MSN, GNP, is a geriatric nurse practitioner and coordinator of the Family Caregiver Project at the Brooklyn Hospital Center. Ms. Borrero has extensive experience in the field of home care. She is also the project coordinator of Redes En Acción, an NCI-sponsored project dedicated to cancer research awareness and training for Hispanics.

Carleen Brenneis, RN, MHSA, is program director, Regional Palliative Care Program, Capital Health Authority. Ms. Brenneis is an oncology nurse who gained interest in palliative care working with Drs. Neil MacDonald and Eduardo Bruera as a nurse in clinical research in pain and symptom management. She completed a master's degree in health service administration to further her interest in community-based programming and palliative care. Ms. Brenneis is also a member of the palliative care working group for the Canadian Strategy for Cancer Control.

David Browning, LICSW, BCD, is a founding partner of the Sturbridge Group <www.sturbridgegroup.com>, a bereavement training and consultation consortium. He is also founder and director of Safe Passage, a bereavement support program located in Harvard, Massachusetts. He is on the faculty of the End-of-Life Care Certificate Program at Smith College School for Social Work, funded by the Project on Death in America. His chapter, "Fragments of Love: Explorations in the Ethnography of Suffering and Professional Caregiving," will be included in a forthcoming textbook on end-of-life care published by Columbia University Press. In his teaching with bereavement and end-of-life care professionals, he focuses on the many levels of meaning at work in the encounter between caregiver and patient, including the centrality of the caregiver's own life experience with loss and suffering.

Christian Juul Busch is a chaplain at Rigshospitalet in Copenhagen, Denmark, where he has worked for more than 15 years with gravely ill patients and bereaved family members. He is an active member of the European Association for Palliative Care and first presented this essay as a plenary talk at the association's biennial conference in Palermo, Italy, in April 2001.

Kathy Carroll, BSN, RN, serves as bereavement services coordinator for both the infant loss program and the system-wide Bereavement Care Track at St. Vincent's Hospital and Health Systems in Indianapolis, Indiana.

Yvette Colón, MSW, ACSW, BCD, is the director of Education & Internet Services at the American Pain Foundation in Baltimore, Maryland <www.painfoundation.org>. Prior to this appointment, she was the program coordinator of Online Services at Cancer Care, Inc., in New York City. Ms. Colón has been facilitating online support groups since 1993 and telephone support groups since 1995. She has been on the Internet for almost 20 years and written, supervised, consulted, and lectured about online group therapy for more than 10 years.

Richard Della Penna, MD, is a geriatrician and has been with the Southern California Permanente Medical Group for 25 years. He has been physician-in-charge of continuing care services, hospice, and home health at Kaiser Permanente's San Diego Medical Center for the past 15 years. He is also the regional elder care co-ordinator for the Southern California region of Kaiser Permanente and the clinical lead for Kaiser Permanente Care Management Institute's Elder Care Initiative. Dr. Della Penna has particular interest in developing and implementing systems that better address the needs of older adults in an integrated managed care environment. His focus has been in the areas of geriatric interdisciplinary team training, dementia, depression, frailty, and end-of-life care. Dr. Della Penna is currently a member of the Institute of Medicine's Committee to Improve Quality in Long Term Care and the National Advisory Committee of The Robert Wood Johnson Foundation's national program office *Promoting Excellence in End-of-Life Care.*

John E. Ellershaw, MA, FRCP, has been medical director at the Marie Curie Centre Liverpool and Consultant in Palliative Medicine at the Royal Liverpool University Hospital since 1994. He earned his master of arts in the philosophy of health care and his areas of research interest include ethical issues in palliative care and care of the dying patient. Dr. Ellershaw is an honorary senior lecturer at the University of Liverpool and is actively involved in the development of the new medical undergraduate curriculum, including the palliative care contribution. Dr. Ellershaw also spends one month every year working in Rotterdam as visiting professor based at the Erasmus University.

Robin L. Fainsinger, MBchB, CCFP, graduated from the University of Cape Town in South Africa in 1981. In 1991, he completed the first fellowship in palliative medicine at the University of Alberta in Edmonton, Canada. He continues to reside in Edmonton, where he has been director of the Palliative Care Program at the Royal Alexandra Hospital since October 1994. He has recently become the director of the Division of Palliative Care Medicine, clinical director for the Regional Palliative Care Program, and director of Palliative Care for the Caritas Health Group. Dr. Fainsinger is an associate professor in the Division of Palliative Care Medicine, Department of Oncology, at the University of Alberta. He is active in education and research and has published articles on a number of palliative care topics, with an interest in dehydration, delirium, sedation at the end of life, and a classification system for cancer pain. He has more than 70 publications in journals and book chapters.

Susie Fitzhugh specializes in documentary photography of people, whether she is working on assignment or on her own, more long-term projects. Her focus has always been the vitality of human interactions. Ms. Fitzhugh has been photographing for nonprofits and foundations in schools, hospitals, and other institutions on the East Coast, where she lived for over twenty-five years, and now in

Seattle. Additionally, Ms. Fitzhugh has been working on a personal project documenting education in other cultures, most recently in Mexico and Nicaragua. An extensive look at the scope of her work can be seen at <www.susiefitzhugh.com>.

Kathleen M. Foley, MD, is an attending neurologist in the Pain and Palliative Care Service at Memorial Sloan–Kettering Cancer Center (MSKCC) in New York City. She is professor of neurology, neuroscience, and clinical pharmacology at Weill Medical College of Cornell University and holds the chair of the Society of Memorial Sloan–Kettering Cancer Center in Pain Research. In 1981, Dr. Foley was appointed chief of the newly formed Pain Service within the Department of Neurology at MSKCC. It was the first designated pain service in a cancer center in the United States. Dr. Foley was elected to the Institute of Medicine of the National Academy of Science for her national and international efforts in the treatment of patients with cancer pain. She is currently director of the Project on Death in America of the Open Society Institute. This project is focused on transforming the culture of death in America through funding initiatives in research, scholarship, and clinical care.

Dr. Foley has focused her career on the assessment and treatment of patients with cancer pain. She has defined the epidemiology, classified the common causes, and defined the common pain syndromes that occur in this patient population. With her colleagues, she has developed scientific guidelines for the treatment of cancer pain with analgesic drug therapy through clinical pharmacologic studies of opioid drugs.

Dr. Foley is a past president of the American Pain Society and a past member of the Board of Directors of the American Academy of Neurology and the International Association of the Study of Pain. She has received numerous awards and honors, including the Distinguished Service Award from the American Cancer Society, the David Karnovsky Award from the American Society of Clinical Oncology, and the Frank Netter Award of the American Academy of Neurology. As an expert consultant to the World Health Organization Cancer and Palliative Care Unit and as past director of a WHO Collaborating Center at Memorial Sloan–Kettering Cancer Center, Dr. Foley chaired three expert committees resulting in the publication of three WHO Monographs: *Cancer Pain Relief* (1986), *Cancer Pain Relief and Palliative Care* (1990), and *Cancer Pain and Palliative Care in Children* (1996).

Julie Griffie, RN, MSN, CS, AOCN, CHPN, received her baccalaureate in nursing from Florida State University, Tallahassee, Florida, and her master's degree in nursing from Marquette University, Milwaukee, Wisconsin. Ms. Griffie has served as the clinical nurse specialist for the Medical College of Wisconsin (MCW) Palliative Care Program since the program's inception in 1993. Her background includes extensive work in oncology nursing, roles in associate degree and BSN nursing education, and management and education in long-term care. In her role at MCW, her focus is to change the culture of end-of-life care through multidiscipline practice changes at Froedtert Hospital. In the community setting, her role has focused on the development and implementation of the project entitled Institutionalizing Improved Pain Management Practices in Long-Term Care Settings both locally and nationally. She also has holds clinical teaching positions at the University of Wisconsin/Milwaukee School of Nursing and the University of Wisconsin/Madison School of Nursing. She was recently recognized by the Delta Gamma Chapter of Sigma Theta Tau with their award for Outstanding Clinical Practice.

Karen S. Heller, PhD, is a senior research associate in the Center for Applied Ethics and Professional Practice at Education Development Center, Inc. (EDC), where she is a co-investigator on a national project, *Enhancing Family-centered Care of Children Living with Life-threatening Conditions*, and serves as associate editor of *Innovations in End-of-Life Care*. At EDC, Dr. Heller formerly directed the national continuing medical education and quality improvement programs *Decisions near the End of Life* and *Decisions near the End of Life: Focus on Cancer Care*. A medical anthropologist with extensive research experience in urban community and clinical settings, Dr. Heller has been a researcher in studies concerning end-of-life decision-making among cancer and AIDS patients from diverse ethnic backgrounds being treated at a large, urban hospital; the management of chronic illness in frail, elderly people living in the community; social interaction among patients and staff in a nursing home; and factors influencing whether HIV-infected adults seek early treatment intervention. She also has worked as a writer and editor and was formerly director of the Communications Office in the Division of Cancer Control, Dana–Farber Cancer Institute. Dr. Heller received her BA from Sarah Lawrence College, her MA from the University of Chicago, and her PhD from the University of California at San Francisco and Berkeley and was a Post-Doctoral Research Scholar at the Stanford University Center for Biomedical Ethics.

Stein Kaasa, MD, PhD, is chair of the Palliative Medicine Unit at the Department of Oncology, Trondheim University Hospital. Additionally, he is a professor of palliative medicine on the faculty of medicine, The Norwegian University of Science and Technology. Dr. Kaasa works as a clinician in the palliative care unit. He specialized in medical oncology and radiotherapy at the Norwegian Radium Hospital. In 1993, he received the first chair in palliative medicine in the Nordic countries and moved to Trondheim, Norway, to establish the university-based Palliative Care Program. Dr. Kaasa has been working in the area of quality of life assessment and clinical trials for more than 15 years. He has published extensively in several areas of clinical research, primarily in palliative oncology and palliative medicine. He served as chairman of the EORTC Study Group on Quality of Life and was one of the investigators of the development of the EORTC QLQ-C30, a well-known instrument for measuring quality of life. Dr. Kaasa was also part of the International Quality of Life Assessment Group (IQOLA) for the international validation of the SF-36. He is an active member of the European Association for Palliative Care (EAPC) Research Network and currently serves as president of the EAPC.

Robin F. Kramer, MS, RN, PNP, has been a clinical nurse specialist/pediatric nurse practitioner at the University of California San Francisco (UCSF) Children's Hospital in the division of pediatric oncology since 1983. She coordinates pediatric outpatient services while also functioning in the clinical nurse specialist/nurse practitioner role. Ms. Kramer is often called on to present on the care of children with cancer. Her most recent focus has been on pediatric palliative care, and she serves on an educational task force involved in planning interdisciplinary end-of-life care workshops for UCSF staff. She recently acted as a clinical collaborator with Betty Davies, PhD, RN, on a research proposal on the influence of cultural beliefs and practices on pediatric end-of-life care. Eight years ago, she initiated the development of the Family Bereavement Retreat Weekend for pediatric oncology and bone marrow transplant families whose children have died. After the June 2000 retreat, she approached several individuals in the pediatric administration with the idea of starting a multidisciplinary pediatric palliative care task force to improve end-of-life care at UCSF. As a result of this task force's ongoing efforts, they launched a pediatric palliative care consultative service in spring 2002.

John Larkin, MD, co-directs the Family Caregiver Initiative at the Brooklyn Hospital Center, where he also serves as an attending in general internal medicine. In addition, Dr. Larkin serves as director of medical student affairs in the Department of General Internal Medicine. Dr. Larkin earned his MD from the Albert Einstein College of Medicine and completed his residency at New York University Medical Center at Bellevue Hospital and Memorial Sloan–Kettering.

Roger Lemoyne began his work in photojournalism with coverage of the crisis in the Horn of Africa in 1991 and has worked regularly for UNICEF and UNHCR (United Nations High Commissioner for Refugees) since then and photographed in more than 30 countries worldwide. His photographs have won multiple awards, including World Press Photo, NPPA (National Press Photographers Association), the Ernst Haas Golden Light Award, and others. Mr. Lemoyne's work has been exhibited in many venues, including an accompaniment to the International Conference on Children in War (2000) and the World Press Photo exhibition (1999), that traveled globally for one year. His photography can be seen online at <www.living-lessons.org> as well as at <www.rogerlemoyne.com>.

Carol Levine is the director of the United Hospital Fund's Families and Health Care Project. She also directs The Orphan Project: Families and Children in the HIV Epidemic, which she founded in 1991. She was the director of the Citizens Commission on AIDS in New York City from 1987 to 1991. As a senior staff associate of The Hastings Center, she edited the *Hastings Center Report*. In 1993, she was awarded the MacArthur Foundation Fellowship for her work in AIDS policy and ethics. Ms. Levine is the editor of *Always on Call: When Illness Turns Families into Caregivers* (2000), published by the United Hospital Fund.

Neil MacDonald, CM, MD, FRCP(C), FRCP(Edin.), LLD(HC), is a medical oncologist and former cancer center administrator who is currently working at the

Centre for Bioethics (Clinical Research Institute of Montreal) and at McGill University. In addition, he works in the Palliative Care Programme of the Royal Victoria Hospital, Montreal. With respect to work in the field of palliative care education, he has edited *The Canadian Palliative Care Curriculum* (in conjunction with the Canadian Palliative Care Education Group) and, more recently, a textbook entitled *Palliative Medicine: A Case-based Manual*, based on the Curriculum. He also serves as a co-editor of the *Oxford Textbook of Palliative Medicine*.

Sandra Matson, BSN, RN, MA, C, received her BSN from Carroll College, Waukesha, Wisconsin, and her MA in bioethics from the Medical College of Wisconsin. She is the clinical MIS/ancillary manager for Lakeland Health Care Center. Ms. Matson has co-authored numerous articles on pain management in long-term care settings and is recognized as a leader in bioethics education in Wisconsin.

Sandra Muchka, RN, MS, CS, CHPN, joined the Palliative Care Program at the Medical College of Wisconsin as a clinical nurse specialist in March 1997. The responsibilities of this role include nursing assessment of patients referred to the Palliative Care Consultation Service, coordinating the grant-funded Roxane Visiting Nurse Scholar Program in Palliative Care, and participating in grant-funded educational programs designed to work with long-term care facilities in the area of pain management. Ms. Muchka's background includes experience as an oncology nurse in the acute care and ambulatory settings and in home hospice nursing. She is a member of the Oncology Nursing Society, Southeastern Wisconsin Oncology Nursing Society, American Association for Cancer Education, American Society of Pain Management Nurses, and Hospice and Palliative Nurses Association. She has co-authored articles related to palliative care, equianalgesic conversion for opioids, and improving pain management practices in the area of long-term care.

Jeffrey N. Nichols, MD, is chief of geriatrics at Cabrini Medical Center in Manhattan, medical director of the Cabrini Center for Nursing and Rehabilitation and the St. Cabrini Nursing Homes as well as the Sr. Josephine Tsieu and Monsignor Terence Attridge Adult Day Health Care Centers, and assistant medical director for geriatrics and palliative care of the Cabrini Hospice. A 1976 graduate of Cornell University Medical College, Dr. Nichols completed his internship and residency in internal medicine at St. Vincent's Hospital in New York. He is board certified in internal medicine and in hospice and palliative care and was awarded a Certificate of Added Qualifications in Geriatrics. He is clinical associate professor of medicine and geriatrics at Mount Sinai Medical School and adjunct assistant professor of medicine (geriatrics and gerontology) at Cornell's Weill Medical College. Additionally, he is co-director of the New York City Long-Term Care Ethics Network and vice-president of the New York Medical Directors Association. Dr. Nichols serves on advisory panels to the Alzheimer's Association.

Mimi Pattison, MD, is board certified in internal medicine, nephrology, and hospice and palliative medicine. She is also an EPEC trained physician (Education for Physicians on End of Life Care). Besides maintaining a busy private medical practice, Dr. Pattison is the medical director for Palliative Care Services and *Improving Care through the End of Life* for Franciscan Health Systems, which includes three hospitals, two long-term care facilities, hospice, and an alliance with seven primary care community clinics. She is chair of the Franciscan Regional Ethics Committee and board president of Compassionate Choices, a statewide, nonprofit, community-based organization that offers referrals to supportive services for patients with serious or life-threatening illness. In addition, Dr. Pattison is medical director for Manor Care, a long-term, skilled nursing, and specialty care unit facility.

Russell K. Portenoy, MD, is chairman, Department of Pain Medicine and Palliative Care, Beth Israel Medical Center, and professor of neurology, Albert Einstein College of Medicine. He is past president of the American Pain Society, current secretary of the International Association for the Study of Pain, and trustee of the American Board of Hospice and Palliative Medicine. He served as co-principal investigator on the American Medical Association's project, Education for Physicians in End-of-Life Care. He is editor-in-chief of the *Journal of Pain and Symptom Management*, associate editor for *Clinical Sciences of Pain*, and editor for the Palliative Care Section for *Cancer Investigation*. In addition, he has been an active clinical investigator in the fields of opioid pharmacology, pain and symptom epidemiology, analgesic trials, and quality-of-life research. Dr. Portenoy is the author or editor of 12 books and more than 350 papers.

Anna L. Romer, EdD, is a senior research associate at the Center for Applied Ethics and Professional Practice at Education Development Center, Inc. (EDC). A developmental psychologist and educator with a strong research background in medical education and physician development, Dr. Romer served on the executive steering committee for the National Task Force on End-of-Life Care in Managed Care, a project conducted by EDC with funding from The Robert Wood Johnson Foundation. In this capacity she was a senior author of the group's report: *Meeting the Challenge: Twelve Recommendations for Improving End-of-Life Care in Managed Care*. She was a member of the faculty at the 1999 seventh annual summer seminar, "Talking Ourselves to Death: Narratives and Caregiving at the End of Life," sponsored by the Center for Literature, Medicine, and the Health Care Professions at Hiram College in Hiram, Ohio. Bilingual in French and English as well as conversant in Polish, she has extensive experience living abroad. Dr. Romer received her BA degree from the University of Massachusetts at Amherst, her MAT from the School for International Training at the Experiment in International Living (now World Learning) in Brattleboro, Vermont, a CAS in counseling and consulting psychology, and her EdD in human development and psychology from the Harvard Graduate School of Education in Cambridge, Massachusetts.

Eleanor Rubin is an artist and a lecturer, whose works can be seen in many permanent collections, from the Museum of Fine Arts, Boston, to the Centrum Masereel, Kesterlee, Belgium. For more than 20 years, her talents have been drawn on at the MFA in Boston as its coordinator of access for audiences with disabilities. Elly is a recipient of a grant from the Massachusetts Council on the Arts and Humanities, which allowed her to create a series of prints for the *Museum Without Walls* project. These commissioned prints circulate to prisons and hospitals and other institutional settings. Additionally, she is a founding artist/contributor to *The Art Connection*, which places the work of older artists in settings such as homeless shelters and elder housing. Her studio and home are in West Newton, Massachusetts.

Alison Ryan was educated at Oxford University in the 1970s, reading philosophy, politics, and economics. She was involved in the disability movement, working as a volunteer in the United Kingdom and in Europe. After leaving Oxford, she worked initially in the UK civil nuclear industry as an economist. In 1983, she met her future husband, a man with complex health and disability problems stemming from severe hemophilia. She decided to change her career track and in 1985 became the chief executive of Horticultural Therapy, a nonprofit organization, working in therapeutic horticulture to benefit people with all kinds of special needs throughout the United Kingdom. At that same time, she married and became the carer of his mother, who had severe dementia and lived with the two of them. At the time, the concept of carers was relatively unknown, and no help was available to support those who were looking after people with such demanding care needs at home. Ms. Ryan was an early member of the Carers National Association, which started to lobby for improvements to this situation. In the 1990s, Ms. Ryan became involved with local mental health services, serving as a member of the board of the Somerset Partnership NHS and Social Care Trust, which provided all National Health Service mental health services in her part of the country. Integrating her life experience as a carer and her administrative experience in the nonprofit sector, she became chief executive of the Princess Royal Trust for Carers in 1999. Founded in 1991, the Princess Royal Trust for Carers is the largest organization providing comprehensive services to carers in the United Kingdom.

Phyllis R. Silverman, PhD, is professor emerita at the Massachusetts General Hospital (MGH) Institute of Health Professions. In addition, she is a lecturer in Social Welfare in the Department of Psychiatry at Massachusetts General Hospital and Harvard Medical School. She has been an active educator, researcher, and clinician focusing on bereavement for more than three decades. Her work is recognized both in the United States and abroad. In her early work she developed the concept of widow-to-widow peer support and directed the project that put this idea into practice. This project demonstrated the value of social support and of mutual help for widows. More recently she was co-principal investigator and project director of the MGH Child Bereavement Study, a longitudinal study of the impact of the death of a parent on dependent children. She is still analyzing data from this study, looking at the data with a more qualitative lens to try to capture what grief looks like in children and how this experience affects their lives. Based on findings from this research, she has challenged the concept of detachment and letting go as necessary aspects of the bereavement process. Dr. Silverman currently serves on the research commit-tee of the National Hospice and Palliative Care Organization and teaches as an adjunct professor in the Smith College School for Social Work End-of-Life Pro-gram. She has just been appointed a visiting scholar at the Brandeis Women's Research Center, where she will continue to pursue her long-held interest in as-pects of experience that are unique to women, such as childbearing and moth-ering, and how these experiences influence women's responses to loss. She was one of the founders of The Children's Room, a program for bereaved children and their families that serves the greater Boston community, for which she serves on the board and facilitates a parent's group. In this work, she finds a real-world opportunity to test out the merit of some of her research findings and to vali-date the importance of volunteers' using some of their own experience with loss to help bereaved children and their parents.

Holly D. Sivec is a research assistant at the Center for Applied Ethics and Pro-fessional Practice at Education Development Center, Inc. (EDC). Prior to joining the *Innovations* staff, Holly worked in both the publishing and the consulting in-dustry as a business and technical editor. She also brings an international aware-ness to her work, stemming from her experience at Harvard Business School co-ordinating executive education programs for executives from across the globe. Holly holds a BA in English and writing from Susquehanna University in Selins-grove, Pennsylvania, as well as a graduate certificate in publishing from Emerson College in Boston. She is an active fiction writer whose projects span such top-ics as family, health, history, psychology, and travel.

Samantha Libby Sodickson was staff editor for *Innovations* from January 2000 to July 2001. She is currently working on a master's degree in broadcast journal-ism from Emerson College.

Mildred Z. Solomon, EdD, is vice-president of Education Development Center, Inc. (EDC), an internationally renowned nonprofit research and development or-ganization based in Newton, Massachusetts, and director of EDC's Center for Ap-plied Ethics and Professional Practice. An expert in adult learning and organiza-tional change, Dr. Solomon has more than 25 years' experience in researching, designing, and evaluating a wide variety of education and quality improvement programs for health professionals, health care organizations, and the public. She is particularly experienced in applying social science research methods to the ex-ploration of values questions and bioethical uncertainty in medicine and public health. Dr. Solomon has served as principal investigator on numerous grants from federal agencies, including the Agency for Health Research and Quality, the Cen-ters for Disease Control and Prevention, and the Health Resources and Services Administration, on topics ranging from end-of-life care to pain management, or-gan donation, and sexually transmitted disease prevention. She co-founded the *De-cisions Near the End of Life program*, which has helped more than 230 health care institutions across the United States improve the care of dying patients and their families and is currently spearheading a national initiative in pediatric palliative care. She was also chair of the National Task Force on End-of-Life Care in Managed Care, which released its report, *Meeting the Challenge: Twelve Recommendations for Improving End-of-Life Care in Managed Care*, in 1999. Dr. Solomon frequently consults to government agencies, foundations, universities, and national organizations, including, for example, the Institute of Medicine and The Robert Wood Johnson Foundation. She received her BA degree from Smith College and her doctorate from Harvard University.

Judith A. Spross, PhD, RN, AOCN, FAAN, is a senior scientist at the Center for Applied Ethics & Professional Practice at Education Development Center, Inc. (EDC). She is a registered nurse with extensive experience in oncology nursing, pain management, institutional change, and health professional education, and has published articles on these topics. She has been co-investigator (1996–2000) and project director (1998–2000) for Mayday PainLink, a virtual community of staff from 60 hospitals whose goal was to improve pain management. She currently serves as project director for the HRSA-funded project, Increasing Organ Donation by Enhancing End-of-Life-Care: A Family-Centered Intervention. She was also co-investigator on an AHRQ-funded intervention to improve cancer pain management in primary care. She received a BSN from Villanova University, an MS in nursing from the Medical College of Virginia, and a doctorate in nursing from Boston College. She is certified in oncology nursing. Honors include the 1985 ONS Schering Award for Excellence in Practice, election to the Academy of Nursing (1992), and the 1993 Distinguished Alumna Award (Villanova University). She is the author of acclaimed textbooks on advanced practice nursing, most recently the *Advanced Practice Nursing: An Integrative Approach*, 2d ed.

James A. Thorson is professor and chairman, Department of Gerontology, University of Nebraska at Omaha. He is a fellow of the Gerontological Society of America. Dr. Thorson is the author or co-author of eight books, 14 book chapters, and more than 70 journal articles on gerontology, death and dying, and psychological coping.

Georganne Trandum, RN, OCN, is a certified oncology and bone marrow transplant registered nurse and has considerable experience in pain management and bedside, end-of-life care. She is a 10-year member of the Franciscan Health Systems West Regional Ethics Committee and is immediate past chair of the Regional Ethics Educational Committee. Ms. Trandum was the collaborative leader of the Improving Care through the End of Life study (July 1997–July 1998) and is now director of the local and nationally expanding program. She has authored a thirteen-chapter training manual and database, both entitled *Improving Care through the End of Life* and both of which are being used in new program settings. She consults, advocates, educates, and speaks to groups of health care professionals and students both regionally and nationally about improving end-of-life care. Ms. Trandum holds degrees in education, sociology, and nursing and is currently studying for a master's degree in business administration.

Vittorio Ventafridda, MD, PhD, MRCP, is retired from the National Cancer Institute of Milan, where he served as head of the Division of Pain Control and Palliative Care. Dr. Ventafridda was one of the founders of IASP (International Association for the Study of Pain) and founder of the EAPC (European Association for Palliative Care), where he currently serves as its honorary president. Additionally, Dr. Ventafridda is currently leading several efforts to shape national and international policies regarding palliative care. These efforts include serving as the director of the WHO collaborating center on cancer control and palliative care at the European Institute of Oncology, scientific director of the Floriani Foundation, president of the Italian School of Palliative Medicine (SIMPA), president of the National Committee on Palliative Care c/o Ministry of Health, president of a research project on the standard of palliative care in Italy, and president of UPSA Institute for Pain Control.

David E. Weissman, MD, is a professor of internal medicine and director of the Medical College of Wisconsin Palliative Care Program. As director of the National Internal Medicine End-of-Life Residency Education Project, he is currently working to introduce an end-of-life curriculum into 210 U.S. internal medicine residency programs. Dr. Weissman co-directs EPERC, End-of-Life Physician Education Resource Center, a Web-based resource for peer-reviewed physician education information, and he is editor-in-chief of the *Journal of Palliative Medicine*.

Nita Winter is an award-winning freelance photographer based in the San Francisco area, where she has been specializing in creating emotion-evoking images of children, teens, families, and seniors in real-life situations for stock or assignments for the past 20 years. Her work has remained closely associated with community organizations. Ms. Winter's multiethnic images have illustrated dozens of books, magazines, and other publications, including the Children's Defense Fund calendar for the past six years. Her fine art images have been purchased by hospitals, corporations, and foundations and can be found in private collections locally and nationally. Currently, Ms. Winter is working on a project commissioned by the Marin Community Foundation that focuses on the need for affordable housing in Marin County, California.

Carol Wogrin, RN, PsyD, is the executive director of the National Center for Death Education and Director of the Bereavement Studies Program at Mount Ida College and the Director of the Massachusetts Compassionate Care Coalition. She is a clinical psychologist and registered nurse who specializes in end-of-life and bereavement issues and has a background working with children, adults, and families in acute care settings, home care, and hospice. She has a private practice in Newton, Massachusetts. Her book, *Matters of Life and Death: Finding the Words to Say Goodbye* was published in August 2001.

Index